Illustrated Coronary Intervention

We shall never learn to feel and respect our real calling and destiny,
unless we have taught ourselves to consider everything as moonshine,
compared with the education of the heart.

JG Lockhart (August 1825),
quoted in Lockhart's *Life of Sir Walter Scott*, volume 6 (1837), chapter 2.

Illustrated Coronary Intervention

A case-oriented approach

David R Ramsdale BSc MB ChB FRCP MD

Consultant Cardiologist
Liverpool Cardiothoracic Centre
Liverpool
UK

MARTIN DUNITZ

© Martin Dunitz Ltd 2001

Although every effort has been made to ensure that all owners of copyright material have been acknowledged in this publication, we would be glad to acknowledge in subsequent reprints or editions any omissions brought to our attention.

First published in the United Kingdom in 2001
by Martin Dunitz Ltd, The Livery House, 7–9 Pratt Street, London NW1 0AE

Reprinted 2001

Although every effort has been made to ensure that drug doses and other information are presented accurately in this publication, the ultimate responsibility rests with the prescribing physician. Neither the publishers nor the authors can be held responsible for errors or for any consequences arising from the use of information contained herein. For detailed prescribing information or instructions on the use of any product or procedure discussed herein, please consult the prescribing information or instructional material issued by the manufacturer.

A CIP record for this book is available from the British Library.

ISBN 1-85317-937-X

Distributed in the USA by:
Fulfilment Center
Taylor & Francis
7625 Empire Drive
Florence, KY 41042, USA
Toll Free Tel: 1 800 634 7064
Email: cserve@routledge_ny.com.

Distributed in Canada by:
Taylor & Francis
74 Rolark Drive
Scarborough
Ontario M1R G2, Canada
Toll Free Tel: 1 877 226 2237
Email: tal_fran@istar.ca

Distributed in the rest of the world by:
ITPS Limited
Cheriton House
North Way, Andover
Hampshire SP10 5BE, UK
Tel: +44 (0) 1264 332424
Email: reception@itps.co.uk

Composition by Scribe Design, Gillingham, Kent
Printed and bound in China by Imago

Contents

Individual contributors

Dr V Abiragi
St John's Hospital, Detroit, Michigan, USA

Dr R Albiero
EMO-Centro-Cuore, Columbus Hospital, Milan, Italy

Dr YEA Appelman
Department of Cardiology, Academic Medical Centre,
Amsterdam, The Netherlands

Dr S Atar
Cedars-Sinai Medical Center, Los Angeles, California, USA

Dr D Baumgart
Department of Cardiology, University Hospital, Essen,
Germany

Dr DH Bennett
Cardiac Centre, Wythenshawe Hospital, Manchester, UK

Dr R Beyar
Rambam Medical Center, Haifa, Israel

Dr R Bonan
Montreal Heart Institute, Montreal, Canada

Dr MH Bowles
HCA Wesley Medical Center, Wichita, Kansas, USA

Dr R Cain
Encino-Tarzana Medical Center, Encino, California, USA

Dr D Carrie
Purpan Hospital, Toulouse, France

Dr P Chandra
Escorts Heart Institute and Research Center, New Delhi, India

Dr M Chester
Cardiothoracic Centre, Liverpool, UK

Dr NAF Chronos
Andreas Gruentzig Cardiovascular Center of Emory University,
Atlanta, Georgia, USA

Dr A Colombo
EMO-Centro-Cuore, Columbus Hospital, Milan, Italy

Dr A Cooper
Regional Cardiac Centre, Wythenshawe Hospital, Manchester,
UK

Dr D Cumberland
Northern General Hospital, Sheffield, UK

Dr M de Belder
Cardiothoracic Unit, South Cleveland Hospital, Middlesbrough, UK

Dr MJ de Boer
Hospital de Weezendlanden, Zwolle, The Netherlands

Dr C Di Mario
EMO-Centro-Cuore, Columbus Hospital, Milan, Italy

Dr BG Denys
Presbyterian University Hospital, Pittsburgh, Pennsylvania,
USA

Dr E Eeckhout
Centre Hospitalier Universitaire Vaudois, Lausanne,
Switzerland

Dr N Eigler
Cedars-Sinai Medical Center, Los Angeles, California, USA

Dr R Erbel
Medical Clinic, Johanes Gutenberg University, Mainz,
Germany

Dr PJ Fitzgerald
Center for Research in Cardiovascular Interventions, Stanford
University School of Medicine, Stanford, California, USA

Dr JA Fleisher
Encino-Tarzana Medical Center, Encino, California, USA

Dr D Foley
Thoraxcenter, Academic Hospital, Rotterdam, The Netherlands

Dr CM Furr
Hamot Medical Center, Erie, Pennsylvania, USA

Dr J Gaspar
Instituto Nacional de Cardiologia, Mexico City, Mexico

Dr A Gershlick
Glenfield Hospital, Leicester, UK

Dr RS Gottleib
The Graduate Hospital, Philadelphia, Pennsylvania, USA

Dr J-J Goy
Centre Hospitalier Universitaire Vaudois, Lausanne,
Switzerland

Dr JA Hall
Cardiothoracic Unit, South Cleveland Hospital,
Middlesbrough, UK

Dr CW Hamm
University of Hamburg, Hamburg, Germany

Dr ZM Hijazi
The University of Chicago Children's Hospital, Chicago,
Illinois, USA

Dr T Hinohara
Sequoia Hospital, Redwood City, California, USA

Dr T Ischinger
Klinik-Bogenhausen, Munich, Germany

Dr CD Ilsley
Department of Cardiology, Royal Brompton and Harefield
NHS Trust, Middlesex, UK

Dr T Joseph
Assistance Publique, Hôpitaux de Paris, Hôpital Ambroise
Pare, Paris, France

Dr K Kent
Washington Heart Hospital Center, Washington, DC, USA

Dr SB King III
Andreas Gruentzig Cardiovascular Center, Emory University
Hospital, Atlanta, Georgia, USA

Dr R Kipperman
HCA Wesley Medical Center, Wichita, Kansas, USA

Dr N Komiyama
Cardiovascular Center, Toranomon Hospital, Toranomon
Minato-ku, Tokyo, Japan

Dr O Kovalenko
EMO-Centro-Cuore, Columbus Hospital, Milan, Italy

Dr T LaLonde
St. John's Hospital, Detroit, Michigan, USA

Dr ME Leimbach
Andreas Gruentzig Cardiovascular Center, Emory University
Hospital, Atlanta, Georgia, USA

Dr P Ludman
Papworth Hospital, Cambridge, UK

Dr H Luo
Cedars-Sinai Medical Center, Los Angeles, California, USA

Dr JM McClure
St. Luke's Hospital, Saginaw, Michigan, USA

Dr ME McIvor
All Children's Hospital, St. Petersburg, Florida, USA

Dr J Marco
Clinique Pasteur, Toulouse, France

Dr M Mason
Department of Cardiology, Royal Brompton and Harefield
NHS Trust, Middlesex, UK

Dr B Meier
University Hospital, Inselspital, Bern, Switzerland

Dr DC Morris
Andreas Gruentzig Cardiovascular Center, Emory University,
Atlanta, Georgia, USA

Dr JL Morris
Cardiothoracic Centre, Liverpool, UK

Dr L Morrison
Cardiothoracic Centre, Liverpool, UK

Dr H Mudra
Klinikum Innenstadt der LMU Medizinische Klinik, Munich,
Germany

Dr T Nagai
Cedars-Sinai Medical Center, Los Angeles, California, USA

Dr Y Nakagawa
Kokura Memorial Hospital, Kitakyushu, Japan

Dr M Nobuyoshi
Kokura Memorial Hospital, Kitakyushu, Japan

Dr MS Norell
Hull Royal Infirmary, Hull, UK

Dr O Ormerod
Cardiac Department, John Radcliffe Hospital, Oxford, UK

Dr JM Parks
University of Alabama, Birmingham, Alabama, USA

Dr IM Penn
University of British Columbia, Vancouver General Hospital,
Vancouver, British Columbia, Canada

Dr RA Perry
Cardiothoracic Centre, Liverpool, UK

Dr JJ Piek
Department of Cardiology, Academic Medical Centre,
Amsterdam, The Netherlands

Dr J Quan
Riverside Community Hospital, Riverside, California, USA

Dr J Rankin
University of British Columbia, Vancouver General Hospital,
Vancouver, British Columbia, Canada

Dr S Ray
Cardiac Centre, Wythenshawe Hospital, Manchester, UK

Dr N Reifart
Ambulantes Herzzentrum, Frankfurt, Germany

Dr CS Rihal
Cardiovascular Diseases and Internal Medicine, Mayo Clinic,
Rochester, Minnesota, USA

Dr G Robertson
Sequoia Hospital, Redwood City, California, USA

Dr U Rosenschein
Department of Cardiology, Tel Aviv Medical Center, Tel Aviv,
Israel

Dr R Safian
William Beaumont Hospital, Royal Oak, Michigan, USA

Dr R Salwan
Escorts Heart Institute and Research Centre, New Delhi, India

Dr I de Scheerder
University Hospital Gasthuisberg, Leuven, Belgium

Dr P Schofield
Papworth Hospital, Cambridge, UK

Dr S Schwarzacher
Center for Research in Cardiovascular Interventions, Stanford
University, Stanford, CA, USA

Dr N Semmler
Ambulantes Herzzentrum, Frankfurt, Germany

Dr A Seth
Escorts Heart Institute and Research Centre, New Delhi, India

Dr RJ Siegel
Cedars-Sinai Medical Center, Los Angeles, California, USA

Dr U Sigwart
Royal Brompton Hospital, London, UK

Dr LDR Smith
Royal Devon and Exeter Hospital, Exeter, UK

Dr A Spring
Washoe Medical Center, Reno, Nevada, USA

Dr JE Tcheng
Duke Medical Center, Durham, North Carolina, USA

Dr P Teirstein
Scripps Clinic and Research Foundation, La Jolla, California, USA

Dr TC Trageser
Hamot Medical Center, Erie, Pennsylvania, USA

Dr P Urban
Cardiology Center, University Hospital, Geneva, Switzerland

Dr N Uren
Department of Cardiology, The Royal Infirmary of Edinburgh, Edinburgh, UK

Dr M Webb-Peploe
St. Thomas's Hospital, London, UK

Dr F Werner
Klinikum Innenstadt der LMU Medizinische Klinik, Munich, Germany

Dr C White
Ochsner Clinic, New Orleans, LA, USA

Dr J Work
Encino-Tarzana Medical Center, Encino, California, USA

Contributors from industry

Advanced Cardiovascular Systems/Guidant Ltd, Temecula, California, USA

Angiodynamics, Glen Falls, New York, USA

Angiosonics Inc, Morrisville, North Carolina, USA

Arterial Vascular Engineering, Santa Rosa, California, USA

Bard/USCI, Galway, Eire

Biocompatibles Ltd, Uxbridge, UK

Biotronik GmbH, Berlin, Germany

Boston Scientific/Scimed Ltd, Maple Grove, Minnesota, USA

Cook Inc, Bloomington, Indiana, USA

Endicor Medical Inc, San Clemente, California, USA

EndoSonics Corporation, Rancho Cordova, California, USA

EndoSonics Europe BV, 2288 EC Rijswijk, The Netherlands

Global Therapeutics Inc, Broomfield, Colorado, USA

Guidant/Advanced Cardiovascular Systems, Santa Clara, California, USA

Interventional Technologies Ltd, San Diego, California, USA

JoMed Intervention AB, Helsingborg, Sweden

Johnson and Johnson Interventional Systems/Cordis Ltd, Warren, New Jersey, USA

Medtronic Interventional Vascular, Kerkrade, The Netherlands

Merit Medical International, Surrey, UK

Novoste Corporation, Norcross, Georgia, USA

Possis Medical Inc, Minneapolis, MN, USA

Progressive Angioplasty Systems Inc, Menlo Park, California, USA

Schneider AG, Bulach, Switzerland

Spectranetics Int, Nieuwegein, The Netherlands

Uni-Cath Inc, Saddle Brook, NJ, USA

(These details were correct at the time of the contributions. Some of these have now changed as a result of takeovers, mergers and restructuring of the industry.)

Preface

Coronary artery intervention began in 1977, when Andreas Gruentzig performed the first PTCA in Zurich. Over the past 23 years, the techniques and knowledge gained by the early pioneers in coronary intervention such as Gruentzig, Myler, Stertzer, King, Simpson and Hartzler have been passed on to another generation of cardiologists. Because of their close collaboration with a wide variety of scientists in industry, PTCA has progressed dramatically alongside developments in material technology, equipment and technique. These have occurred perhaps as a result of simultaneous improvements in imaging methods, such as digital angiography.

Besides PTCA, other innovative techniques such as mechanical atherectomy, laser devices and stents have been developed and introduced into clinical practice in an attempt to optimize short- and long-term clinical results, with each technique demanding new clinical skills to be learned and new clinical trials to be performed. In parallel with these advances, and perhaps because of them, a better understanding of the pathophysiology of atherosclerosis and the pathobiology of coronary thrombosis and restenosis after arterial injury has developed. Intracoronary angioscopy, intracoronary ultrasound and techniques for measuring coronary blood flow have all proved helpful to cardiologists in their assessment of patients undergoing interventional procedures and in their achievement of optimal outcomes.

Since 1977, much information and education about the practical aspects of interventional techniques for the treatment of coronary artery disease have come from meetings and symposia held all over the world. The courses in Emory University in Atlanta, the San Francisco Heart Institute in California and The Mid-America Heart Institute in Kansas, USA and Geneva in Switzerland were responsible for most of the early teaching in this specialty. The highlights of such meetings were the live case demonstrations, in which the experts' strategy and technique during simple and complex procedures were observed, questioned, discussed and criticized. Such cases proved highly instructive and memorable to those of us who were to be closely involved with the practice and teaching of coronary intervention and it is with this concept in mind that the current book was planned and developed.

A picture is worth a thousand words and it is the intention of this book to have limited text and to teach by the presentation of numerous illustrated cases. Although it is impossible to present every conceivable case within a single book, I have tried to illustrate a wide range of coronary interventional techniques that are currently available to us for a variety of clinical and anatomical challenges. The book is intended to be easy and quick to read so that the reader can learn much without too much effort and as quickly as possible. I would certainly have liked to have had such a book available to me during my introduction to interventional cardiology and I hope that it will be of benefit to junior and senior fellows training in cardiology, nurses, catheter laboratory technicians, physiological measurement technicians and radiographers as well as to our colleagues in industry who work alongside us for the benefit of our patients.

David R Ramsdale
Liverpool, UK
October 2000

Acknowledgements

I would like to acknowledge the help of my friend and colleague, Dr John Morris, who shared many of the cases presented here. His expertise, wit and good humour made the work most enjoyable. I am grateful to Sister Jill Stanistreet and her catheter laboratory nursing staff for their expert day-to-day skills and assistance. I thank my cardiac radiographers at the Cardiothoracic Centre in Liverpool and in particular Janette Rekitas and Christopher Abell for help in preparing the images from digital tape and CD, and Jackie Hyland, Tony Hanmer, Julian Johnson and Ken Maddock in the Department of Medical Photography for their invaluable assistance in producing the illustrations for publication. I greatly appreciate the constant support of my personal secretary Samantha Kelly to whom I turned frequently for help with this project.

My thanks are particularly due to colleagues and friends from around the world who have provided many additional interesting cases. Their contributions have been acknowledged individually in the relevant figure legends and are a tribute to their skill and expertise in this specialty. I am indebted to Gary Kelly of Interventional Technologies Inc, San Diego, California, USA for helping to provide interesting cases involving transluminal extraction catheter atherectomy and to the various manufacturers of interventional equipment for providing illustrations of their devices.

Finally, I must specifically acknowledge Boston Scientific-Scimed, Cordis/Johnson and Johnson, Biocompatibles, Endosonics, S-Pace, JoMed and Guidant for their assistance during the production of this work, the personal efforts and technical expertise of Clive Lawson, Robert Whittle and colleagues at Martin Dunitz Ltd and in particular the commissioning editor there, Mr Alan Burgess, for his enthusiastic support and advice.

Glossary of terms and abbreviations

AVCx	Atrioventricular branch of the circumflex coronary artery
CABG	Coronary artery bypass graft
CFR	Coronary flow reserve
DCA	Directional coronary atherectomy
DG	Diagonal coronary artery
ECG	Electrocardiogram
ELCA	Excimer laser coronary atherectomy
FFR	Fractional flow reserve
GP	Glycoprotein
INT	Intermediate coronary artery
IVUS	Intravascular ultrasound
LAD	Left anterior descending coronary artery
LAO	Left anterior oblique
LLAT	Left lateral
LCx	Left circumflex coronary artery
MI	Myocardial infarction
MLD	Minimal lumenal diameter
OMCx	Obtuse marginal branch of circumflex coronary artery
PA	Posteroanterior
PDA	Posterior descending artery
PLCx	Posterolateral branch of the circumflex coronary artery
psi	Pounds per square inch
PTCA	Percutaneous transluminal coronary (or balloon) angioplasty
PTFE	Polytetrafluorethylene
QCA	Quantitative coronary arteriography
RAO	Right anterior oblique
RCA	Right coronary artery
rpm	Revolutions per minute
rtPA	Recombinant tissue plasminogen activator
SVG	Saphenous vein graft
TEC	Transluminal extraction catheter
TIMI	Thrombolysis in myocardial infarction
TLR	Target lesion revascularization

Dedication

This book is dedicated first and foremost to my wife, Bernie, and to my children, Christopher, Mark and Kathryn, for their love and support during its production, and secondly to all my previous junior medical colleagues, nursing and technical staff with whom I have worked for many hours in our catheter laboratories. It has been a joy and a pleasure to work with them and I hope they will recall and remember some of the events and lessons learned from the illustrated cases presented here.

1

Single-vessel PTCA

PTCA may be performed using monorail or rapid-exchange balloon catheters or with 'over-the-wire' systems. Although the 'over-the-wire' systems predominate in North America, in the rest of the world rapid-exchange catheters are the more popular type because of their ease and speed of use. Fixed-wire balloon catheters are no longer available because their advantages ceased to exist with the advent of the newer 'ultra-low-profile' balloon catheters of today. A wide variety of balloon catheters is available with balloons of various sizes, lengths, profile, compliance, trackability, pushability and conformability (Fig. 1.1).

There is a range of intracoronary guidewires; various coatings and different characteristics (flexibility, diameter, radio-opacity and torquability) give the operator a wide choice of equipment for particular lesion subsets. Their structure and design are an engineering feat in themselves (Fig. 1.2). Guiding catheters have large internal lumens, come with and without side holes, have non-traumatic soft tips, are available in many shapes and French sizes and are designed to provide improved back-up for the delivery of guidewires, balloons and other devices compared to those of 5 years ago (Fig. 1.3). Although PTCA is most commonly performed via the femoral artery, the procedure can be performed via the brachial or radial arteries using 6F large-lumen guiding catheters.

Indeflators are generally ergonomic, hand-held, disposable devices that use dilute contrast media to deliver inflation pressures of over 20 atmospheres to the balloon (Fig. 1.4).

High-quality fluoroscopic imaging, preferably with a biplane system in a state-of-the-art, spacious catheter laboratory, is essential for performing coronary intervention (Fig. 1.5). Road-mapping of several optimal angiographic views is most helpful in cases in which there are overlapping vessels, tortuous anatomy and bifurcation lesions, and the facility to provide magnified images during the procedure is ideal.

Generally the best clinical results from PTCA are obtained in short, discrete, concentric, proximal lesions in non-tortuous main vessels, although more typically one is challenged by multiple lesions in single vessels or lesions in branch vessels and tortuous arteries.

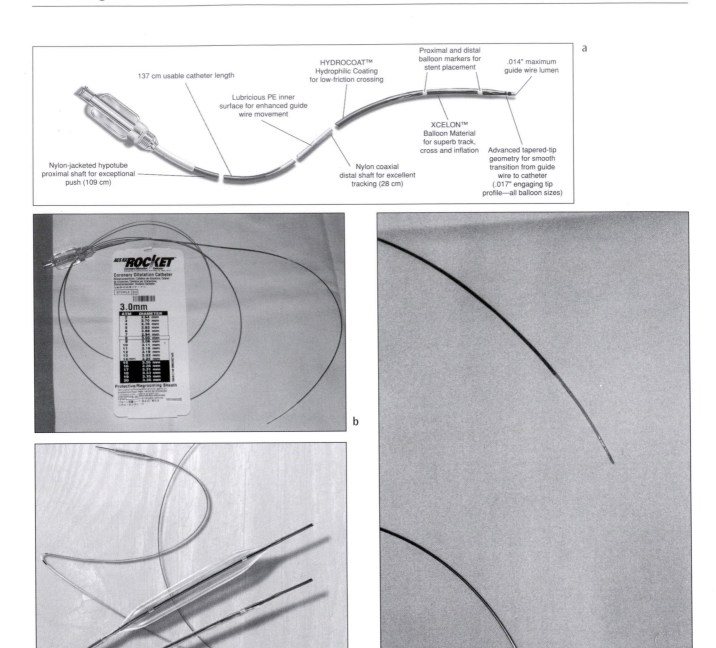

Figure 1.1

(a) A modern, low-profile balloon catheter has a tapered tip with a crossing profile of less than 0.02 inches, good pushability, good trackability and special inner and outer coatings that reduce friction to enhance wire movement and crossing of the lesion by the balloon.

(b) The Rocket™ balloon catheter (Guidant) is a modern, low-profile, rapid-exchange catheter with radio-opaque markers at the proximal and distal ends of the balloon. Catheters are accompanied by a balloon-compliance chart, which indicates the approximate diameter of the balloon when it is inflated at various inflation pressures. A small plastic 'regrooming' sheath aids rewrapping of the balloon when a lesion in another vessel is to be addressed with the same balloon.

(c) This close-up view shows the two gold markers within the balloon and the excellent low-profile of the balloon that exists before it is inflated.

(d) The Omnipass® (Cordis/Johnson and Johnson) balloon catheter is shown inflated and deflated.

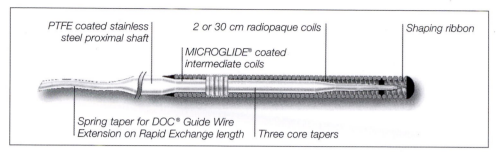

PTFE coated stainless steel proximal shaft

2 or 30 cm radiopaque coils

Shaping ribbon

MICROGLIDE® coated intermediate coils

Spring taper for DOC® Guide Wire Extension on Rapid Exchange length

Three core tapers

a

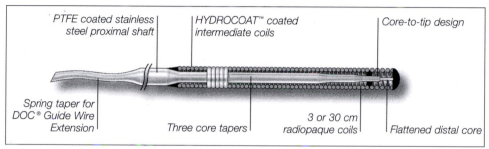

PTFE coated stainless steel proximal shaft

HYDROCOAT™ coated intermediate coils

Core-to-tip design

Spring taper for DOC® Guide Wire Extension

Three core tapers

3 or 30 cm radiopaque coils

Flattened distal core

b

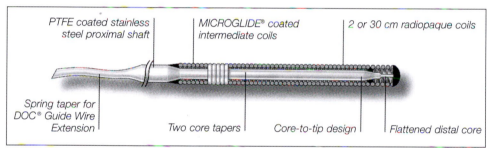

PTFE coated stainless steel proximal shaft

MICROGLIDE® coated intermediate coils

2 or 30 cm radiopaque coils

Spring taper for DOC® Guide Wire Extension

Two core tapers

Core-to-tip design

Flattened distal core

c

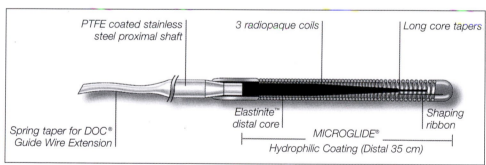

PTFE coated stainless steel proximal shaft

3 radiopaque coils

Long core tapers

Elastinite™ distal core

Shaping ribbon

Spring taper for DOC® Guide Wire Extension

MICROGLIDE®

Hydrophilic Coating (Distal 35 cm)

d

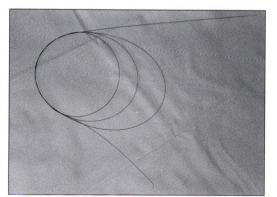

e

Figure 1.2
Internal structure of 0.014-inch (a) high-torque Floppy® guidewire (Guidant), (b) Intermediate® guidewire (Guidant), and (c) Standard® guidewire (Guidant). These guidewires are available in 190cm and 300cm lengths. The 190cm guidewire can be extended using the DOC® extension wire (Guidant).
(d) The 0.014-inch Balance® guidewire (Guidant) has an Elastinite® distal core, which tends to retain its integrity, shape and torque control more than stainless steel. This is quite important in tortuous coronary anatomy and when one is accessing multiple lesions. Guidewires are coated with PTFE/Teflon® for reduced resistance, reduced fibrin-platelet adhesion and enhanced trackability. Some have hydrophilic coatings (e.g. Hydrocoat™) in order to reduce friction further and provide smooth tracking and optimum wire movement.
(e) The 190cm long, 0.014-inch high torque Floppy® guidewire.

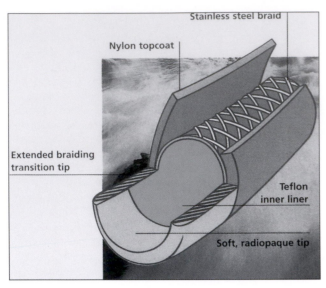

a

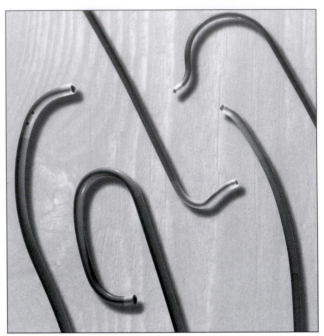

b

Figure 1.3

(a) Guiding catheters are specially designed to provide back-up support to enable safe delivery of guidewires, balloon catheters, stents and other interventional devices down the coronary arteries.

(b) A wide variety of shapes is available, and catheters come with and without side holes. The Vista Brite Tip® guide catheters from Cordis/Johnson and Johnson are shown.

(c) Modern guide catheters such as the Wiseguide™ from SCIMED/Boston Scientific consists of several 'zones' (denoted by change in colour) which is designed to have specific characteristics in order to optimize pushability, torquability and flexibility in the correct place along the shaft of the catheter. They are also designed to have a safe, atraumatic distal end.

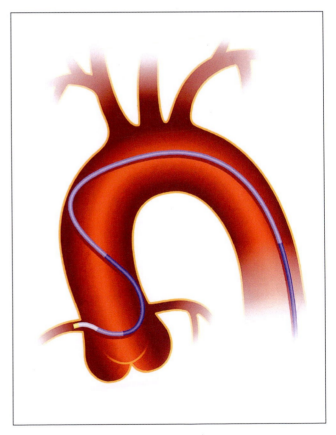

c

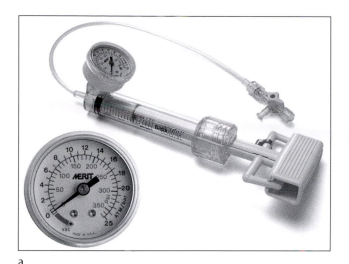

a

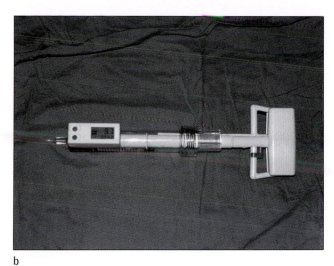

b

Figure 1.4

The indeflator inflates and deflates the balloon catheter when necessary. High pressure can be provided with ease using such an ergonomic device, and the amount of pressure and the duration of inflation is displayed on the device.

(a) The BasixCOMPAK™ indeflator (Merit Medical) has an angled pressure gauge with a luminescent dial to assist the operator.

(b) The Monarch™ indeflator (Merit Medical) provides a digital readout of pressure (in psi or atmospheres), the duration of inflation, the previous inflation pressure and the previous deflation time.

(c) The Encore™ 26 inflation device from SCIMED/Boston Scientific.

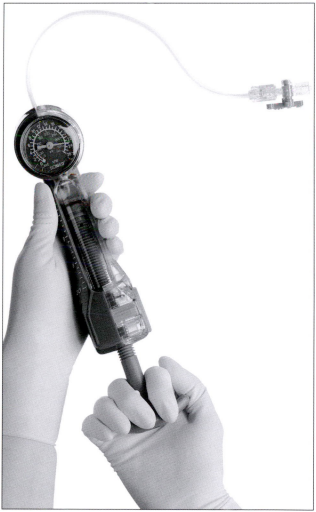

c

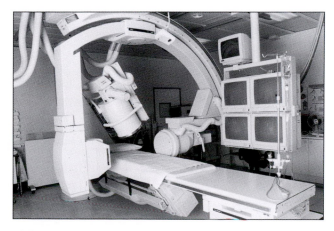

Figure 1.5

High-quality fluoroscopic imaging, preferably using a biplane system in a state-of-the-art catheter laboratory, is essential for performing coronary intervention. A bank of four monitors – providing two fixed 'road-map' images and two 'live' images – is ideal.

Left anterior descending coronary artery lesions

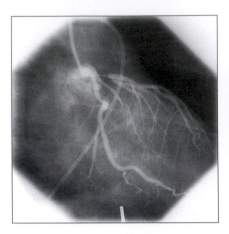
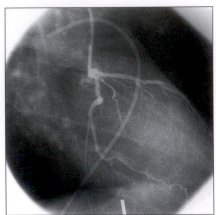

a   b

Figure 1.6
Proximal stenosis in LAD (a) before and (b) after PTCA with a 3.0mm Picolino™ monorail (Schneider) balloon catheter in a 38-year-old glazing manager with a 4-week history of severe angina. He remained asymptomatic 8 years after the PTCA.

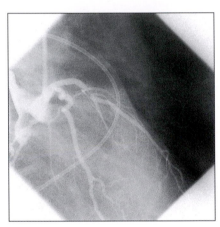
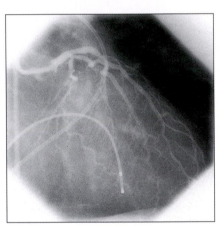

a   b

Figure 1.7
A more complex lesion in a high take-off LAD (a) before and (b) after PTCA with a 3.5mm Micross™ balloon catheter (Datascope).

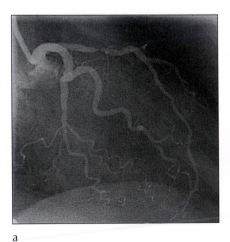
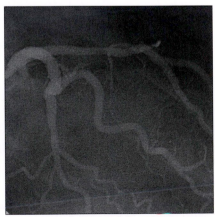

a   b

Figure 1.8
(a) A proximal LAD stenosis that was causing severe angina in a 63-year-old woman.

The lesion was dilated with a 3.0mm Goldie™ balloon (Schneider), giving an excellent angiographic result (b) and symptomatic relief.

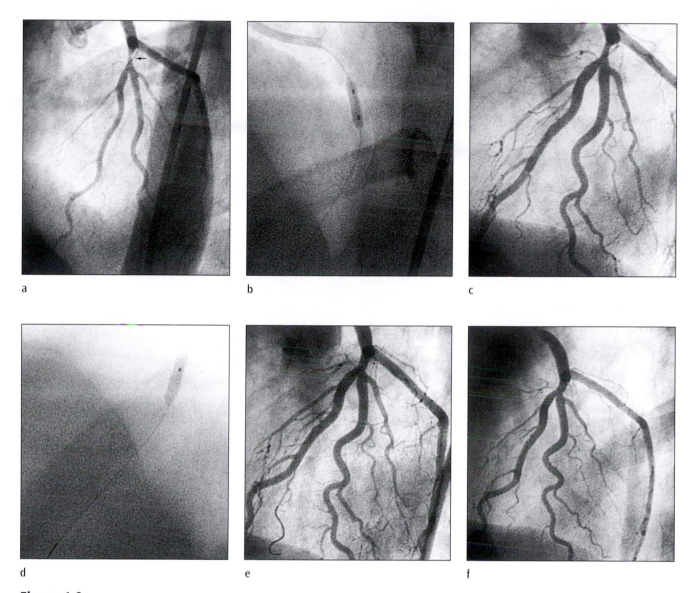

a   b   c

d   e   f

Figure 1.9

(a) A 34-year-old man had angina during long-distance running and was found to have a severe stenosis in the proximal LAD (arrow). Elective stent implantation was considered in order to reduce the likelihood of restenosis. However, it was decided to perform PTCA alone on the premise that in-stent restenosis may be more difficult to deal with, especially if it was diffuse and involved the nearby large diagonal branch.

After PTCA with a 3.0mm, 12mm long Cruiser (Nycomed) balloon (b), a residual stenosis remained (c).

Further PTCA with a 3.5mm, 20mm long Worldpass™ balloon (Cordis) (d) produced a satisfactory angiographic result (e), and IVUS showed an MLD of 3.2mm.

(f) The angiographic result persisted at 3 months. After 24 months, the patient remains asymptomatic when running long distances and has a negative exercise stress test.

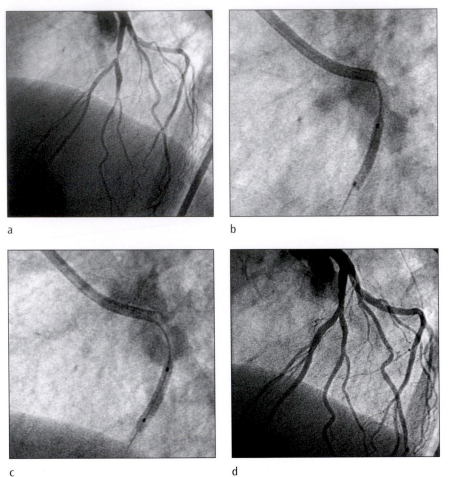

a

b

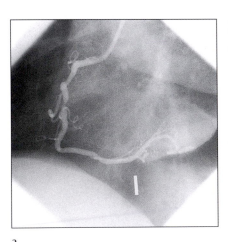

c

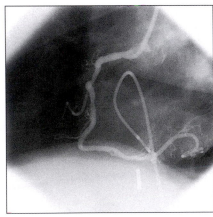

d

Figure 1.10
(a) A severe stenosis in the proximal LAD just above but not involving the diagonal branch in a 57-year-old barman who had severe, limiting angina. The strategy was to perform PTCA alone unless the angiographic result was poor in order to avoid the need to cover the ostium of the diagonal branch with a stent and, of course, the difficult-to-treat in-stent restenosis.

The lesion was crossed with a 0.014-inch Floppy® guidewire and dilated with (b) a 2.5mm Worldpass™ balloon and then (c) a 3.0mm Worldpass™ balloon.

(d) The angiographic result was excellent.

Right coronary artery lesions

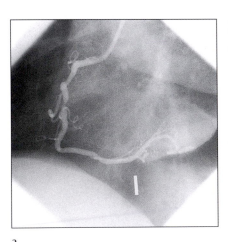

a

b

Figure 1.11
(a) Dominant RCA with a severe mid-third stenosis before PTCA. (b) After PTCA with a 3.0mm Low Profile Plus® (USCI) balloon catheter. Note the temporary pacing wire placed prophylactically in the right ventricle of this 69-year-old retired nursing sister who had moderate angina.

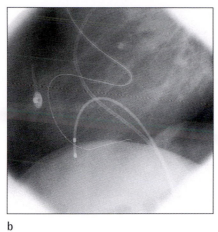

a

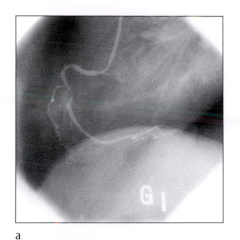

b

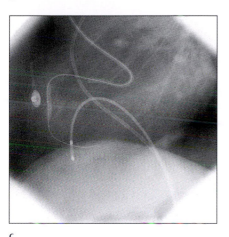

c

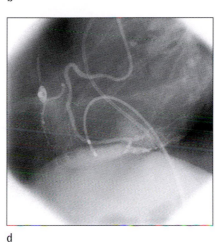

d

Figure 1.12
A 71-year-old woman with unstable angina. (a) The tortuous RCA with shepherd's crook anatomy has a severe proximal/mid-third stenosis.

A left Amplatz guide catheter is used to provide back-up support for crossing (b) with the guidewire and (c) with a 3.0mm Low Profile Plus® balloon catheter.

(d) Result after PTCA.

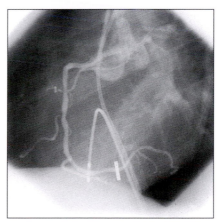

a

b

Figure 1.13
A 71-year-old woman with unstable angina. (a) Coronary arteriography showed a tight proximal and mid-third stenosis in RCA.
(b) Result after PTCA with a 3.0mm Express™ balloon catheter (Scimed).

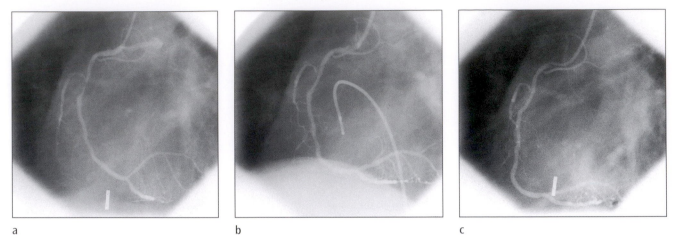

a   b   c

Figure 1.14
(a) Proximal stenosis in RCA before PTCA. (b) Result immediately after PTCA. (c) Result at 6 months.

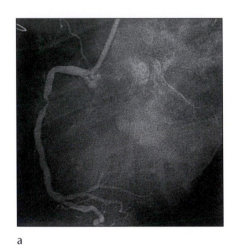
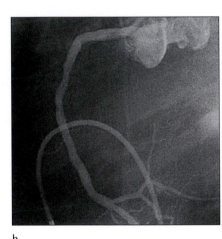

Figure 1.15
(a) Eccentric stenosis in the proximal RCA in a 72-year-old woman with severe angina before PTCA. (b) After PTCA with a 3.0mm Gold Ex® (Medtronic) balloon.

a   b

Left circumflex artery lesions

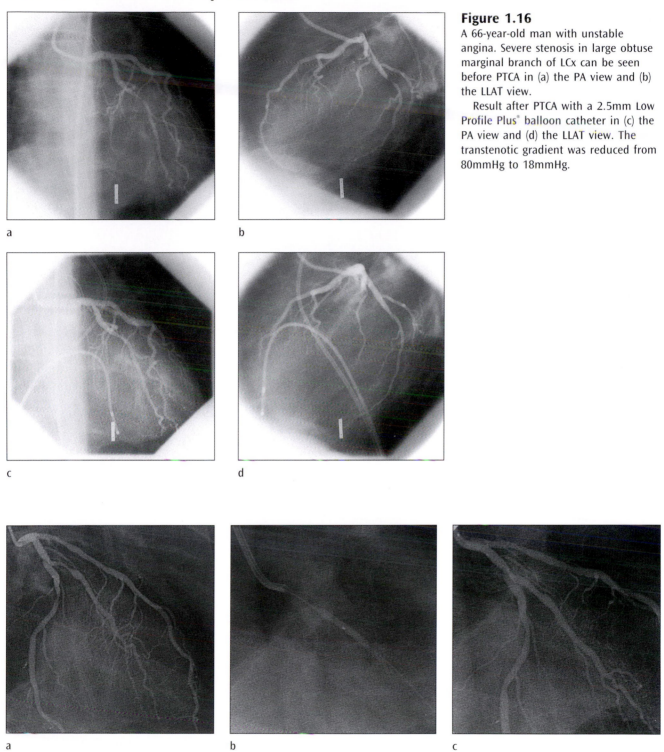

Figure 1.16
A 66-year-old man with unstable angina. Severe stenosis in large obtuse marginal branch of LCx can be seen before PTCA in (a) the PA view and (b) the LLAT view.

Result after PTCA with a 2.5mm Low Profile Plus® balloon catheter in (c) the PA view and (d) the LLAT view. The transtenotic gradient was reduced from 80mmHg to 18mmHg.

Figure 1.17
A 65-year-old man. (a) Significant stenosis in proximal OMCx before PTCA. (b) During and (c) after PTCA with a 3.0mm Elipse™ balloon (Guidant).

Lesions in series

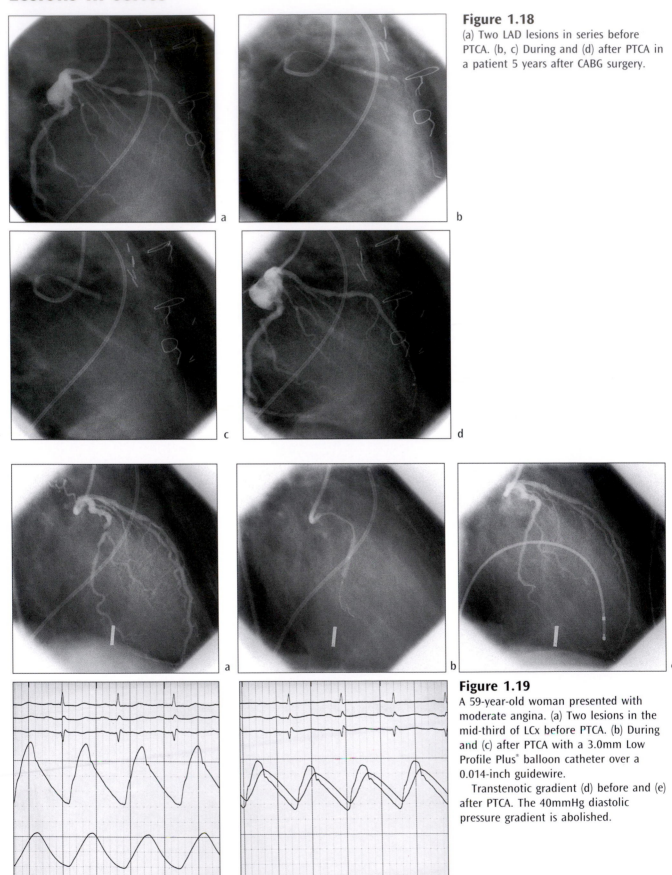

Figure 1.18
(a) Two LAD lesions in series before PTCA. (b, c) During and (d) after PTCA in a patient 5 years after CABG surgery.

Figure 1.19
A 59-year-old woman presented with moderate angina. (a) Two lesions in the mid-third of LCx before PTCA. (b) During and (c) after PTCA with a 3.0mm Low Profile Plus® balloon catheter over a 0.014-inch guidewire.

Transtenotic gradient (d) before and (e) after PTCA. The 40mmHg diastolic pressure gradient is abolished.

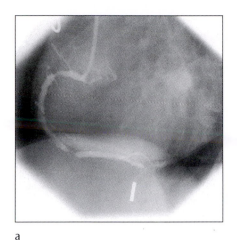

a

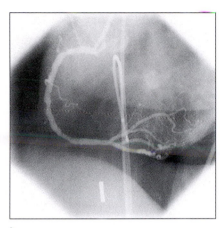

b

Figure 1.20
(a) Proximal and mid-third lesions in RCA before PTCA. (b) Result after PTCA.

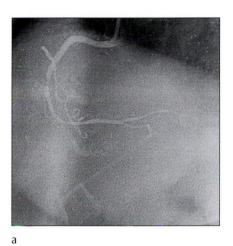

a

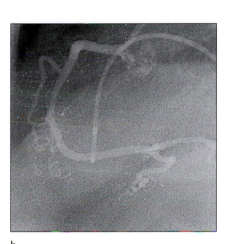

b

Figure 1.21
(a) Two mid-third lesions in RCA before PTCA. (b) Result after PTCA.

Lesions in branch vessels

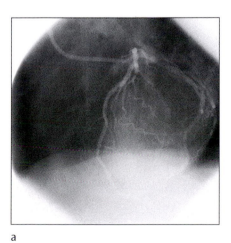

a

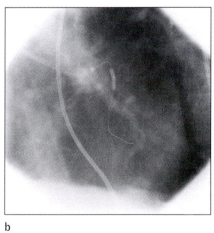

b

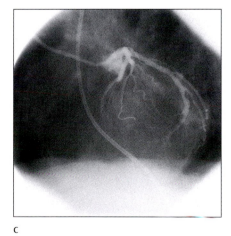

c

Figure 1.22
(a) Stenosis in a diagonal branch of the LAD before PTCA. (b) During and (c) after PTCA with a 2.5mm Gold Ex® balloon catheter.

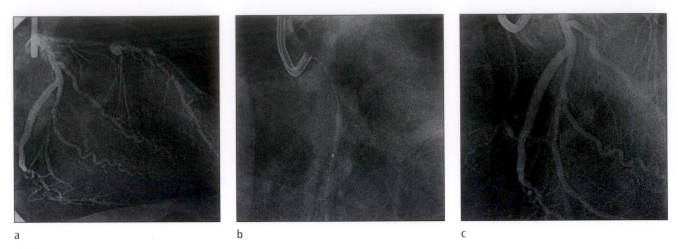

a   b   c

Figure 1.23
(a) Subtotal occlusion of obtuse marginal branch of the LCx in a 60-year-old company director who had moderately severe angina and significant two vessel coronary artery disease. (b) The vessel was reopened by PTCA with a 2.0mm Express™ balloon (Scimed) and then a 2.5mm, 30mm long Elipse™ balloon catheter. (c) Final result.

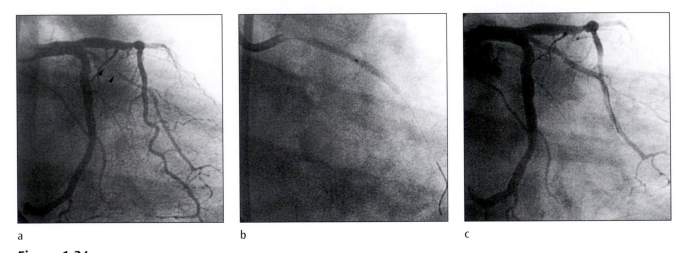

a   b   c

Figure 1.24
(a) This intermediate artery had a subtotal occlusion proximally (arrowheads) and the artery appeared relatively small.
However, after PTCA with a 2.5mm, 30mm long Elipse™ balloon (b), the angiographic result was excellent and the vessel appeared much larger (c).

Reading

Baim DS, ed. Interventional cardiology 1987: a symposium. Am J Cardiol 1988;61:1G-86G.

Detre K, Holubkov R, Kelsey S, et al for the co-investigators of the NHLBI's PTCA Registry. Percutaneous transluminal coronary angioplasty in 1985-1986 and 1977-1981. N Engl J Med 1988;318:265-70.

Faxon DP, ed. Practical Angioplasty. New York: Raven Press; 1994.

Finci L, Meier B, Roy P, et al. Clinical experience with the monorail balloon catheter for coronary angioplasty. Cathet Cardiovasc Diagn 1988;14:206-12.

Gershlick AH, Smith LS. Angiography for the interventional cardiologist. In: Grech ED, Ramsdale DR, eds. Practical Interventional Cardiology. London: Martin Dunitz; 1997:11-30.

Grech ED, Ramsdale DR, eds. Practical Interventional Cardiology. London: Martin Dunitz; 1997.

Gruentzig AR, Senning A, Siegenthaler WE. Non-operative dilatation of coronary artery stenosis: percutaneous transluminal coronary angioplasty. N Engl J Med 1979;301:61-8.

Gruentzig AR. Transluminal dilatation of coronary artery stenosis. Lancet 1978;1:263.

Hubner PJB. Guide to Coronary Angioplasty and Stenting. Amsterdam: Harwood Academic; 1998.

Kiemeneij F, Laarman GJ, Oderkerken D, et al. A randomized comparison of percutaneous transluminal coronary angioplasty by the radial, brachial and femoral approaches: the ACCESS study. J Am Coll Cardiol 1997;29:1269-75.

Kimura T, Kaburagi S, Tamura T, et al. Remodelling of human coronary arteries undergoing coronary angioplasty or atherectomy. Circulation 1997;96:475-83.

Meier B. How to treat small coronary vessels with angioplasty. Heart 1998;79:215-16.

Mooney MR, Douglas JS Jr, Mooney JF, et al. Monorail picolino catheter: a new rapid exchange/ultralow profile coronary angioplasty system. Cathet Cardiovasc Diagn 1990;20:114-19.

Myler RK, Gruentzig AR, Stertzer SH. Coronary angioplasty. In: Rapaport E, ed. Cardiology Update. New York: Elsevier Biomedical; 1983:1-66.

Myler RK, Mooney MR, Stertzer SH, et al. The balloon on a wire device: a new ultra-low-profile coronary angioplasty system/concept. Cathet Cardiovasc Diagn 1988;14:135-40.

O'Murchu B, Myler RK. Percutaneous transluminal coronary angioplasty: history, techniques, indications and complications. Unstable angina: pathophysiology and treatment with angioplasty. In: Grech ED, Ramsdale DR, eds. Practical Interventional Cardiology. London: Martin Dunitz; 1997:31-48.

Popma JJ, Kuntz RE. The practical application of quantitative angiographic methods for investigating newer coronary interventions and balloon angioplasty. In: White CJ, Ramee SR, eds. Interventional Cardiology: New Techniques and Strategies for Diagnosis and Treatment. New York: Marcel Dekker; 1995:79-112.

Rozenman Y, Sapoznikov D, Mosseri M, et al. Long-term angiographic follow-up of coronary balloon angioplasty in patients with diabetes mellitus. J Am Coll Cardiol 1997;30:1420-5.

Simpson JB, Baim DS, Robert EW, et al. A new catheter system for coronary angioplasty. Am J Cardiol 1982;49:1216-22.

Stertzer SH. Brachial approach to transluminal coronary angioplasty. In: Jang GD, ed. Angioplasty. New York: McGraw-Hill; 1986:260-94.

ten Berg JM, Gin TJ, Ernst SMPG, et al. Ten-year follow-up of percutaneous transluminal coronary angioplasty for proximal left anterior descending coronary artery stenosis in 351 patients. J Am Coll Cardiol 1996;28:82-8.

White CJ, Ramee SR, eds. Interventional Cardiology: New Techniques and Strategies for Diagnosis and Treatment. New York: Marcel Dekker; 1995.

2

Multivessel PTCA

Multivessel PTCA is now common practice but it is still less commonly performed than single-vessel PTCA. Even in this era of coronary stents, multivessel PTCA demands careful strategic planning, an experienced interventionist and surgical back-up. Generally, the most difficult or the most important lesion should be approached first, and staged procedures may be appropriate. Complication rates including the mortality rate, are not significantly higher in multivessel PTCA than in single-vessel PTCA but in multivessel PTCA fewer patients are rendered asymptomatic by a single procedure. A good long-term clinical result may require multiple angioplasty procedures instead of a single CABG operation.

Nevertheless, PTCA is less invasive and better than a partially successful surgical procedure and it may delay CABG surgery for several years. The in-hospital stay is shorter, the morbidity is less and the return to work and leisure activities is quicker after PTCA than after CABG surgery.

Although observational studies have demonstrated safety and clinical efficacy of PTCA in selected patients with multivessel disease, the role of PTCA compared with CABG surgery has also been recently evaluated by several randomized trials - RITA, BARI, CABRI, EAST, GABI and ERACI. These trials showed that both procedures were effective and had similar rates of myocardial infarction and mortality at 1-3 years of follow-up. However, owing to restenosis, both recurrent angina and further revascularization procedures were more common in those who underwent PTCA.

Coronary artery stenting has made multivessel coronary intervention (see Chapter 11) safer and more predictable than PTCA and has also reduced the incidence of repeat intervention for restenosis.

Two-vessel PTCA

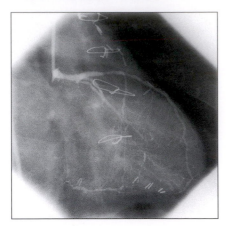

a

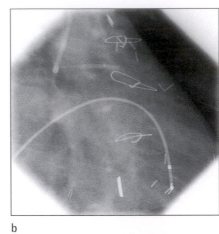

b

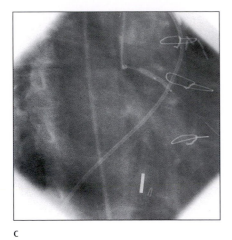

c

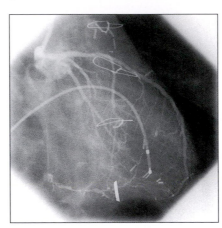

d

Figure 2.1
(a) Two-vessel PTCA in a 50-year-old mechanic with unstable angina. The proximal LAD and the obtuse marginal artery have significant stenoses.

PTCA to (b) the proximal LAD and (c) the obtuse marginal artery.

(d) Result after PTCA.

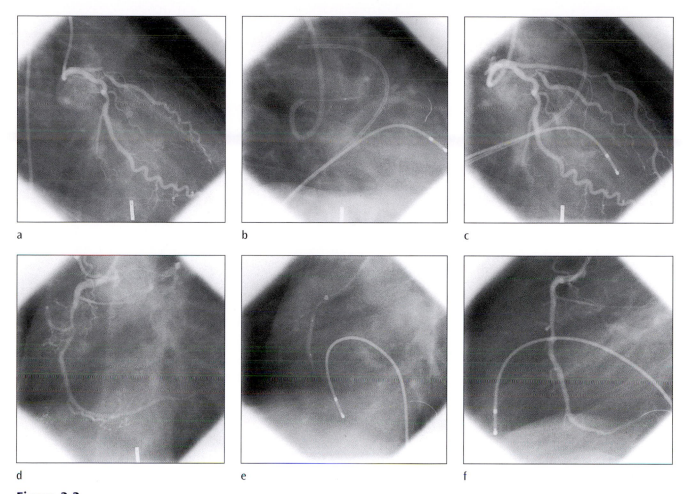

a   b   c

d   e   f

Figure 2.2

A 46-year-old joiner presented 8 months after an inferior myocardial infarct with a 3-week history of unstable angina. Angiograms showed significant three-vessel coronary artery disease, including significant stenoses in OMCx and the mid-RCA and (a) a proximally occluded LAD.

(b, c) The LAD occlusion was opened by PTCA with a 2.0mm Low Profile Plus® balloon and then a 3.0mm Low Profile Plus® balloon.

(d, e) The RCA stenosis was dilated by a 2.5mm Monorail® (Schneider) balloon over a 0.014-inch Standard® guidewire.

(f) The final result in the RCA. The LAD lesion subsequently restenosed twice before PTCA was finally successful (see Fig. 15.58).

Three-vessel PTCA

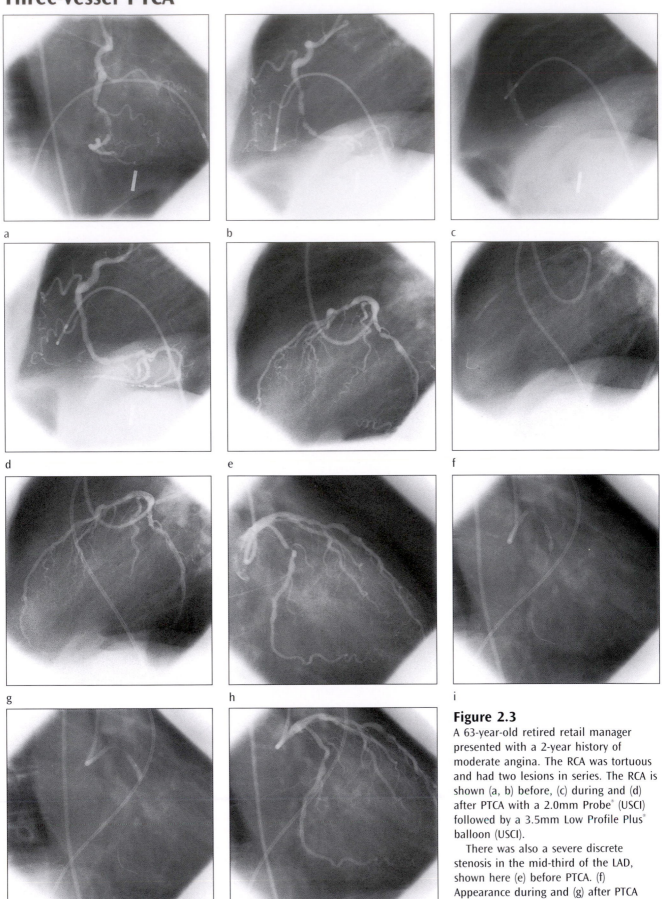

a

b

c

d

e

f

g

h

i

j

k

Figure 2.3

A 63-year-old retired retail manager presented with a 2-year history of moderate angina. The RCA was tortuous and had two lesions in series. The RCA is shown (a, b) before, (c) during and (d) after PTCA with a 2.0mm Probe® (USCI) followed by a 3.5mm Low Profile Plus® balloon (USCI).

There was also a severe discrete stenosis in the mid-third of the LAD, shown here (e) before PTCA. (f) Appearance during and (g) after PTCA with a 3.0mm Micross™ balloon.

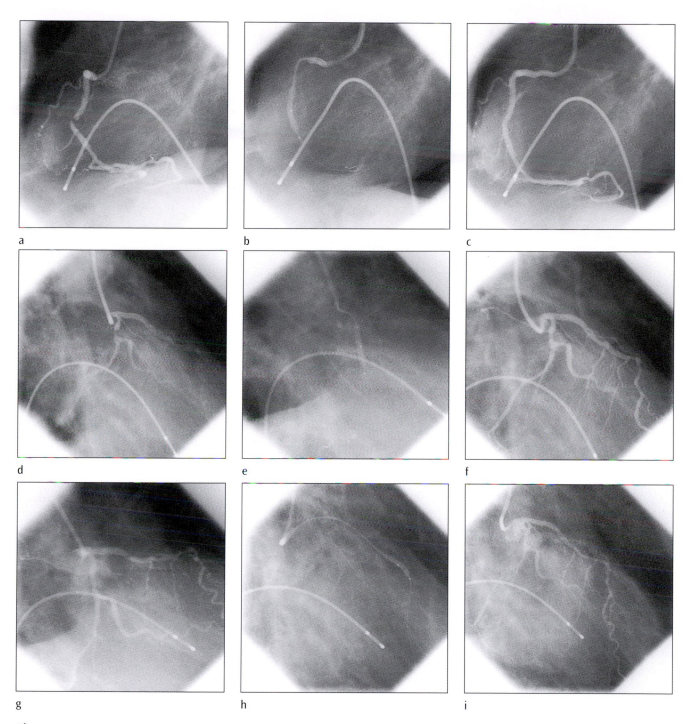

Figure 2.4

Three-vessel PTCA in 1985 in a 68-year-old man who had unstable angina and three-vessel disease. Angulated stenosis in the mid-third of the RCA (a) before, (b) during and (c) after PTCA with a 3.0mm Low Profile Plus® balloon catheter. There was an 80mmHg pressure gradient across this lesion before PTCA, which was abolished after dilatation.

There was also stenosis in the proximal LCx, shown here (d) before, (e) during and (f) after PTCA with the same balloon catheter. Here the transtenotic pressure gradient fell from 50mmHg to 10mmHg after PTCA.

A further stenosis in the mid-third of LAD is shown here (g) before, (h) during and (i) after PTCA.

Figure 2.3 *continued*

There was also a stenosis in the mid-third of the LCx, shown here (h), (i) during lesion rupture (note the indentation of the balloon by the hard stenosis), (j) after lesion rupture at 9 atmospheres and (k) after PTCA with the same 3.0mm Micross™ balloon.

The LAD occluded 2 months later and required further PTCA (see Figs 15.18 and 15.57).

Much commitment is required from both patient and interventional cardiologist if multivessel and multilesion PTCA is to be successful in the long term. Staged or multiple procedures, or both, may be necessary, as in this case.

Reading

BARI, CABRI, EAST, GABI and RITA: coronary angioplasty on trial. Lancet 1990;335:1315-16.

Berger PB, Holmes DR Jr. Dilation strategies in patients with multivessel disease. In: Faxon DP, ed. Practical Angioplasty. New York: Raven Press; 1994:71-87.

Berger PB. Randomized trials comparing percutaneous transluminal coronary angioplasty and coronary artery bypass surgery. In: Topol EJ, Serruys PW, eds. Current Review of Interventional Cardiology, 2nd ed. Philadelphia: Current Medicine; 1995:259-78.

Cowley MJ, Vetrovec GW, DiSciascio G, et al. Coronary Angioplasty of Multiple Vessels: Short-Term Outcome and Long-Term Results. Circulation 1985;72:1314-20.

Deligonul U, Vandormael MG, Kern MJ, et al. Coronary angioplasty: a therapeutic option for symptomatic patients with two and three vessel coronary disease. J Am Coll Cardiol 1988;11:1173-9.

Dorros G, Stertzer SH, Cowley MJ, et al. Complex coronary angioplasty: multiple coronary dilatations. Am J Cardiol 1984;53:126C-130C.

Ellis SE, Vandormael MG, Cowley MJ, et al and the Multivessel Angioplasty Prognosis Group. Coronary morphology and clinical determinants of procedural outcome with angioplasty for multivessel coronary disease: implications for patient selection. Circulation 1990;82:1193-202.

Hartzler GO. Percutaneous coronary angioplasty in patients with multivessel disease. In: Jang GD, ed. Angioplasty. New York: McGraw-Hill; 1986:321-36.

Meyer BJ, Kaufmann UP, Meier B. Single-vessel and multivessel percutaneous transluminal coronary angioplasty. In: Grech ED, Ramsdale DR, eds. Practical Interventional Cardiology. London: Martin Dunitz; 1997:49-66.

Myler RK, Topol EJ, Shaw RE, et al. Multiple vessel coronary angioplasty: classification, results and patterns of restenosis in 494 consecutive patients. Cathet Cardiovasc Diagn 1987;13: 1-15.

Raco D, Rihal CS, Yusuf S. Randomized trials of percutaneous transluminal coronary angioplasty: comparison of medical and surgical therapy. In: Grech ED, Ramsdale DR, eds. Practical Interventional Cardiology. London: Martin Dunitz; 1997:317-326.

3

Complex PTCA

Complex PTCA demands careful strategic planning and an experienced interventional cardiologist. Today's equipment enables many challenging lesions, such as ostial and bifurcation lesions, long lesions and distal lesions, to be addressed without too much difficulty. However, procedures are likely to be more prolonged and to demand the use of other technologies if the short- and long-term clinical outcomes are to be improved. As with intervention in multivessel disease, complex PTCA usually involves more than one balloon, guidewire and guiding catheter, a greater volume of contrast media and more radiation exposure to the operator than single-vessel PTCA. It is inevitably more expensive than single-vessel PTCA.

Ostial lesions

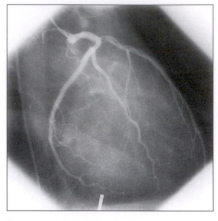

a

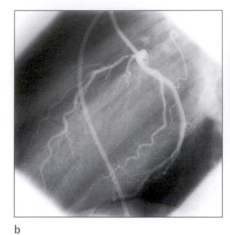

b

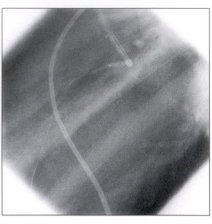

c

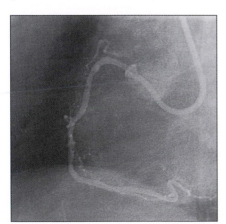

d

Figure 3.1

(a) RAO view and (b) LLAT view of a severe ostial LAD lesion before PTCA.

The same lesion, (c) during and (d) after PTCA with a 2.5mm RX® balloon (ACS).

Lesions such as this have a high rate of restenosis (see Fig. 15.55), as occurred in this 45-year-old insurance agent who developed restenosis three times within 14 months of this first procedure. The final PTCA (8 years ago) was successful.

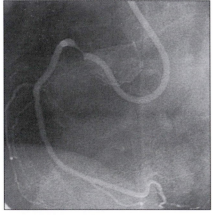

a

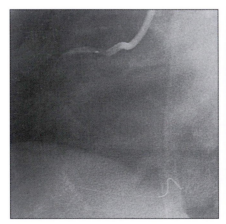

b

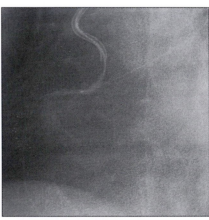

c

d

Figure 3.2

(a) Severe ostial stenosis in a large dominant RCA in a 57-year-old woman with severe angina.

The stenosis was first dilated with (b) a 2.5mm Gold Ex® balloon followed by (c) a 3.0mm RX® perfusion balloon. Note the position of the tip of the Amplatz guiding catheter, which often has to be disengaged from the ostium in such procedures.

(d) Final result.

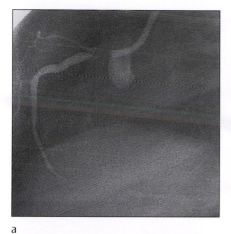

a

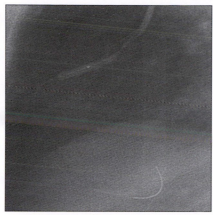

b

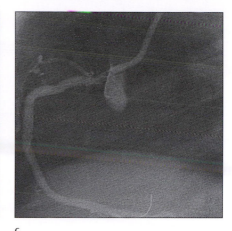

c

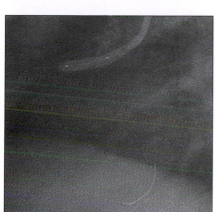

d

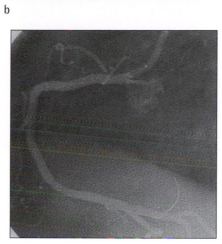

e

Figure 3.3
(a) A severe, flow-limiting, ostial stenosis in the RCA of a 58-year-old woman.
(b) PTCA with a 3.0mm Passage® (Cordis) balloon.
(c) This resulted in an improvement but the result was angiographically unacceptable and prevented stent delivery.
After dilatation with a 3.5mm Viva™ balloon (Scimed), a 3.5mm, 12mm long Microstent™ II (AVE) (d) was deployed.
(e) The final result was excellent.

Bifurcation lesions

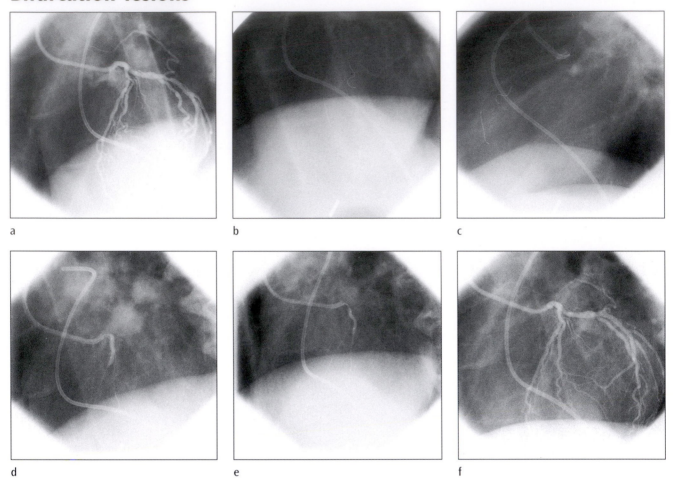

a b c

d e f

Figure 3.4
A 57-year-old man with severe angina. (a) An LAD/DG bifurcation stenosis.
(b, c) Both vessels were wired with 0.014-inch high-torque Floppy® guidewires.
(d) A 3.0mm balloon catheter dilated the stenosis in the LAD, and (e) a 2.5mm Monorail® balloon dilated the stenosis in the proximal/mid-third of the DG.
(f) Final result after PTCA.

Kissing balloons

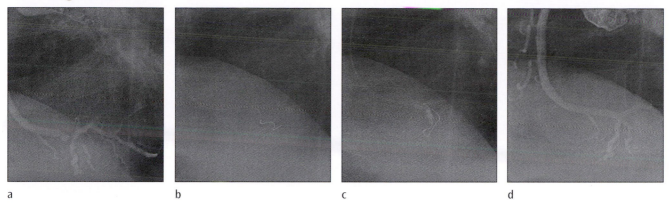

a   b   c   d

Figure 3.5
A 39-year-old computer engineer with recurrence of angina 3 months after multivessel PTCA. (a) Angiography revealed a severe restenosis at the crux of the RCA. The patient's obesity made it difficult to visualize the lesion.
(b) A 0.014-inch Floppy® guidewire was placed down the posterolateral branch and a 0.014-inch Intermediate® guidewire down the posterior descending branch.
A 2.5mm Passage® balloon was used to dilate both lesions in turn, followed by a kissing balloon technique (c) with a 2.5mm balloon in the posterolateral artery and a 3.0mm Passage® balloon in the PDA.
(d) Final result after 3.0mm Passage® balloon used in the posterolateral branch.

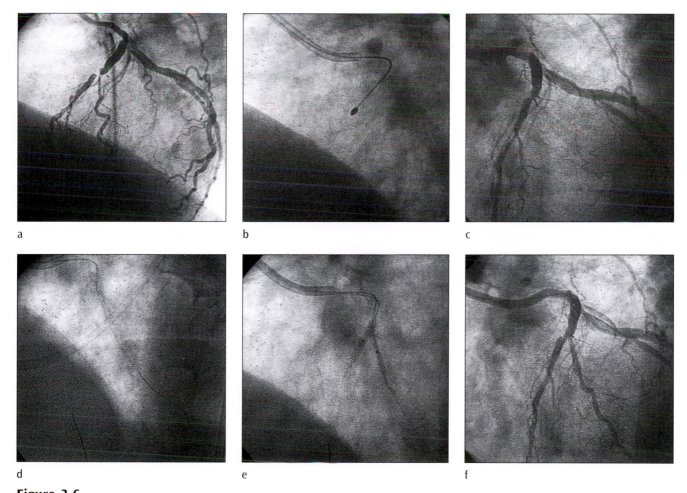

a   b   c

d   e   f

Figure 3.6
(a) A severe calcific stenosis in the mid-LAD at the bifurcation with the DG that also involves the origin of the DG. It was not possible to enter DG with a guidewire. After (b) Rotablator® atherectomy of the LAD stenosis, (c) the DG artery occludes. (d) The DG is then easily entered with a guidewire, and (e) simultaneous inflations are performed with two 2.5mm balloon catheters (kissing balloon technique). (f) Result after PTCA.

Hugging balloons

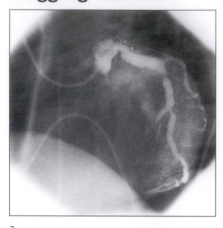

a

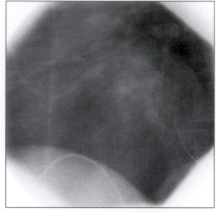

b

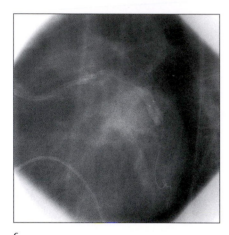

c

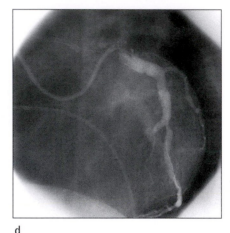

d

Figure 3.7
A 50-year-old man with severe hypertension and renal failure was awaiting renal transplantation when he developed worsening angina on minimal effort. (a) Severe proximal stenosis in a large (8mm diameter) LCx coronary artery.
(b) Two guidewires were placed down the LCx using two Amplatz guide catheters via right and left femoral arteries.

A 3.5mm and a 4.25mm Monorail® balloon catheter were inflated in turn but made no impression on the stenosis. (c) A 3.5mm Monorail® and a 4.0mm RX® balloon were therefore inflated side-by-side (hugging balloon technique) across the stenosis.

(d) The result after PTCA.

The patient underwent successful renal transplantation and the post-PTCA result persisted 7 years later.

Distal disease

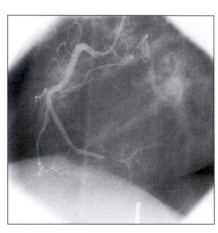

a

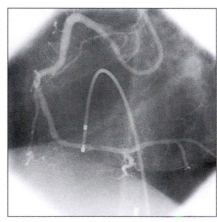

b

Figure 3.8
(a) A severe distal stenosis in a dominant RCA in a 51-year-old politician with moderately severe angina. (b) Result after PTCA with a 2.0mm Monorail® balloon catheter followed by a 3.7mm low profile Monorail® balloon.

Good back-up support from the guide catheter and low-profile balloon catheters enhance success in distal lesions.

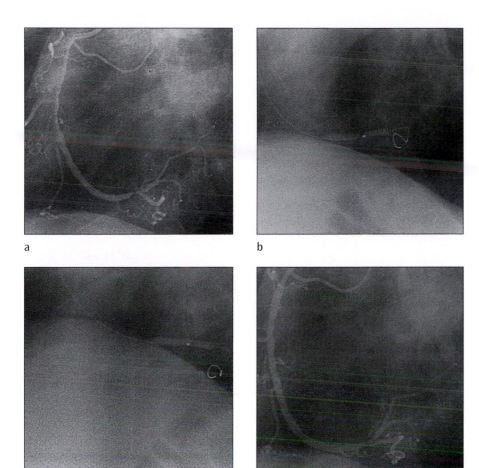

a

b

c

d

Figure 3.9
(a) A severe stenosis in the distal RCA.
(b) The stenosis indents the balloon at 8 atmospheres but (c) dilates at 10 atmospheres.
(d) Final result.

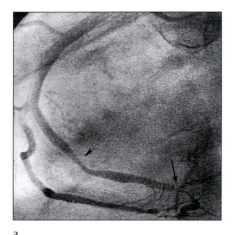

a

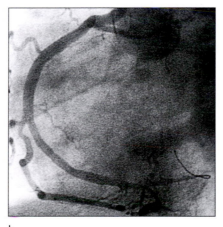

b

Figure 3.10
A 46-year-old car salesman with mild angina. (a) A tight stenosis was found at the distal trifurcation point of the RCA (arrow), with a less severe stenosis more proximally. The posterior descending and posterolateral branches were entered with 0.014-inch Floppy® guidewires and the distal lesion was dilated in turn using a 2.0mm Passage® balloon placed first in the posterior descending branch and then in the posterolateral branch. The more proximal lesion (arrowhead) was dilated with a 3.0mm Elipse™ balloon and stented with a 3.0mm, 15mm long Multilink™ stent (Guidant).
(b) Final result.

Long lesions

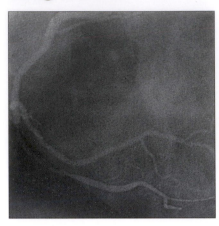
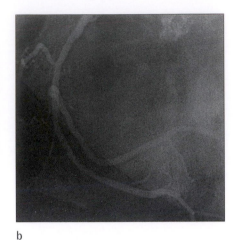

a   b

Figure 3.11
(a) A long lesion in the RCA.
(b) The lesion responded well to PTCA with a 2.5mm, 30mm long balloon.

Diffuse disease

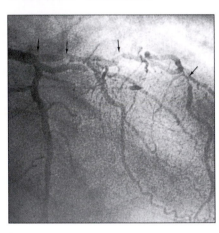
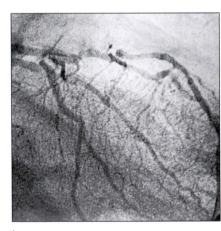

a   b

Figure 3.12
A 65-year-old man with hypertension, hypercholesterolemia and severe angina was found to have significant three-vessel disease, including (a) diffuse disease along the length of the LAD (arrows).
The series of LAD lesions were ablated with a 1.5mm followed by a 1.75mm Rotablator® burr (Boston Scientific) and then post-dilated with a 2.0mm Supercrosse® balloon (Progressive Angioplasty Systems) and subsequently a 2.5mm Express™ balloon. (b) The angiographic result was acceptable, and the lesions in the OMCx and RCA were dilated during the same procedure.

PTCA in patients with poor left ventricular function

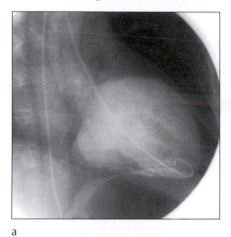

a

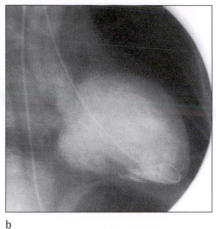

b

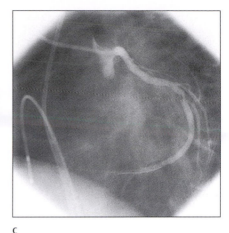

c

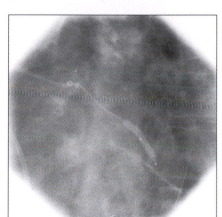

d

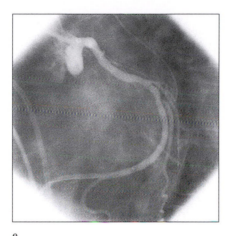

e

Figure 3.13
Left ventricular angiogram in a 54-year-old man with poor left ventricular function and severe angina during (a) systole and (b) diastole.

A severe mid-third LCx lesion (c) before, (d) during and (e) after PTCA with a 3.0mm Low Profile Plus balloon.

Short-duration (15-second) inflations were used in this case to avoid precipitous falls in blood pressure. Perfusion balloon technology is useful in this situation, and circulatory support (e.g. intra-aortic balloon counterpulsation) may lower the risks involved during PTCA in high-risk cases such as this.

This good clinical result was found to persist at 8 years, when the patient underwent oesophagogastrectomy for adenocarcinoma of the oesophagus.

GP IIb-IIIa inhibitors in high-risk, complex lesion PTCA

The CAPTURE and EPIC studies demonstrated the efficacy of abciximab (Reopro®, Eli Lilly), a glycoprotein IIb-IIIa inhibitor, in reducing complications in patients who are at high risk during coronary intervention because of unstable ischaemic syndromes or unfavourable lesion morphology, albeit at the expense of a small increase in the risk of bleeding. The EPILOG study showed that abciximab together with weight-adjusted heparin markedly reduced the risk of acute ischaemic complications in patients undergoing percutaneous coronary revascularization without increasing the risk of haemorrhage.

Reading

Brymer JF, Khaja F, Kraft PL. Angioplasty of long or tandem coronary artery lesions using a new longer balloon dilatation catheter: a comparative study. Cathet Cardiovasc Diagn 1991;23:84-8.

Ellis SG, Topol EJ. Results of percutaneous transluminal coronary angioplasty of high-risk angulated stenoses. Am J Cardiol 1990;66:932-7.

George BS, Myler RK, Stertzer SH, et al. Balloon angioplasty of coronary bifurcation lesions: the kissing balloon technique. Cathet Cardiovasc Diagn 1986;12:124-38.

Goudreau E, DiSciascio G, Kelly K, et al. Coronary angioplasty of diffuse coronary artery disease. Am Heart J 1991;121:12-19.

Hartzler GO. Coronary angioplasty of bifurcation lesions. In: Faxon DP, ed. Practical Angioplasty. New York: Raven Press; 1994:89-100.

Holmes DR Jr. Complex coronary interventions: chronic total occlusions and bifurcation disease. In: Beyar R, Keren G, Leon MB, Serruys PW. Frontiers in Interventional Cardiology. London: Martin Dunitz; 1997:21-7.

King SB III. Angioplasty, stenting or surgery? In: Beyar R, Keren G, Leon MB, Serruys PW, eds. Frontiers in Interventional Cardiology. London: Martin Dunitz; 1997:2-7.

Kohli RS, DiSciascio G, Cowley MJ, et al. Coronary angioplasty in patients with severe left ventricular dysfunction. J Am Coll Cardiol 1990;16:807-11.

Lee BI, Schwartz MB, Seides SF. Balloon angioplasty of lesions beyond extremely angulated bends. J Invas Cardiol 1996;8:157-60.

Lincoff AM, Califf RM, Anderson KM, et al. for the EPIC Investigators. Evidence for prevention of death and myocardial infarction with platelet membrane glycoprotein IIb/IIIa receptor blockade by abciximab (c7e3 fab) among patients with unstable angina undergoing percutaneous coronary revascularization. J Am Coll Cardiol 1997;30:149-56.

Mathias DW, Mooney JF, Lange HW, et al. Frequency of success and complications of coronary angioplasty of a stenosis at the ostium of a branch vessel. Am J Cardiol 1991;67:491-5.

Meier B. Kissing balloon coronary angioplasty. Am J Cardiol 1984;54:918-20.

Myler RK, Shaw RE, Stertzer SH, et al. Lesion morphology and coronary angioplasty: current experience and analysis. J Am Coll Cardiol 1992;19:1641-52.

O'Murchu B, Myler RK. Percutaneous transluminal coronary angioplasty: history, techniques, indications and complications. Unstable angina: pathophysiology and treatment with angioplasty. In: Grech ED, Ramsdale DR, eds. Practical Interventional Cardiology. London: Martin Dunitz; 1997:31-48.

Pande AK, Gosselin G, Rashdan I, et al. Coronary angioplasty in the treatment of post-cardiac transplant coronary artery disease. J Invas Cardiol 1996;8:252-6.

Tan K, Sulke N, Taub N, et al. Clinical and morphologic determinants of coronary angioplasty success and complications: current experience. J Am Coll Cardiol 1995;25:855-65.

The CAPTURE Investigators. Randomised placebo-controlled trial of abciximab before and during coronary intervention in refractory unstable angina: the CAPTURE study. Lancet 1997;349:1429-35.

The EPIC Investigators. Use of monoclonal antibody directed against the platelet glycoprotein IIb/IIIa receptor in high-risk coronary angioplasty. N Engl J Med 1994;330:956-61.

The EPILOG Investigators. Platelet glycoprotein IIb/IIIa receptor blockade and low-dose heparin during percutaneous coronary revascularization. N Engl J Med 1997;336:1689-96.

Topol EJ, Ellis EG, Fishman J, et al. Multicenter study of percutaneous transluminal angioplasty for right coronary artery ostial stenosis. J Am Coll Cardiol 1987;9:1214-18.

Weinstein JS, Baim DS, Sipperly ME, et al. Salvage of branch vessels during bifurcation lesion angioplasty: acute and long-term follow-up. Cathet Cardiovasc Diagn 1991;22:1-6.

Zidar JP, Tanaglia AN, Jackman JD Jr, et al. Improved acute results for PTCA of long coronary lesions using long angioplasty balloon catheters. J Am Coll Cardiol 1992;19:34A.

4

Chronic total occlusions

PTCA for chronic total occlusions is indicated for relief of angina and as part of a strategy for safe intervention in multivessel PTCA.

The shorter the duration of occlusion, the higher the success rate, with the success rate being highest in arteries occluded for less than 3 months compared with those occluded for more than 3 months. Success rates vary from 55 to 80%. Favourable features include:

- a tapered-tip or 'nipple' at the point of occlusion;
- the absence of side-branches at the occlusion site;
- the absence of 'bridging' collaterals; and
- a short length of occlusion.

Adverse features include:

- the absence of a tapered-tip;
- the occlusion being flush at the origin of a vessel or at a bend point;
- side-branches exiting from the point of occlusion;
- the presence of bridging collaterals; and
- the presence of long occlusions (more than 10mm in length).

Success rates are lower in occluded SVGs than in occluded native vessels.

Adequate visualization of the distal vessels via collateral vessels is a significant help in achieving success, and contrast injection down the contralateral artery may be warranted if retrograde filling is provided by this vessel. A pre-occlusion angiogram, if available, is very useful for mapping the course of the vessel to be recanalized.

Floppy 0.014-inch guidewires tend to buckle and curl up against true chronic total occlusions; intermediate- or standard-stiffness guidewires (Fig. 4.1) are usually required, often 'backed up' or supported by a balloon catheter close to the occlusion in order to aid crossing. Larger (0.018-inch) guidewires (Fig. 4.2) and the Magnum™ (0.021-inch) guidewire (Schneider) (Fig. 4.3) can be useful for difficult, chronic occlusions. Care should be taken not to enter a false lumen with the guidewire or balloon catheter by frequently injecting small boluses of contrast media down the guide catheter or through the lumen of an over-the-wire balloon catheter. The guidewire usually moves freely once the true lumen beyond the occlusion is reached. 'Grittiness' or 'resistance' despite apparent advancement of the wire suggests that the guidewire is not in the true lumen of the vessel. The Spectranetics 0.018-inch Prima™ laser guidewire (Fig. 4.4) can recanalize chronic total occlusions by using excimer laser energy emitted from its tip placed up against the occlusion point.

Restenosis or reocclusion occurs in up to 50% of cases treated by PTCA, but this high rate may be reduced by debulking with mechanical or laser atherectomy and/or by coronary stent implantation.

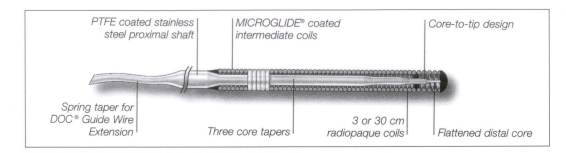

PTFE coated stainless steel proximal shaft

MICROGLIDE® coated intermediate coils

Core-to-tip design

Spring taper for DOC® Guide Wire Extension

Three core tapers

3 or 30 cm radiopaque coils

Flattened distal core

Figure 4.1
Structure of the 0.014-inch Intermediate® guidewire.

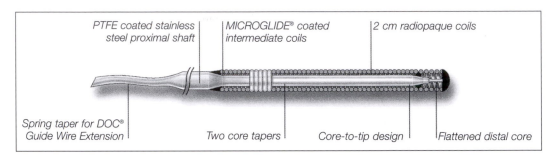

PTFE coated stainless steel proximal shaft

MICROGLIDE® coated intermediate coils

2 cm radiopaque coils

Spring taper for DOC® Guide Wire Extension

Two core tapers

Core-to-tip design

Flattened distal core

Figure 4.2
Structure of the 0.018-inch Standard® guidewire. This is a stiff guidewire that is useful for crossing chronic total occlusions. However, care must be taken to avoid dissection or perforation with such a guidewire and one must ensure that a suitable balloon or exchange catheter is available to accommodate a 0.018-inch guidewire before beginning to use it!

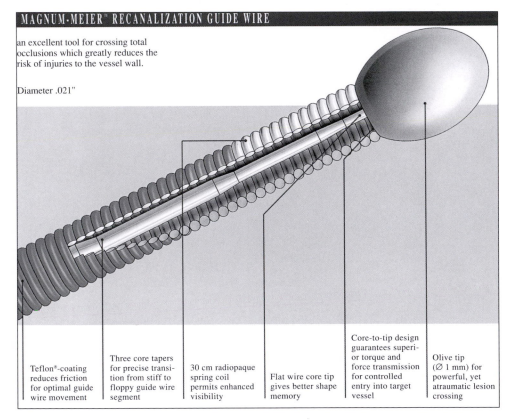

MAGNUM·MEIER® RECANALIZATION GUIDE WIRE

an excellent tool for crossing total occlusions which greatly reduces the risk of injuries to the vessel wall.

Diameter .021"

Teflon®-coating reduces friction for optimal guide wire movement

Three core tapers for precise transition from stiff to floppy guide wire segment

30 cm radiopaque spring coil permits enhanced visibility

Flat wire core tip gives better shape memory

Core-to-tip design guarantees superior torque and force transmission for controlled entry into target vessel

Olive tip (Ø 1 mm) for powerful, yet atraumatic lesion crossing

Figure 4.3
Structure of the 0.021-inch diameter Magnum-Meier™ guidewire, which has a 1mm diameter olive-shaped tip.

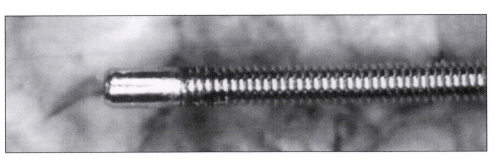

Figure 4.4
The Prima™ laser wire (Spectranetics) can recanalize chronic total occlusions by using excimer laser energy.

Right coronary artery lesions

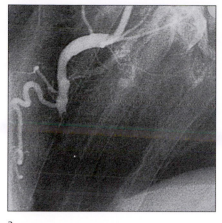
a

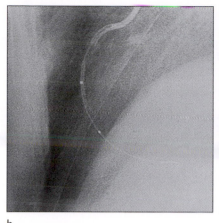
b

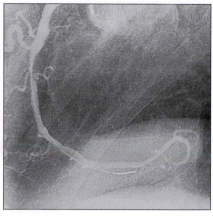
c

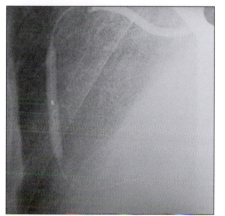
d

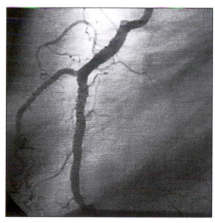
e

Figure 4.5
(a) Totally occluded RCA (of 5 months' duration) showing a tapered distal tip – a favourable feature for successful PTCA.
(b) Occlusion crossed with a 0.014-inch Intermediate® guidewire and a 2.0mm RX® perfusion (ACS, Guidant) balloon catheter, resulting in reperfusion of the RCA but (c) a suboptimal angiographic result.
(d) A 30mm long, 3.0mm Elipse™ balloon catheter is used to obtain (e) a satisfactory appearance.

a

b

Figure 4.6
Proximal RCA occlusion in a 77-year-old man (a) before and (b) after PTCA with a 3.5mm Express Supra™ balloon and 3.5mm Wiktor® (Medtronic) stent implantation. The angiographic result is excellent.

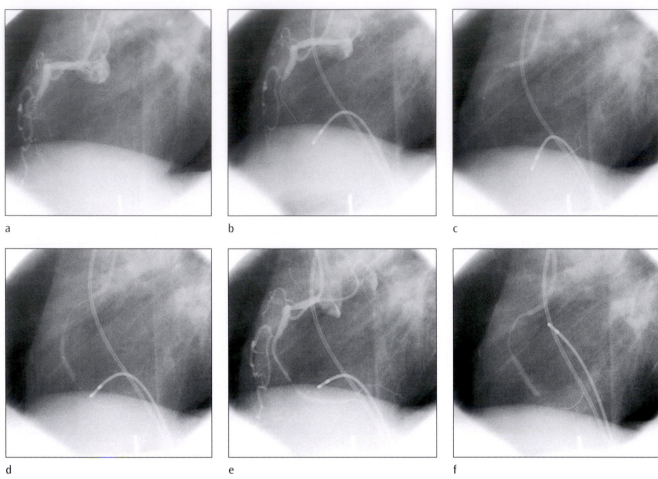

a   b   c

d   e   f

Figure 4.7
(a) Proximal RCA occlusion in a 59-year-old actress with a 7 month history of angina.
(b) A guidewire was advanced across the occlusion and (c) into the distal vessel with some difficulty.
(d) A 3.0mm balloon catheter was inflated to reopen the RCA.
(e) This revealed a further, more distal stenosis.
(f) The more distal lesion was also dilated successfully.
(g) The angiographic result was excellent, as was the clinical result.

g

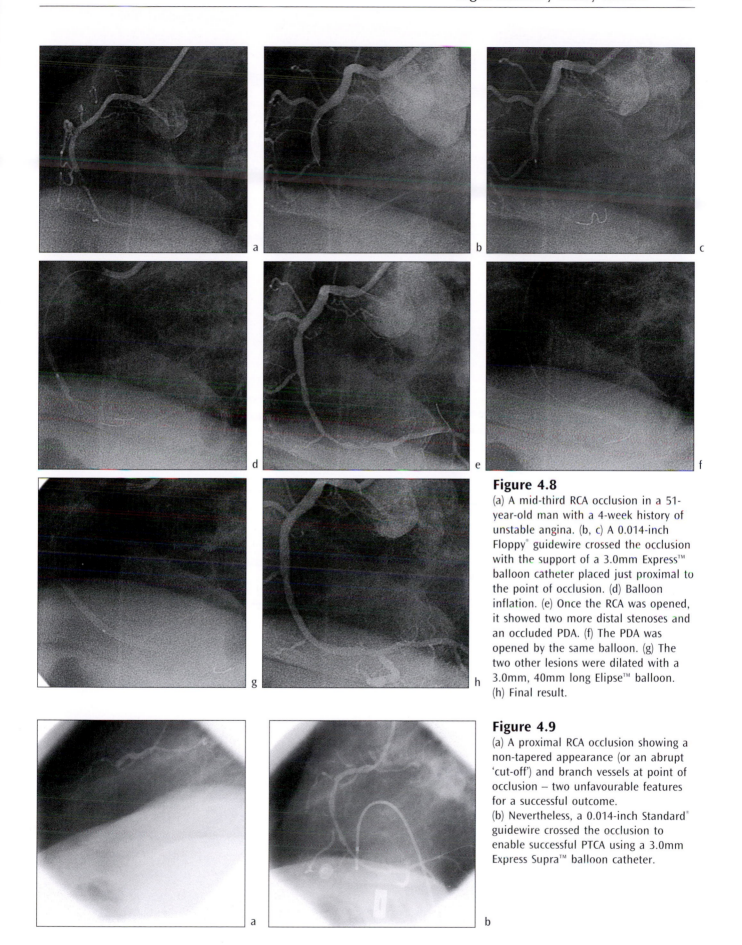

Figure 4.8
(a) A mid-third RCA occlusion in a 51-year-old man with a 4-week history of unstable angina. (b, c) A 0.014-inch Floppy® guidewire crossed the occlusion with the support of a 3.0mm Express™ balloon catheter placed just proximal to the point of occlusion. (d) Balloon inflation. (e) Once the RCA was opened, it showed two more distal stenoses and an occluded PDA. (f) The PDA was opened by the same balloon. (g) The two other lesions were dilated with a 3.0mm, 40mm long Elipse™ balloon. (h) Final result.

Figure 4.9
(a) A proximal RCA occlusion showing a non-tapered appearance (or an abrupt 'cut-off') and branch vessels at point of occlusion – two unfavourable features for a successful outcome.
(b) Nevertheless, a 0.014-inch Standard® guidewire crossed the occlusion to enable successful PTCA using a 3.0mm Express Supra™ balloon catheter.

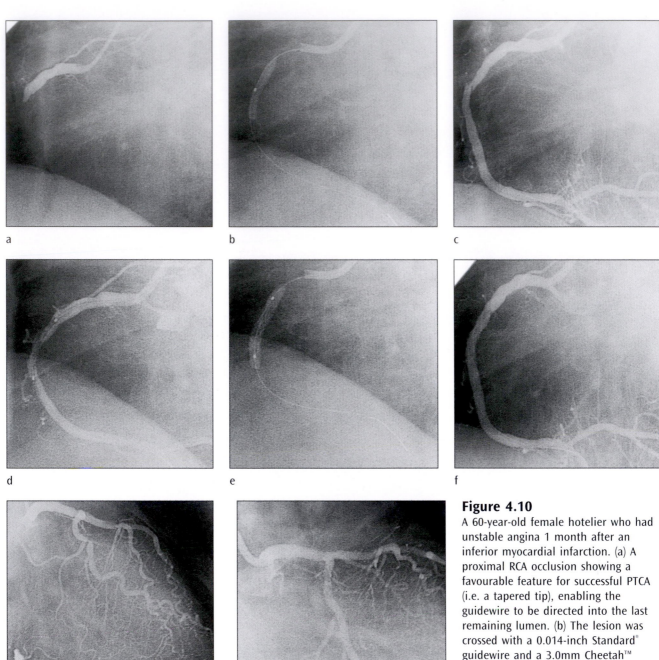

Figure 4.10

A 60-year-old female hotelier who had unstable angina 1 month after an inferior myocardial infarction. (a) A proximal RCA occlusion showing a favourable feature for successful PTCA (i.e. a tapered tip), enabling the guidewire to be directed into the last remaining lumen. (b) The lesion was crossed with a 0.014-inch Standard® guidewire and a 3.0mm Cheetah™ balloon catheter (Medtronic). (c) The occlusion was then reopened to reveal a large dominant RCA. The angiogram, however, showed a suboptimal result owing to a local intimal, non-occlusive dissection. (d, e) A 3.5mm, 18mm long Microstent II™ coronary stent was deployed to produce (f) an excellent angiographic result. In this patient, injection of the left coronary artery initially showed (g) retrograde filling of the distal RCA. There was also a severe stenosis in the LCx. Once the RCA was recanalized, the retrograde filling disappeared. (h) The LCx stenosis was also dilated by PTCA alone using a 3.0mm Cheetah™ balloon over a 0.014-inch Floppy® guidewire.

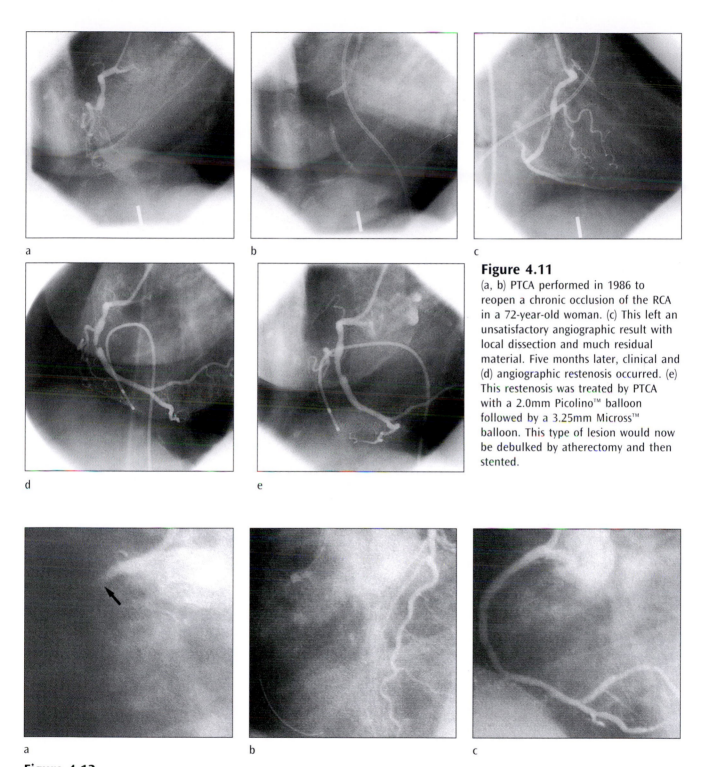

Figure 4.11

(a, b) PTCA performed in 1986 to reopen a chronic occlusion of the RCA in a 72-year-old woman. (c) This left an unsatisfactory angiographic result with local dissection and much residual material. Five months later, clinical and (d) angiographic restenosis occurred. (e) This restenosis was treated by PTCA with a 2.0mm Picolino™ balloon followed by a 3.25mm Micross™ balloon. This type of lesion would now be debulked by atherectomy and then stented.

Figure 4.12

A 39-year-old man. (a) The RCA was proximally occluded (arrow) 16 months after an inferior myocardial infarction.

(b) A stiff Miracle™ guidewire (Asahi®) crossed the occlusion with the help of a contralateral contrast injection into the left coronary artery.

(c) Final result after IVUS-guided implantation of a 32mm long, 7-cell NIR™ stent (Scimed/Boston Scientific).

Courtesy of Dr C Di Mario, EMO-Centro-Cuore, Columbus Hospital, Milan, Italy.

Left anterior descending artery

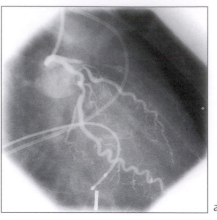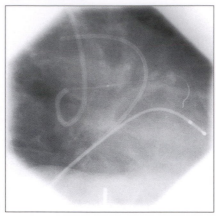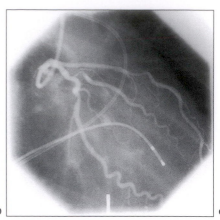

Figure 4.13

A 46-year-old man with unstable angina. (a) A proximal occlusion of the LAD of 4 months' duration. (b) This was crossed with a 0.014-inch Intermediate® guidewire with support from a 2.0mm balloon catheter and 'Amplatzing' of the Judkins guide catheter. (c) Result after PTCA with a 3.0mm balloon catheter.

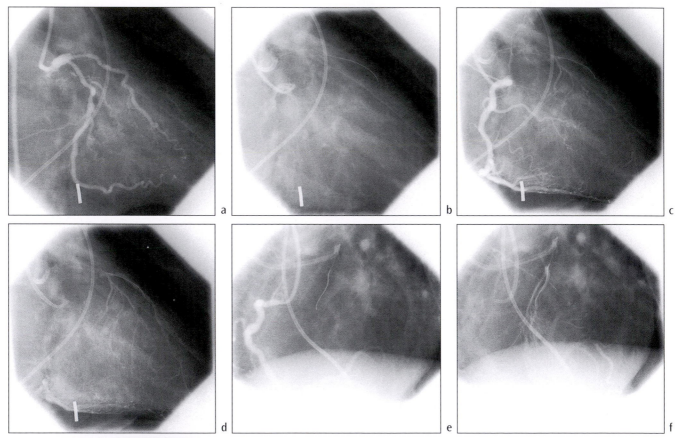

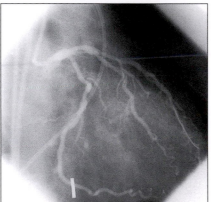

Figure 4.14

A 63-year-old man with moderate angina of 18 months' duration. (a) A proximal occlusion of the LAD; the distal vessel is not visualized.

(b) A guidewire crossed the occlusion.

However, in order to be certain that the wire is in the lumen of the LAD, (c) early- and (d) late-phase right coronary angiography is used to show retrograde filling of LAD up to point of occlusion.

(e, f) This confirms that the guidewire is indeed in the LAD.

(g) Final result after PTCA to point of occlusion with a 3.0mm balloon catheter.

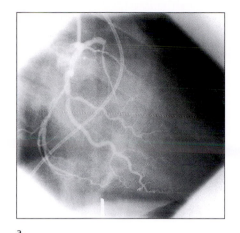

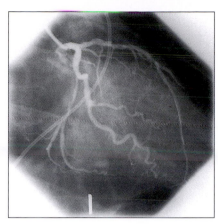

a   b

Figure 4.15
(a) LAD occlusion before PTCA. Note the abrupt 'cut-off' to the LAD, which had probably been occluded for 6 months. (b) Despite this abrupt 'cut-off', a good result was obtained by PTCA after crossing the occlusion with a 0.014-inch Intermediate® guidewire.

Left circumflex artery lesions

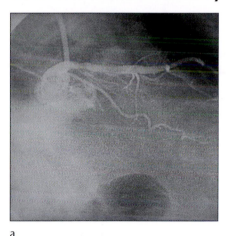

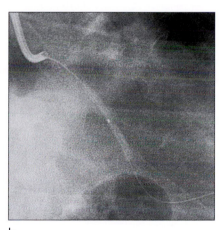

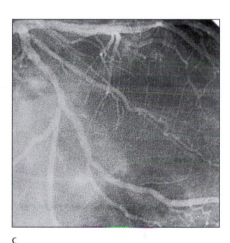

a   b   c

Figure 4.16
(a) A proximal LCx occlusion of 3.5 months' duration.
(b) The occlusion was crossed with a 0.014-inch Intermediate® guidewire and a 3.0mm, 30mm long Elipse™ balloon catheter.
(c) Result after PTCA.

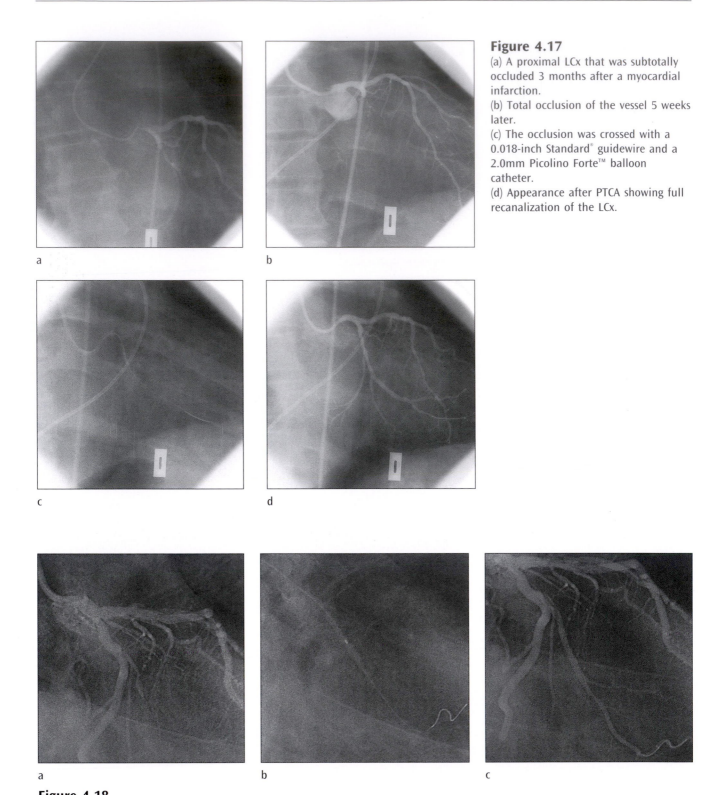

Figure 4.17
(a) A proximal LCx that was subtotally occluded 3 months after a myocardial infarction.
(b) Total occlusion of the vessel 5 weeks later.
(c) The occlusion was crossed with a 0.018-inch Standard® guidewire and a 2.0mm Picolino Forte™ balloon catheter.
(d) Appearance after PTCA showing full recanalization of the LCx.

Figure 4.18
(a) A chronically occluded OMCx.
   The artery was opened using a 0.014-inch high torque Intermediate® guidewire supported by a 2.0mm Express™ balloon. (b) It was subsequently dilated with a 2.5mm, 30mm long Elipse™ balloon.
   (c) A satisfactory result was obtained but local dissection occurred proximally.

Magnum wire for recanalization of chronic total occlusions

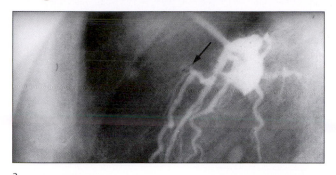

a

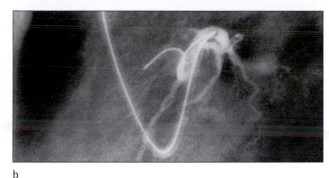

b

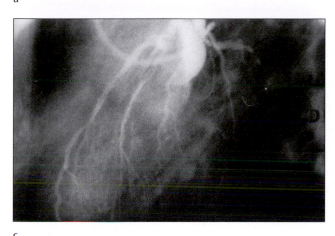

c

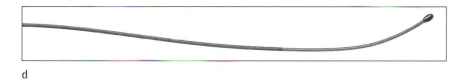

d

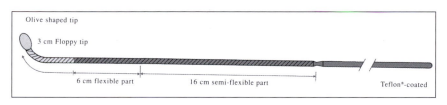

Olive shaped tip

3 cm Floppy tip

6 cm flexible part   16 cm semi-flexible part   Teflon®-coated

e

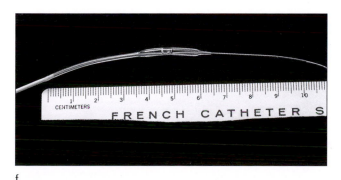

f

Figure 4.19
A 71-year-old woman with exertional angina 9 months after an anterior myocardial infarction was found to have (a) a tortuous LAD that was occluded just beyond the second diagonal branch (arrow).

The excellent trackability of the 0.021-inch Magnum™ wire was advantageous when approaching the lesion. (b) The wire was supported by a balloon catheter advanced up to the occlusion point in order to stiffen the wire.

(c) Final result showing patency of the LAD.

(d, e) The Magnum-Meier™ wire has an olive-shaped tip of approximately 1mm diameter and is backed-up by either the Magnarail™ probing catheter (Schneider) or a balloon catheter such as the Magnarail™ balloon catheter (Schneider) when crossing chronic total occlusions (f).

Courtesy of Dr B Meier, University Hospital, Bern, Switzerland.

Recanalization of chronic total occlusions by laser wire

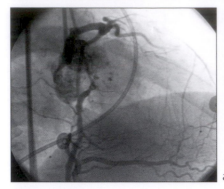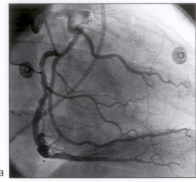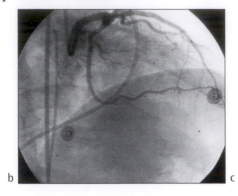

Figure 4.20
A 41-year-old seafarer was known to have had an occluded LAD artery for at least 8 months (10 months after an anterior myocardial infarction) when an attempt to reopen the vessel by PTCA failed (a). The occlusion was approached with a 0.018-inch laser wire supported by its probing catheter. The occlusion was crossed using nine laser bursts of 3 seconds each (energy 50mJ; repetition rate 25Hz). The J-tip of the laser wire was carefully reoriented between each firing, as judged by simultaneous contrast injection into both the right and left coronary arteries. (b) The laser wire was then severed from its hub and used as a conventional exchange guidewire to treat the occlusion with a single pass of an over-the-wire 1.4mm diameter laser catheter (energy 50mJ; repetition rate 25Hz). The laser wire was then replaced by a conventional 0.014-inch wire and the area of previous occlusion dilated by a 3.0mm Europass™ balloon (Cordis) before deploying a 3.0mm, 39mm long Microstent II™ (11 atmospheres). (c) Final result. **Courtesy of Dr M Webb-Peploe, St. Thomas's Hospital, London, UK.**

The TOTAL randomized trial compared the effectiveness of the Prima™ Laser guidewire with conventional guidewires for crossing chronic total occlusions.

Stent implantation for chronic total occlusions

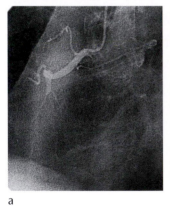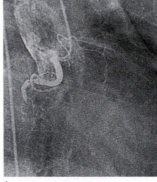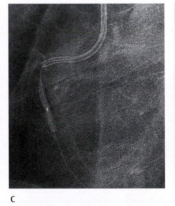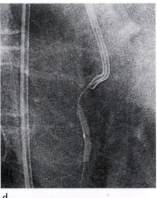

a   b   c   d

Figure 4.21
A 51-year-old storekeeper presented with severe unstable angina 1 month after an inferior myocardial infarction treated with rtPA. (a, b) The RCA is very tortuous and occluded in its middle third. (c, d) The occlusion was crossed with a 0.014-inch Intermediate® guidewire supported by a deeply engaged Amplatz AR2 guide catheter and a 3.0mm Express™ balloon catheter. (e) Once the RCA had

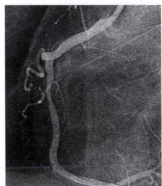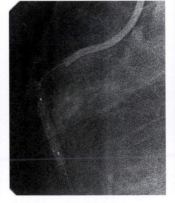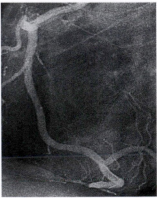

e   f   g

been opened with a 3.0mm balloon, a residual stenosis and local dissection was visible. (f) This was treated by implantation of a 3.5mm, 18mm long Microstent II™. (g) Final result.

The SICCO trial showed that stenting chronic total occlusions results in superior angiographic and clinical outcomes at 6 months compared with PTCA (restenosis rate 32% versus 74%; rate of angina 43% versus 76%; TLR rate at 6 months 22% versus 42%). These findings are supported by the Italian GISSOC study.

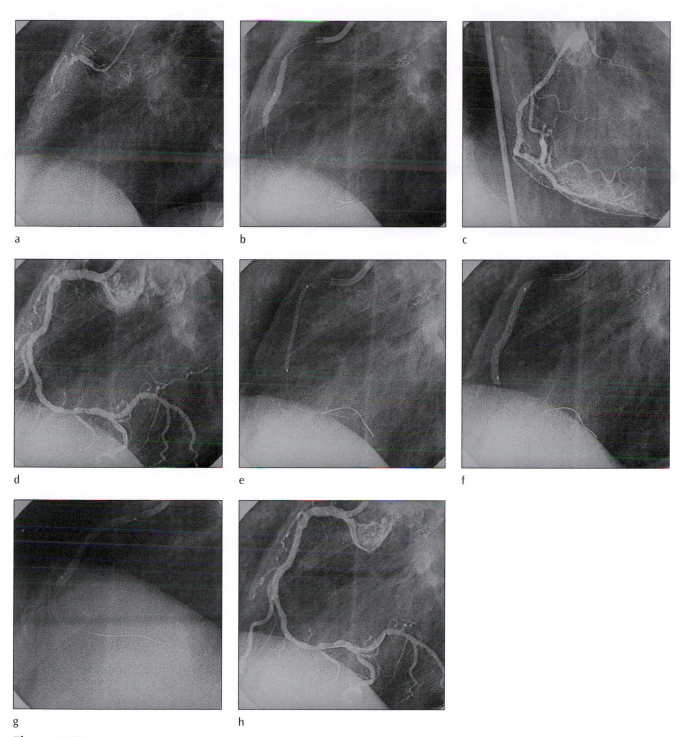

a   b   c

d   e   f

g   h

Figure 4.22

A 60-year-old man who was a retired schoolteacher complained of easily provoked angina 2 months after a suspected inferior myocardial infarction. (a) The RCA was totally occluded over a long segment. The distal vessel was seen to fill retrogradely from the left coronary artery.

(b) The occlusion was easily crossed with a 0.014-inch Intermediate® guidewire and the RCA was reopened with a 3.0mm, 30mm long Elipse™ balloon catheter.

(c) This revealed a severe stenosis in the middle third of the RCA.

(d) Further dilatation produced a satisfactory result.

However, because of some visible recoil, a 3.0mm, 39mm long Microstent II™ was implanted (e–g).

(h) The final result was good.

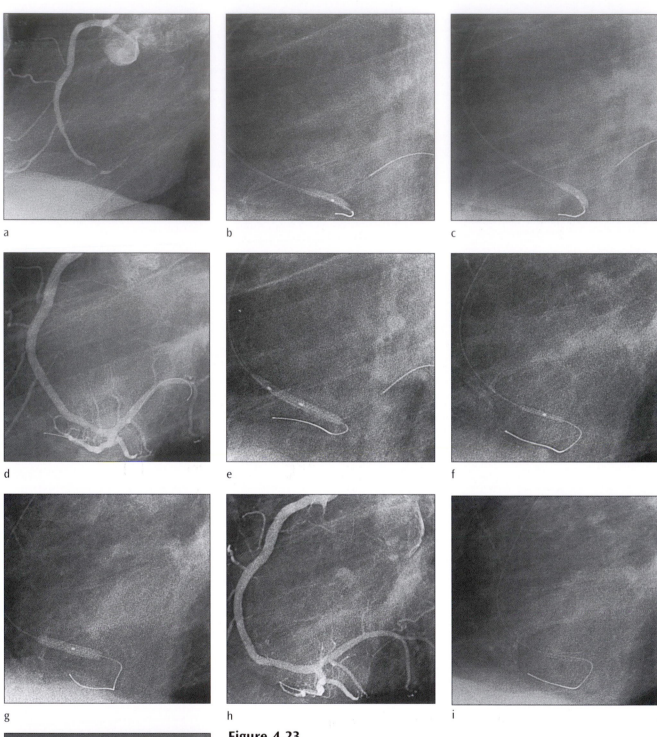

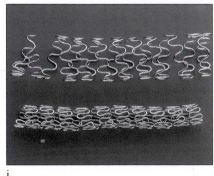

Figure 4.23

A 58-year-old banker presented with chest pain and dyspnoea. (a) A dominant RCA was occluded at the crux.

(b, c) Two 0.014-inch Intermediate® guidewires were used to cross the lesion into the posterior descending and posterolateral branches, and a 2.5mm Passage® balloon was used along the posterior descending wire to reopen the RCA.

(d) Once the RCA was reopened, a more proximal lesion was revealed.

(e) A 3.0mm, 30mm long Samba™ balloon (USCI) then dilated both lesions.

(f, g) A 3.0mm, 15mm long Crossflex™ stent (Cordis) was then implanted at the crux.

(h) The angiographic result was excellent. The stent is (i) radio-opaque and (j) configured into sinusoidal wavelets and wound into a helical coil.

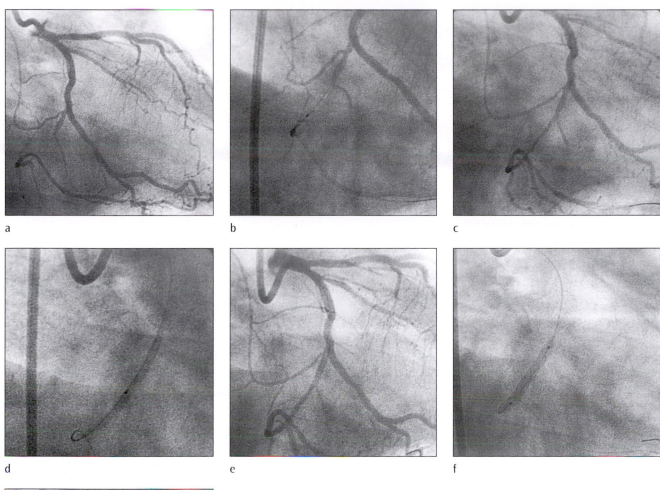

a   b   c

d   e   f

g

Figure 4.24
A 50-year-old man with a 2-year history of post-infarct angina had (a) an occluded LCx.
(b, c) The occlusion was crossed with a 0.014-inch Intermediate® guidewire supported by a 2.0mm Worldpass™ balloon and dilated.
(d, e) It was then dilated with a 2.5mm, 30mm long Elipse™ balloon, resulting in marked improvement.
(f, g) The lesion was then stented with a 3.0mm, 24mm long Microstent II™ , with a good final result.

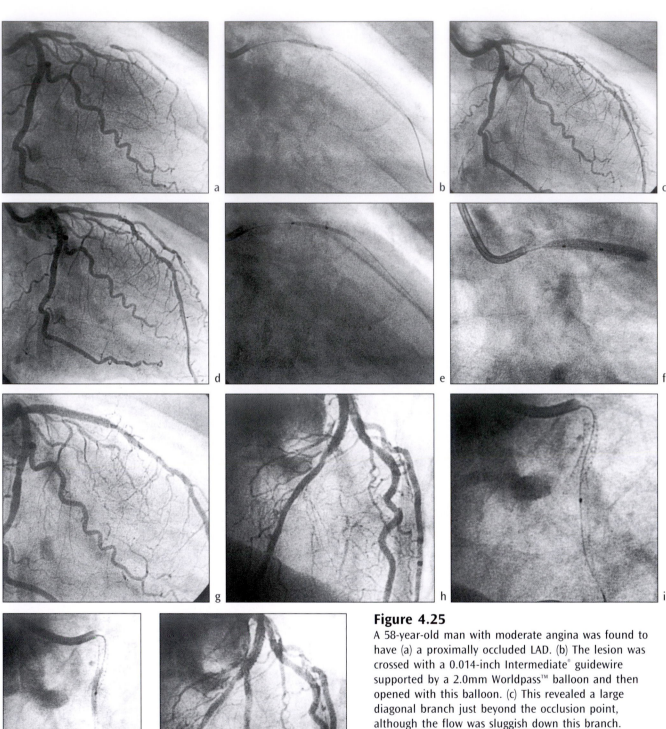

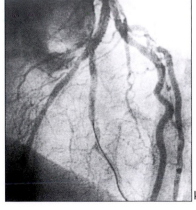

Figure 4.25

A 58-year-old man with moderate angina was found to have (a) a proximally occluded LAD. (b) The lesion was crossed with a 0.014-inch Intermediate® guidewire supported by a 2.0mm Worldpass™ balloon and then opened with this balloon. (c) This revealed a large diagonal branch just beyond the occlusion point, although the flow was sluggish down this branch.

After further dilatation with a 3.0mm Cruiser II balloon (d), the lesion was stented with a 3.0mm, 25mm long Crossflex™ stent (e, f).

This gave an excellent angiographic result in the LAD. However, the diagonal branch covered by the stent became virtually occluded (g, h).

(i) The diagonal branch was entered with a 0.014-inch Floppy® guidewire via the side wall of the stent.

(j) It was then reopened with a 2.0mm followed by a 2.5mm Worldpass™ balloon.

(k) Final result.

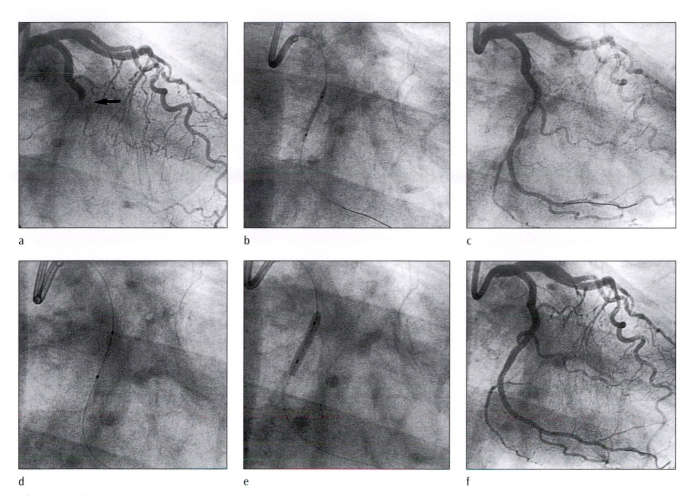

a   b   c

d   e   f

Figure 4.26

A 65-year-old man with moderate angina had (a) a proximal occlusion of the LCx (arrow).

(b) The LCx was crossed with a 0.014-inch Intermediate® guidewire supported by a 2.0mm Rocket™ balloon catheter, and the vessel was recanalized by dilatation with the Rocket™ balloon at 8 atmospheres.

(c) This produced a good result.

(d, e) A 3.0mm, 15mm long Multilink™ stent was then implanted,

(f) giving an excellent final result, and relief of symptoms.

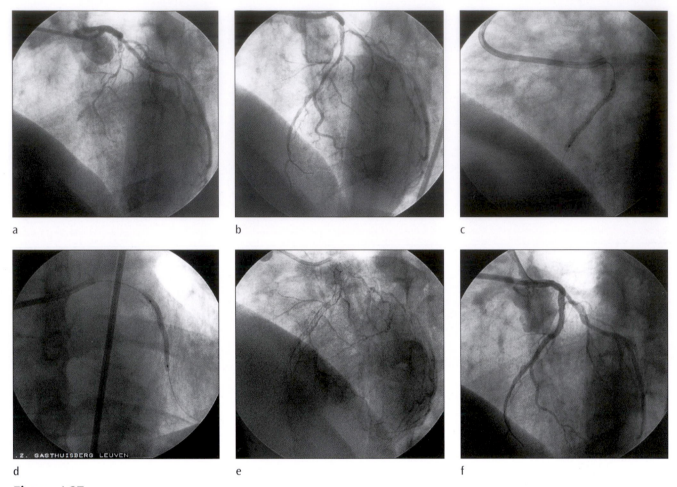

Figure 4.27

An 82-year-old lady with unstable angina was found to have (a) an occluded LAD.

(b) The vessel was recanalized using a 0.014-inch Floppy® guidewire and a 2.5mm Goldie™ balloon.

(c, d) A 40mm long Freedom™ stent (Global Therapeutics) was mounted on a 3.0mm, 40mm long Schneider® balloon and implanted in the LAD.

The stent is radio-opaque (e) and the final angiographic result is excellent (f). The patient remained angina-free 3 years later.

Courtesy of Dr I de Scheerder, University Hospital Gasthuisberg, Leuven, Belgium.

Stents in series for long segments of disease in totally occluded vessels

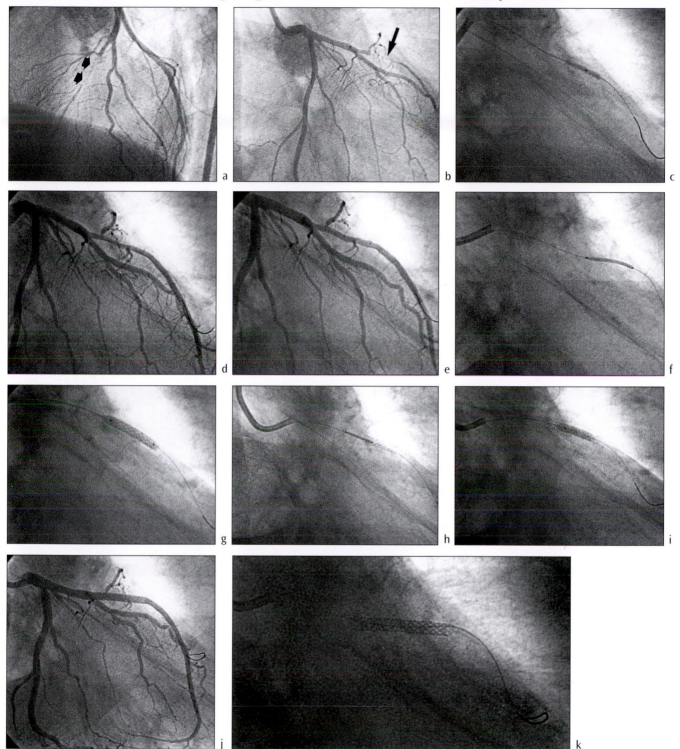

Figure 4.28

A 45-year-old support worker with a history of anterior myocardial infarction 2 years earlier had mild angina of effort despite medical therapy. Seven months before undergoing intervention he had been shown to have (a, b) an occluded LAD (arrows).
(c) The occlusion was crossed with a 0.014-inch Intermediate® guidewire supported with a 2.0mm Adante™ balloon (Scimed/Boston Scientific) and opened by PTCA after forcing the low-profile balloon across the occlusion. (d) The post-PTCA result was very good.
(e) However, this was further improved by dilatation with a 3.0mm Adante™ balloon. (f, g) A 3.5mm, 25mm long NIRoyal™ stent (Scimed/Boston Scientific) was deployed in the distal half of the lesion. A second 3.5mm, 16mm long NIRoyal™ stent was then placed proximally.

Care was taken to overlap the two stents and leave none of the lesion uncovered and the radio-opacity of these gold-plated stents helps to achieve this (h). (i) The stent 'overlap' was then post-dilated at high pressure (16 atmospheres) and (j) an excellent angiographic result was obtained. (k) The radio-opaque NIRoyal™ stents are clearly visible on fluoroscopy.

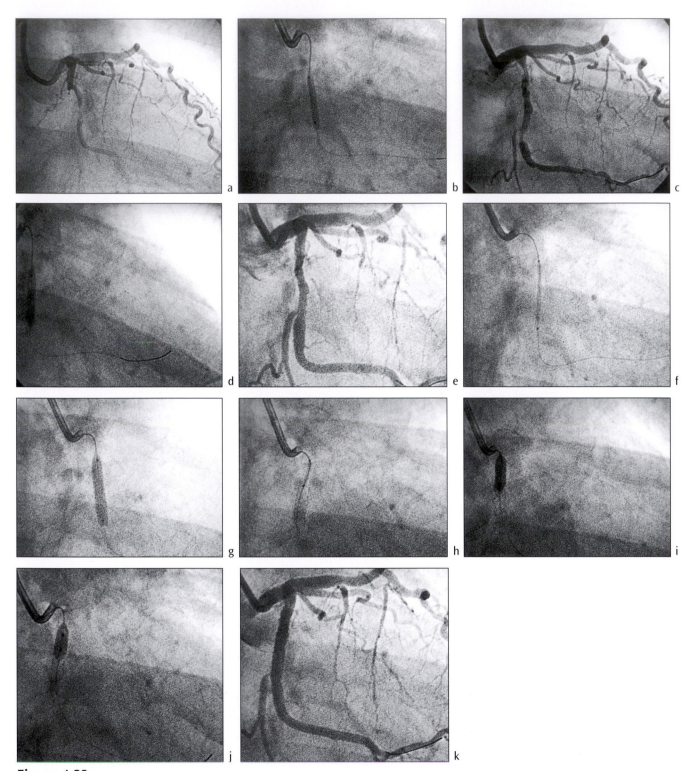

Figure 4.29

A 61-year-old man with angina of moderate severity had (a) an occluded LCx.

(b) The occlusion was crossed with a 0.014-inch Floppy® guidewire and opened with a 2.5mm Vital (Blue Medical) balloon. This revealed extensive disease (c).

Further dilatations with a 3.0mm Vital balloon (d) produced significant improvement (e).

A 4.0mm, 25mm long Phytis® (Phytis) stent was then deployed in the distal half of the lesion (f, g) and a 4.0mm, 16mm long Phytis® stent was deployed in the proximal half of the lesion (h, i). Care was taken to ensure that the stents overlapped.

(j) The stents were then post-dilated with a 4.0mm, 9mm long Maxxum™ balloon (Boston Scientific) up to 16 atmospheres.

(k) This gave an excellent final result.

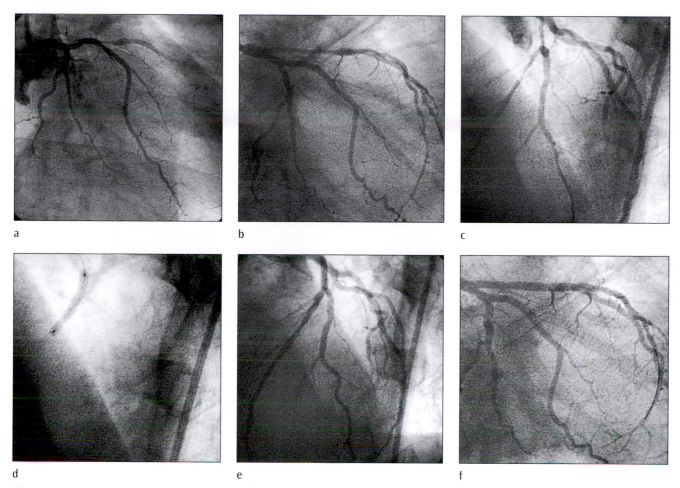

a

b

c

d

e

f

Figure 4.30

(a) An occluded LAD of approximately 10 months' duration in a 36-year-old man with limiting angina. This angiogram shows occlusion at the ostium (arrow), although some of the mid-third segment can be seen from collateral vessels.

It was possible to cross the occlusion with a 0.014-inch Intermediate® guidewire with back-up support from a 2.0mm Rocket™ balloon. The long occlusion was opened with three sequential dilatations from the mid-LAD back to the ostium using the 2.0mm Rocket™ followed by a 2.5mm, 30mm long Worldpass™ balloon.

(b, c) This produced significant improvement but there was a residual stenosis.

(d) A 3.0mm, 33mm long Velocity™ stent (Cordis/Johnson and Johnson) was deployed in the distal/mid-LAD segment and a 3.0mm, 23mm long Velocity™ stent was deployed from the mid-LAD back to the ostium. The stents were overlapped and post-dilated to high pressure.

(e, f) The final result was excellent.

The 'FlexSegment'-multicellular design of the recently released Velocity™ stent provides for flexibility and conformability while maintaining radial strength and good wall coverage on bend sites. Stent flaring at the edges of the balloon is minimized and the shoulders of the stent delivery balloon do not dilate more than the rest of the balloon, so reducing the chance of edge dissection.

The SPACTO trial showed that, after successful recanalization, chronic total occlusions treated with Wiktor® coil stents demonstrated reduced restenosis rates and adverse cardiac events when compared to PTCA alone.

The Canadian TOSCA trial compared the long-term clinical and angiographic outcome of patients with a chronic total occlusion who were treated with the heparin-coated Palmaz-Schatz® stent with the outcome of those patients treated with PTCA alone. The trial showed improved patency and a lower need for revascularization at 6 months in the stented patients compared with those who had undergone PTCA.

Use of non-balloon catheter for guidewire support and confirmation of guidewire position in true lumen

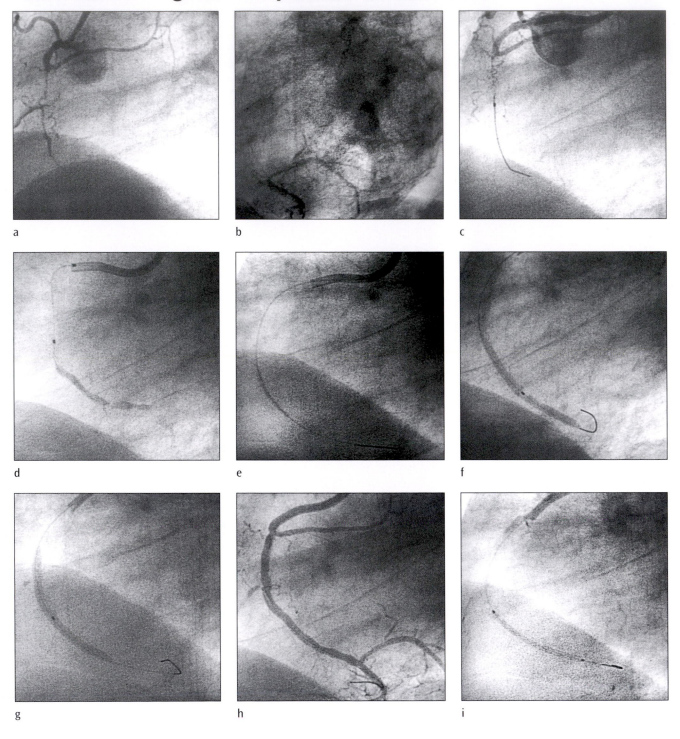

a

b

c

d

e

f

g

h

i

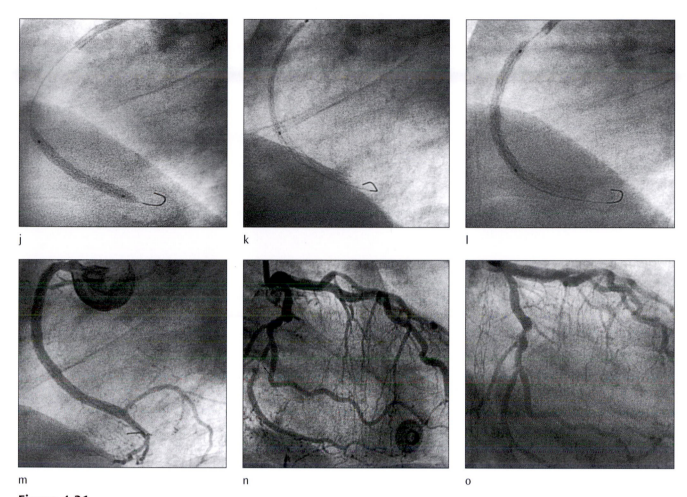

j   k   l

m   n   o

Figure 4.31

A 61-year-old woman with moderately severe angina had an occluded RCA and a severe stenosis in the OMCx. (a) The RCA looked unfavourable for PTCA with 'bridging collaterals', the absence of a 'nipple' and the presence of side-branches at the site of occlusion.

(b) The occlusion was long with little distal vessel filling retrogradely from the left coronary artery.

The 0.014-inch Floppy® and Intermediate® guidewires could not be passed even with support of a Bullet™ catheter (Cardiovascular Dynamics). (c) However, a 0.014-inch Standard® guidewire was passed progressively into the distal vessel with the Bullet™ catheter supporting the wire. A radio-opaque marker is present at the tip of the Bullet™ catheter.

(d) Contrast injection down the Bullet™ showed the distal lumen, confirming that the guidewire was within the true lumen and that significant stenoses lay ahead.

(e) A 1.5mm Worldpass™ balloon was passed over the guidewire and inflated serially from the distal to the proximal RCA.

(f-h) A 3.0mm, 40mm long Elipse™ was then inflated along its length with a good angiographic result.

(i, j) A 3.0mm, 30mm long Microstent™ was placed distally beginning at the crux.

(k, l) A 3.0mm, 39mm long Microstent™ was placed proximally (overlapping).

(m) This gave an excellent angiographic result.

(n) Once the RCA was opened, the OMCx stenosis (arrow) was dilated with a 1.5mm followed by a 2.5mm Worldpass™ balloon.

(o) This produced an excellent angiographic result.

Therapeutic ultrasound to recanalize a chronic total occlusion using the Sonicross® device

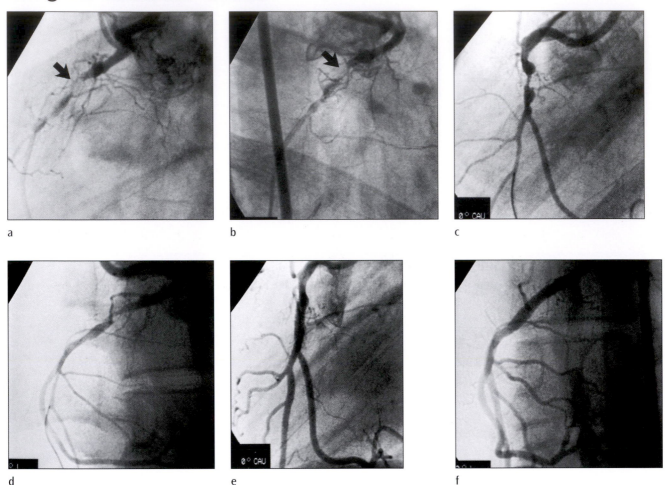

a   b   c

d   e   f

Figure 4.32

A 31-year-old man was found to have an occluded RCA of 15 weeks' duration. PTCA failed to reopen the vessel. (a, b) The coronary angiogram demonstrates a proximal occlusion of the RCA with bridging collaterals that provide antegrade filling of the distal RCA. An 8F Amplatz guiding catheter was used.

However, a 0.014-inch guidewire (HiTorque Super Sport™, ACS) failed to cross the occlusion despite support with a 1.5mm balloon catheter. The balloon catheter was then exchanged for the therapeutic ultrasound catheter, which was placed gently at the beginning of the occlusion.

(c, d) After the first treatment of 30 seconds, the guidewire easily passed the occlusion and the vessel reopened with PTCA using the 1.5mm balloon catheter.

With additional ultrasound treatment and following PTCA and stent deployment with a 3.0mm Multilink™ stent, the angiographic result appeared excellent with full recanalization.

(e, f) There was minimal residual stenosis and good distal run-off.

IVUS imaging confirmed the successful angiographic result and showed a well expanded stent, no dissection and no thrombus in the RCA.

Courtesy of Drs T Nagai, N Eigler, H Luo, S Atar and R J Siegel, Cedars-Sinai Medical Center, Los Angeles, California, USA.

Use of the Terumo® Crosswire™ for crossing difficult chronic total occlusions

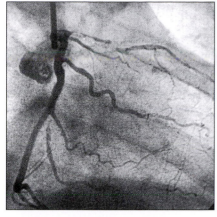

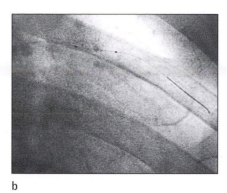

b

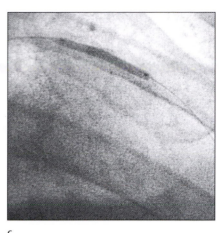

a

c

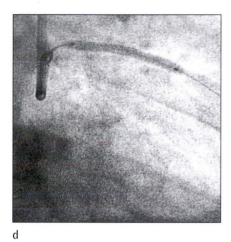

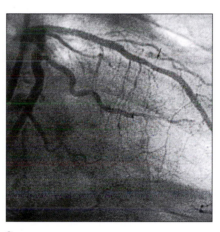

d

e

The lubricious hydrophilic coating of the Terumo® Crosswire™ (Terumo Medical Corporation) may permit a smooth passage through the most challenging occlusions. Its nickel and titanium core offers less risk of kinking.

Figure 4.33

(a) A long chronic total occlusion of the LAD in a 55-year-old journalist with severely limiting angina.

Neither a 0.014-inch Intermediate® nor a Standard® guidewire would cross the occlusion, even with support from a 2.0mm balloon catheter. However, a 0.014-inch Terumo® Crosswire™ crossed into the distal LAD without too much difficulty.

(b) This enabled a 2.0mm Worldpass™ balloon to be advanced across the occlusion and to re-establish flow.

(c, d) The proximal and mid-LAD were then dilated with a 2.5mm Worldpass™ balloon and stented with a 3.0mm, 33mm long Multilink Tristar™ stent (Guidant).

(e) The final angiographic result was excellent. The mid-section (arrow) was intramyocardial and compressed in systole, but it was not stented.

Note the Amplatz guiding catheter that was chosen to provide the back-up support required when chronic total occlusions are being crossed with a balloon catheter.

Reading

Buller CE, Dzavik V, Carere RG, *et al*. Primary stenting versus balloon angioplasty in occluded coronary arteries. The Total Occlusion Study of Canada (TOSCA). Circulation 1999;100:236-42.

Chronos N, King SB III. Chronic total occlusions. In: Grech ED, Ramsdale DR, eds. Practical Interventional Cardiology. London: Martin Dunitz; 1997:67-81.

Dick RJL, Haudenschild CC, Popma JJ, *et al*. Directional coronary atherectomy for total coronary occlusions. Coronary Artery Dis 1991;2:189-99.

Hamburger JN, Serruys PW. Laser guidewire for recanalization of chronic total occlusions. In: Beyar R, Keren G, Leon MB, Serruys PW. Frontiers in Interventional Cardiology. London: Martin Dunitz; 1997:47-53.

Hoher M, Grebe O, Woehrle J, *et al*. Wiktor stent implantation in chronic total occlusions reduces restenosis rate: initial results of the SPACTO trial. Circulation 1997;96(Suppl I):I-268.

Ivanhoe RJ, Weintraub WS, Douglas JS Jr. Percutaneous transluminal coronary angioplasty of chronic total occlusions: primary success, restenosis and long-term clinical follow-up. Circulation 1992;85:106-15.

Maiello L, Colombo A, Gianrossi R, *et al*. Coronary angioplasty of chronic occlusions: factors predictive of procedural success. Am Heart J 1992;124:581-4.

Medina A, Melian F, deLozo JS, *et al*. Effectiveness of coronary stenting for the treatment of chronic total occlusions in angina pectoris. Am J Cardiol 1994;73:1222-4.

Meier B, Carlier M, Finci L, *et al*. Magnum wire for balloon recanalization of chronic total occlusions. Am J Cardiol 1989;64:148-54.

Meier B. Total occlusion. In: Faxon DP, ed. Practical Angioplasty. New York: Raven Press; 1994:101-19.

Sirnes PA, Golf S, Myreng Y, *et al*. Stenting In Chronic Coronary Occlusion (SICCO): a randomized, controlled trial of adding stent implantation after successful angioplasty. J Am Coll Cardiol 1996;28:1444-51.

5

Percutaneous coronary intervention in acute myocardial infarction

Primary PTCA

Primary PTCA is probably the best technique for restoring coronary artery patency after acute occlusion has caused an acute myocardial infarction. Prompt recanalization can usually be achieved within minutes of the patient's arrival at the catheter laboratory and obtaining the angiograms. Recurrent ischaemia, myocardial infarction, in-hospital and long-term mortality have been shown to be lower after primary PTCA than after thrombolytic therapy.

However, logistic difficulties currently prevent this service from being offered 24 hours a day in the majority of communities around the world. Specific complications are associated with PTCA in acute myocardial infarction and it should be practised only by experienced interventional cardiologists in a catheter laboratory with experienced staff and surgical back-up. Ancillary means of cardiac support, such as intra-aortic balloon counterpulsation or percutaneous bypass, should be available for patients with cardiogenic shock after extensive acute myocardial infarction.

Rescue PTCA

Rescue PTCA can be performed when thrombolysis fails to reperfuse the myocardium after 90 minutes and in patients who have persisting angina despite successful recanalization.

Immediate PTCA

Immediate PTCA, performed routinely after successful thrombolytic therapy, has been thought to offer little additional benefit and possibly to be associated with an increased complication rate. However, whether this negative outcome is true when stenting and modern antiplatelet drugs are used in this situation is doubtful; further study is required.

Stent implantation

In recent times, coronary stent implantation in acute myocardial infarction has proved to be of great benefit in improving the angiographic result after successful recanalization by PTCA. With antiplatelet agents, stenting does not cause increased thrombosis and it is associated with a low incidence of in-hospital recurrent ischaemia, reinfarction, early and late reocclusion and late restenosis.

Thrombectomy devices

Newer devices such as the AngioJet® Thrombectomy catheter enable the destruction and removal of unorganized thrombus from native coronary arteries and from bypass grafts.

Rescue PTCA

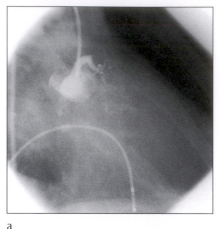

a

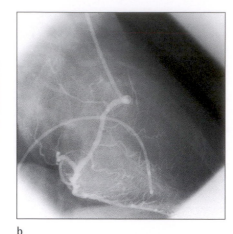

b

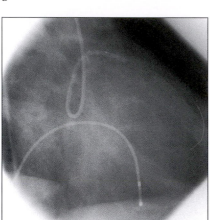

c

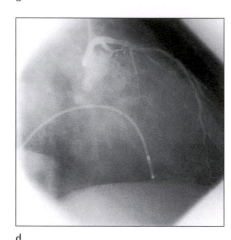

d

Figure 5.1

A proximal LAD occlusion in a 49-year-old woman with cardiogenic shock after thrombolysis. (a, b) Angiograms show an acutely occluded LAD, as well as (a) chronic occlusion of LCx and (b) a normal RCA with retrograde filling of LAD to the point of occlusion.
(c) The LAD occlusion was crossed by a 0.014-inch Floppy® guidewire and a 3.0mm RX® balloon catheter with enhanced guide catheter support.
(d) An angiogram showing the post-PTCA result and a fully patent LAD. The recanalization resulted in normalization of the blood pressure without complication. The LCx could not be reopened even with a 0.018-inch Standard® guidewire and was assumed to be a chronic occlusion.

The CORAMI study demonstrated 90% angiographic success, 96% hospital survival and a 7% angiographic reocclusion rate in patients undergoing rescue PTCA for failed thrombolysis.

Immediate PTCA after a myocardial infarction

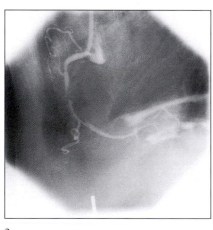

a

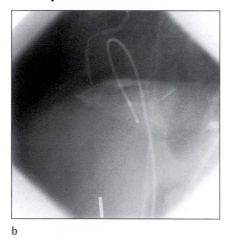

b

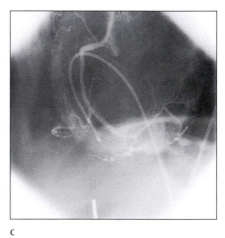

c

Figure 5.2

Successful thrombolysis after acute myocardial infarction often leaves behind a severe residual stenosis, as occurred in this patient after rtPA therapy. (a) The RCA has a severe residual stenosis in its middle third. (b) The lesion was easily crossed with a guidewire and balloon catheter and dilated. (c) This yielded an excellent angiographic result. Note the presence of a temporary pacing electrode.

Immediate PTCA after thrombolysis was originally reported to be associated with a significant complication rate, especially an increased reocclusion rate, and PTCA was therefore reserved for patients who had persisting angina. However, coronary stenting after successful thrombolysis has been shown to be safe and effective and to prevent early major cardiac events. Thus there is a need to reappraise this stent strategy for patients after thrombolysis.

Primary PTCA in acute myocardial infarction

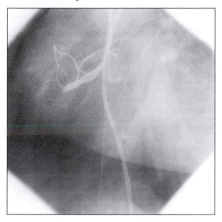

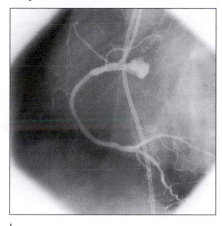

a

b

Figure 5.3

(a) Acute occlusion of an RCA in a 65-year-old woman who presented with an acute inferior myocardial infarction.
(b) The post-PTCA angiogram showing full recanalization of a dominant vessel.

The PAMI and ZWOLLE randomized trials showed significantly greater infarct artery patency, lower reocclusion and reinfarction rates and improved morbidity and mortality in patients treated with primary PTCA compared with those treated with thrombolytic therapy.

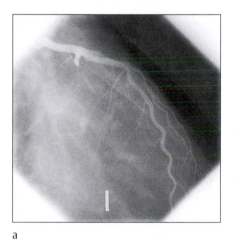

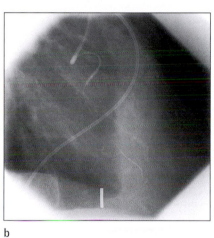

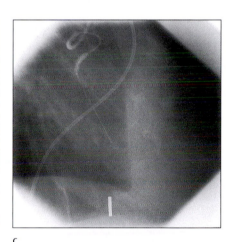

a

b

c

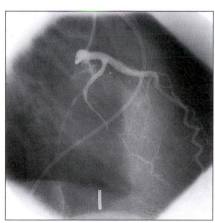

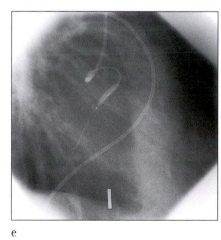

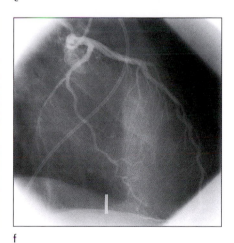

d

e

f

Figure 5.4

(a) Acute occlusion of the LCx in a 50-year-old man who presented with an acute inferolateral myocardial infarction and ventricular fibrillation.

The occlusion was easily crossed with a 0.014-inch Floppy® guidewire placed into the obtuse marginal branch. (b) A 2.0mm balloon catheter followed by (c) a 3.0mm balloon catheter was used to recanalize the vessel.

(d) This revealed a further stenosis just beyond the bifurcation.

(e) The guidewire was then placed in the true LCx and the second stenosis was dilated.

(f) This produced a satisfactory result.

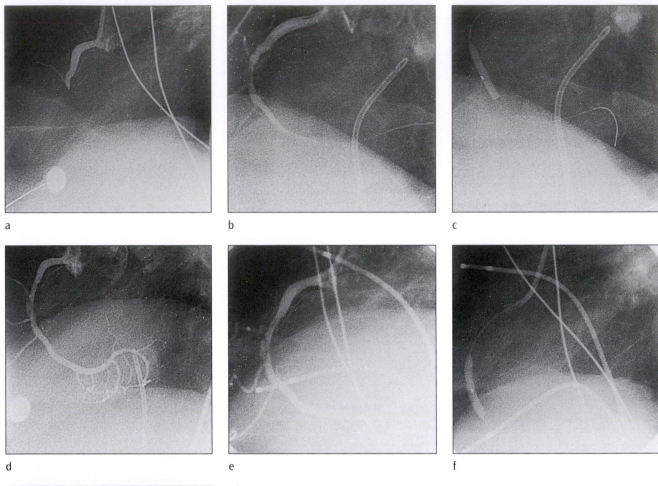

a   b   c

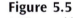

d   e   f

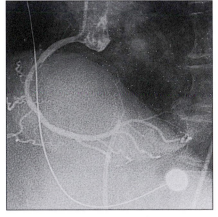

g

Figure 5.5

A 65-year-old man presented with an acute inferior myocardial infarction. (a) There was acute occlusion of an RCA that showed a favourable 'nipple' or 'tapered tip'.
(b) Successful recanalization was achieved by a floppy guidewire placed into the distal posterolateral branch, which then revealed a severe stenosis in the middle third of the RCA.
(c) PTCA with a 3.5mm Express™ balloon catheter produced (d) a local intimal dissection and (e) a less than satisfactory result.
(f) Prolonged (15-minute) inflation sealed the dissection.
(g) This produced an acceptable angiographic result.

   This patient developed severe hypotension and idioventricular rhythm immediately after the RCA had been reopened. The patient required an intracardiac adrenaline infusion and atrioventricular pacing. Note the atrial and ventricular pacing electrodes in situ (e, f).

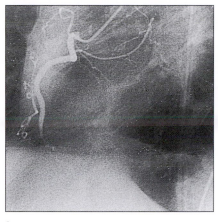

a

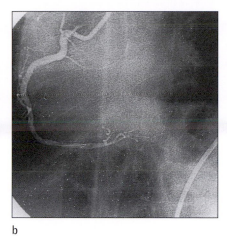

b

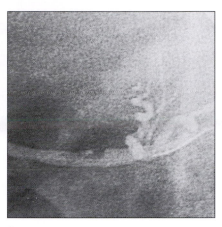

c

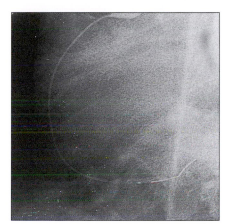

d

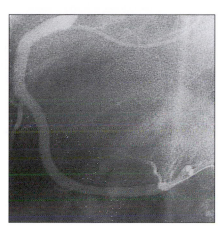

e

Figure 5.6

(a) Acute occlusion of the middle third of the RCA in a 60-year-old general practitioner who presented within 3 hours of an acute inferior myocardial infarction. Thrombus is visible.

(b, c) The thrombus became more obvious after recanalization by a floppy guidewire and a 3.0mm balloon catheter.

(d) The thrombus was dilated and crushed by PTCA.

(e) After 15mg of intracoronary rtPA, an excellent result was produced without complication.

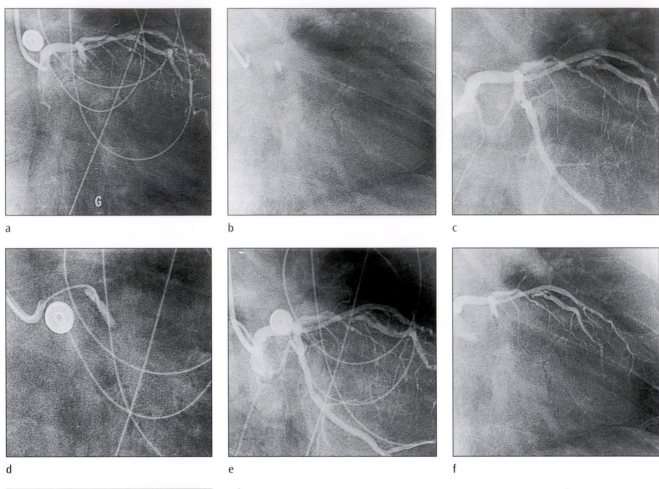

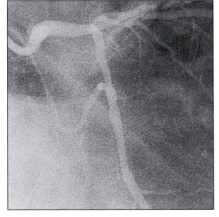

Figure 5.7

(a) Acute occlusion of the proximal LCx in a patient who presented 2.5 hours after the onset of an acute inferolateral myocardial infarction.

(b) Contrast persisted in the short occluded segment.

(c) The vessel was easily reopened by a 0.014-inch Floppy˚ guidewire to reveal a severe underlying stenosis.

(d) Balloon dilatation showed indentation by the hard lesion.

(e) Result after PTCA.

   Two hours later, further chest pain was associated with a return of ST-segment elevation in the inferolateral leads. (f) Angiography revealed reocclusion of the LCx. (g) The LCx was easily reopened by PTCA using a prolonged inflation with a 3.0mm balloon catheter without further complication.

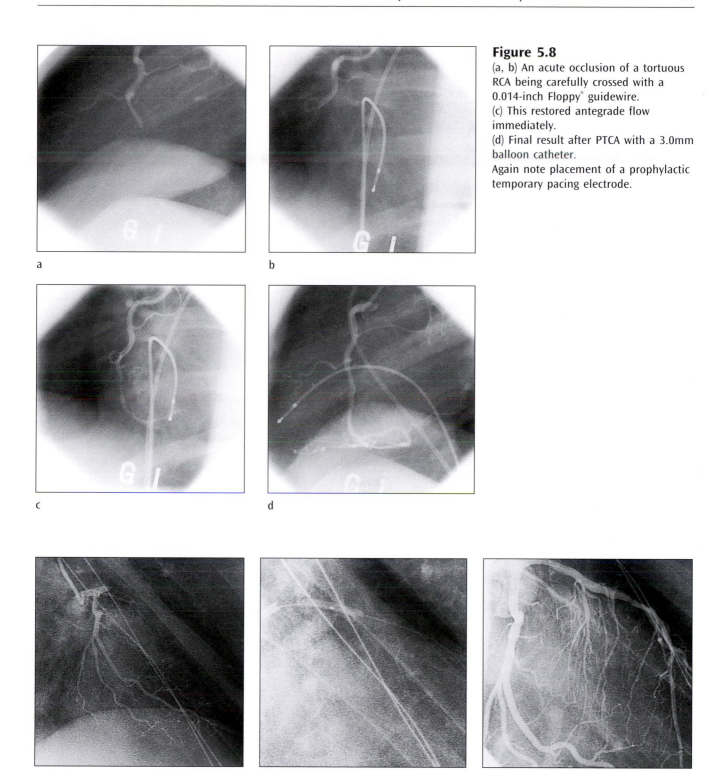

Figure 5.8
(a, b) An acute occlusion of a tortuous RCA being carefully crossed with a 0.014-inch Floppy® guidewire.
(c) This restored antegrade flow immediately.
(d) Final result after PTCA with a 3.0mm balloon catheter.
Again note placement of a prophylactic temporary pacing electrode.

Figure 5.9
A 61-year-old man who presented within 65 minutes of onset of an acute anterior myocardial infarction. (a) Angiography showed acute occlusion of the LAD.
(b) The vessel was opened by a 3.0mm balloon.
(c) An excellent angiographic result was achieved, with prompt improvement in left ventricular contractility.

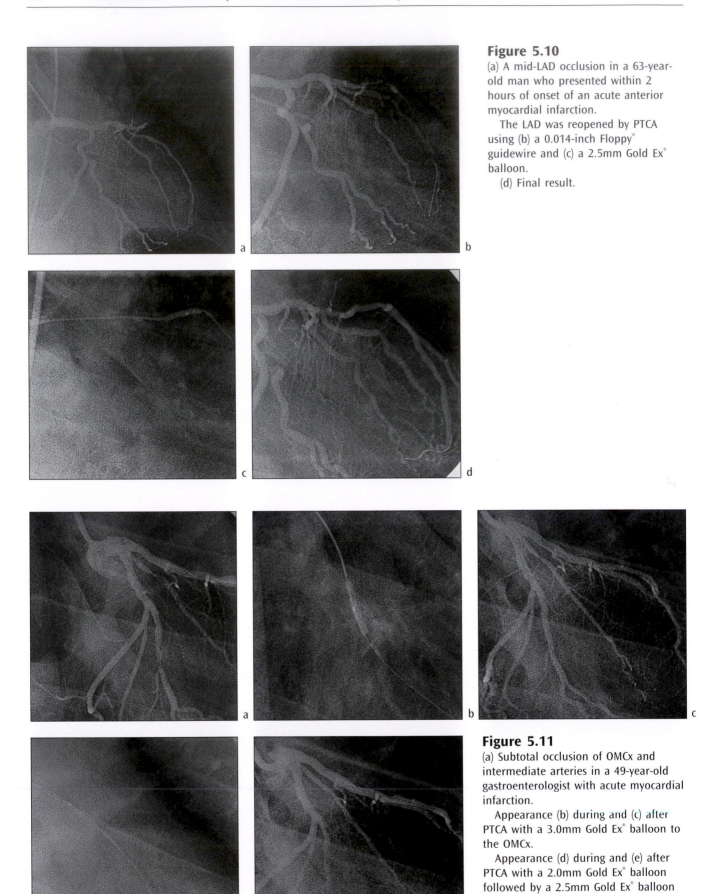

Figure 5.10
(a) A mid-LAD occlusion in a 63-year-old man who presented within 2 hours of onset of an acute anterior myocardial infarction.

The LAD was reopened by PTCA using (b) a 0.014-inch Floppy® guidewire and (c) a 2.5mm Gold Ex® balloon.

(d) Final result.

Figure 5.11
(a) Subtotal occlusion of OMCx and intermediate arteries in a 49-year-old gastroenterologist with acute myocardial infarction.

Appearance (b) during and (c) after PTCA with a 3.0mm Gold Ex® balloon to the OMCx.

Appearance (d) during and (e) after PTCA with a 2.0mm Gold Ex® balloon followed by a 2.5mm Gold Ex® balloon to the intermediate artery.

Primary PTCA and stent implantation in acute myocardial infarction

The FRESCO randomized trial showed that primary stenting in acute myocardial infarction resulted in a lower rate of major adverse cardiac events and a lower rate of restenosis or reocclusion compared with optimal PTCA alone. Findings from the GRAMI study also indicated that there were higher TIMI III flow rates and fewer acute complications after primary stenting in acute myocardial infarction than after PTCA alone. The PASTA randomized trial in acute myocardial infarction reported greater procedural success, fewer in-hospital events and a lower target lesion revascularization rate at 6 months in patients treated with primary Palmaz-Schatz stenting than in those treated with PTCA alone.

The STENTIM-2, STENT PAMI and ESCOBAR randomized trials compared early and late clinical outcomes in patients with acute myocardial infarction who were treated with either primary stent implantation or PTCA alone. STENT-PAMI showed a primary success rate of over 99% and a lower reocclusion rate with stenting than with PTCA alone. TIMI III flow was associated with a 6.4% reocclusion rate. Late results showed a lower revascularization rate for stenting and hence greater cost-effectiveness than PTCA alone.

The GRAPE Pilot study suggested that abciximab could aid reperfusion in patients with acute myocardial infarction who were awaiting primary PTCA.

The ADMIRAL trial showed that abciximab before primary PTCA and stenting improved TIMI III flow and reduced death, recurrent myocardial infarction and urgent target-vessel revascularization at 30 days.

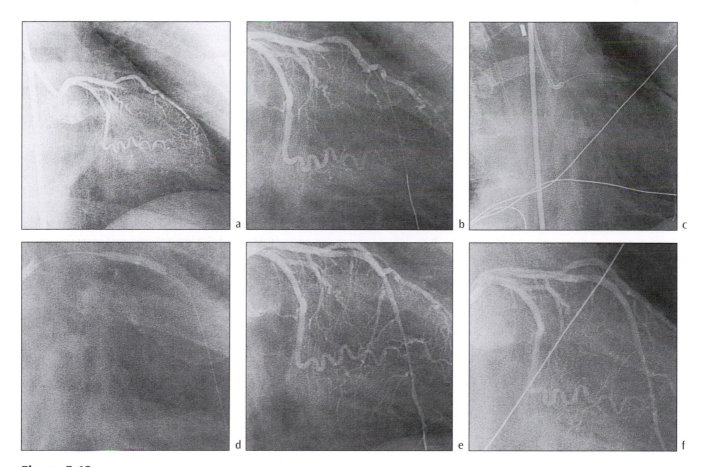

Figure 5.12
(a) An acute occlusion of the proximal/mid-LAD, which was associated with cardiogenic shock in this 64-year-old woman within 2 hours of an acute anterior myocardial infarction.
(b) The occlusion was easily crossed by a guidewire but there was little antegrade flow. (c) The intra-aortic balloon can be seen to be inflated and it proved to be essential for providing some haemodynamic stability once the vessel was reopened and some blood pressure was restored. (d) After PTCA with a 3.0mm Samba™ balloon, it became evident that there was (e) antegrade flow with distal spasm. (f) After intracoronary glyceryl trinitrate, the spasm resolved and the flow improved.   *continued*

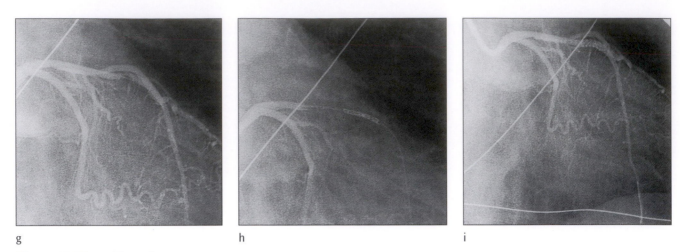

g h i

Figure 5.12 *continued*

(g) A residual stenosis was evident and this became suboptimal (owing to recoil) within 5 minutes of the last inflation. (h) A 3.0mm Wiktor® stent was carefully placed at the lesion site. This stent was deployed successfully to produce (i) an excellent angiographic and clinical result.

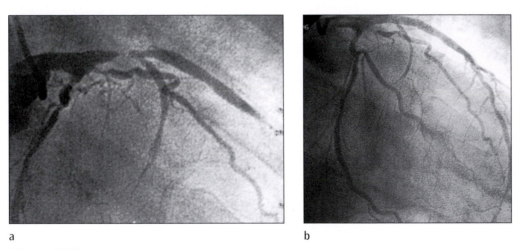

a b

Figure 5.13

A 76-year-old man with previously well-controlled angina presented with an acute anterior myocardial infarction and cardiogenic shock. (a) Coronary angiography showed an occluded RCA, moderate disease in the LCx and a subtotal occlusion of the LAD above the first septal artery.

Left ventricular angiography showed poor left ventricular contractility with an ejection fraction of 38%.

An intra-aortic balloon pump was inserted via the opposite femoral artery. A 0.014-inch Floppy® guidewire crossed the LAD stenosis and the lesion was dilated with a 3.5mm Quantum™ balloon (Cook) at 8 atmospheres. A Palmaz-Schatz™ stent (Johnson and Johnson) was then mounted on the same balloon and deployed at the lesion site at a pressure of 12 atmospheres.

(b) The angiographic appearance was excellent and the haemodynamic recovery was immediate.

The patient continued on heparin and was supported by the intra-aortic balloon pump for 36 hours. Repeat left ventricular angiography at 48 hours revealed an ejection fraction of 55%. Eighteen months later he remained asymptomatic on no anti-anginal medication.

Courtesy of Dr LDR Smith, Royal Devon and Exeter Hospital, Exeter, UK.

Randomized trials such as the SHOCK trial are comparing a policy of early revascularization with PTCA and stenting versus medical stabilization and late revascularization as clinically indicated. Intervention appears to improve outcome and survival and stenting appears to improve angiographic and clinical success over PTCA alone.

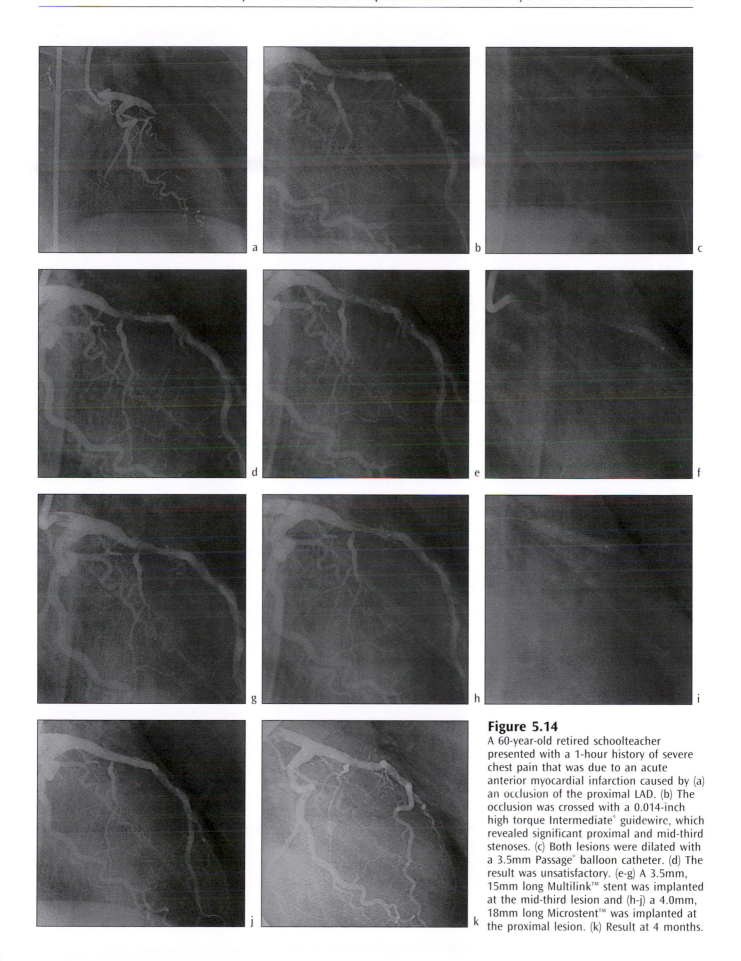

Figure 5.14
A 60-year-old retired schoolteacher presented with a 1-hour history of severe chest pain that was due to an acute anterior myocardial infarction caused by (a) an occlusion of the proximal LAD. (b) The occlusion was crossed with a 0.014-inch high torque Intermediate® guidewire, which revealed significant proximal and mid-third stenoses. (c) Both lesions were dilated with a 3.5mm Passage® balloon catheter. (d) The result was unsatisfactory. (e-g) A 3.5mm, 15mm long Multilink™ stent was implanted at the mid-third lesion and (h-j) a 4.0mm, 18mm long Microstent™ was implanted at the proximal lesion. (k) Result at 4 months.

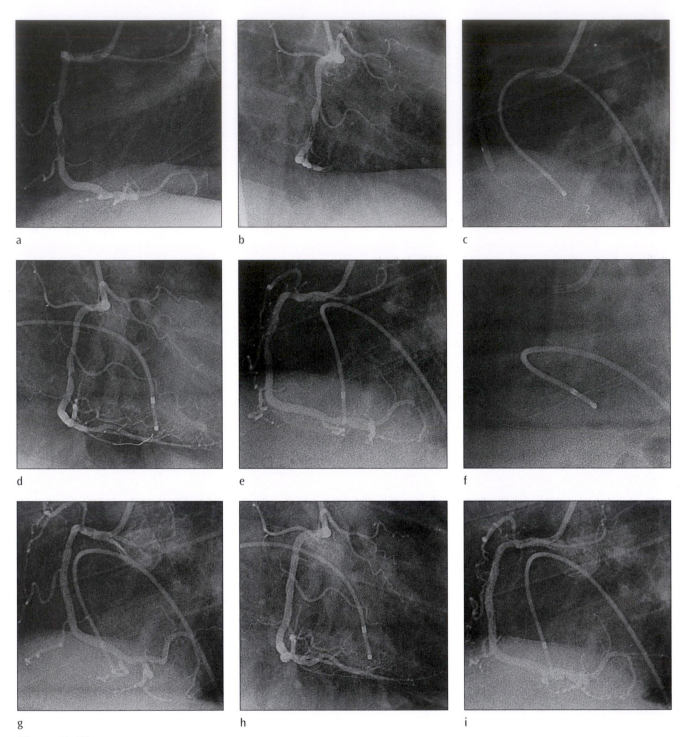

Figure 5.15

A 41-year-old social worker developed acute inferior myocardial infarction while pushing his car. An ECG showed ST-elevation in the inferior leads and (a, b) angiography showed acute subtotal occlusion of a dominant RCA with a large thrombus that was producing severe flow limitation.

(c) The lesion was crossed with a 0.014-inch Floppy® guidewire and dilated with a 3.0mm Cheetah™ balloon.

(d) A significant residual stenosis was evident.

(e) Thrombus was also seen to have embolized into the distal posterolateral branch of the RCA.

(f) A 3.5mm, 30mm long Microstent II™ was implanted at the lesion site.

(g, h) This gave a good angiographic result.

(i) The distal thrombus resolved with the aid of 20mg of intracoronary rtPA. The result persisted at 4 months.

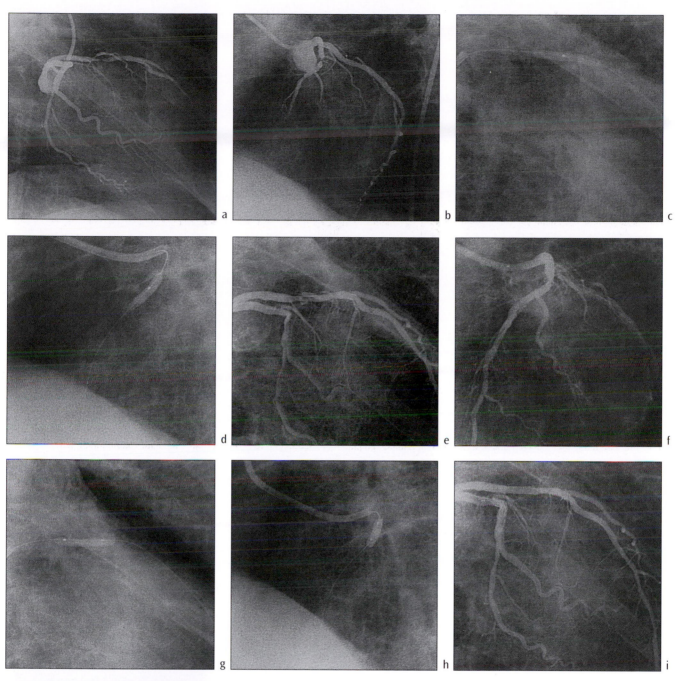

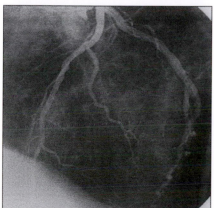

Figure 5.16

A 70-year-old retired pharmacist presented within 2 hours of onset of an acute anterior myocardial infarction. An ECG showed extensive ST-elevation in the anterior leads. (a, b) Angiography showed that the LAD was subtotally occluded proximally. (c, d) The lesion was crossed with a 0.014-inch Floppy® guidewire and dilated with a 3.0mm Elipse™ balloon.

Because of a suboptimal angiographic result (e, f), the lesion was stented with a 3.5mm, 15mm long Multilink™ stent (g, h).

(i, j) This produced a good result. Note the temporary loss of the first diagonal branch that exits just above the stenosis.

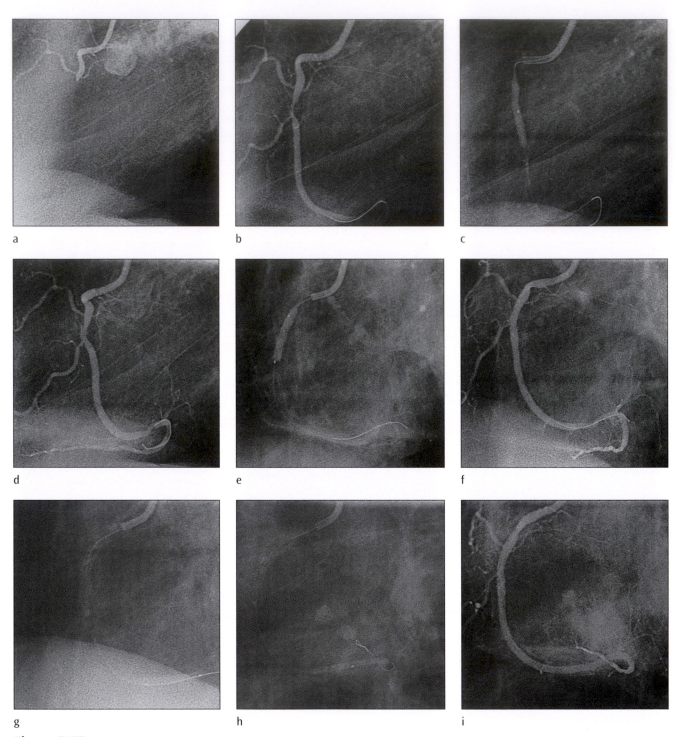

Figure 5.17
A 51-year-old unemployed man presented with a 2-hour history of severe chest pain that was due to acute inferior myocardial infarction. (a) Angiography showed the RCA to be occluded proximally above a bend.
(b) A 0.014-inch Intermediate® guidewire was necessary to cross the occlusion, and the vessel was reperfused, revealing a distal stenosis.
(c, d) A 3.0mm Elipse™ was used to dilate the proximal stenosis.
(e, f) A 3.0mm, 18mm long Microstent II™ was implanted with a good result.
(g) Dilatation of the distal stenosis with a 3.0mm balloon at 4 atmospheres caused occlusive dissection of the distal vessel.
(h) The vessel was successfully reopened with a 2.5mm, 30mm long Elipse™ balloon inflated for 20 minutes.
There were no further sequelae after producing an excellent angiographic result (i).

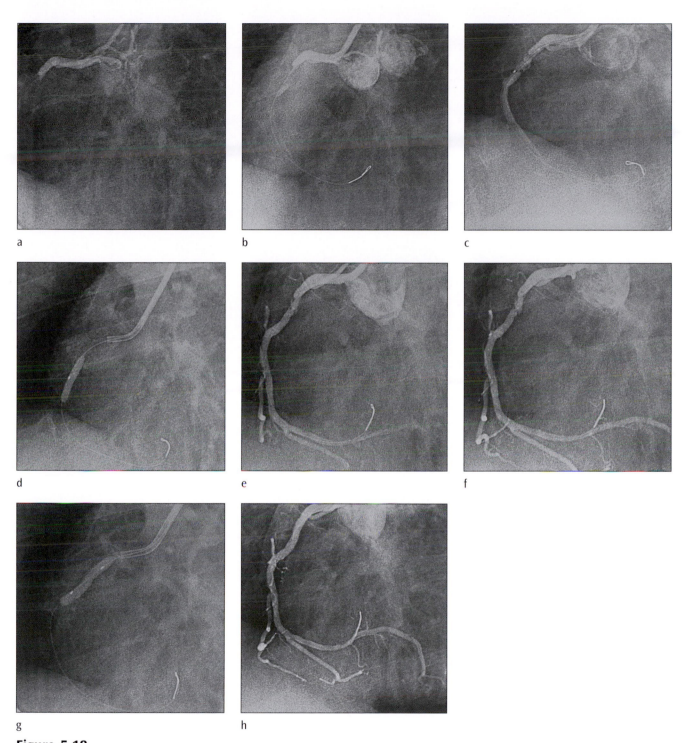

Figure 5.18

A 47-year-old man with an acute inferior infarction was found at emergency angiography to have (a) an occluded RCA and severe three-vessel disease.

The strategy was to open the RCA and to plan elective PTCA to the LCx and the LAD at another session.

The RCA occlusion was crossed with (b) a 0.014-inch Floppy® guidewire and then (c) a 3.5mm Elipse™ balloon. Some antegrade flow was achieved.

(d) Balloon dilatation produced reperfusion with (e) distal embolization/spasm in both distal branches.

(f) After treatment with intracoronary nitrates this rapidly normalized.

(g) Residual stenosis and local dissection was treated with a 3.5mm, 15mm long Multilink™ stent.

(h) This gave an excellent final result.

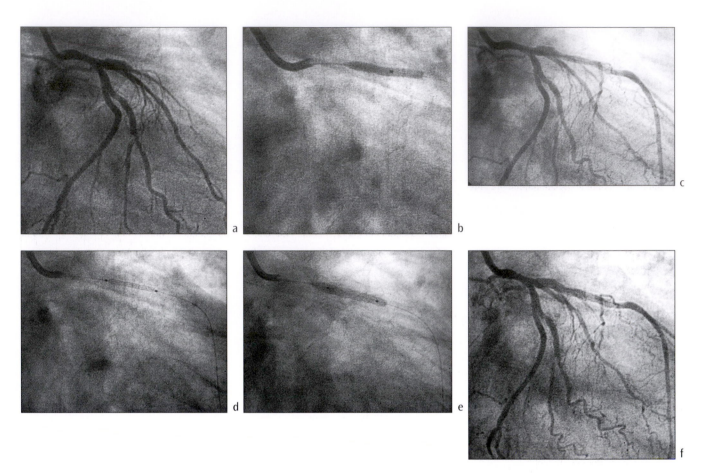

Figure 5.19

A 70-year-old retired glass worker presented 2 hours after onset of an acute anterior myocardial infarction. An ECG showed extensive ST-segment elevation in leads V1-V6, I and aVL. (a) The LAD was found to be occluded proximally.
(b, c) The occlusion was crossed with a 0.014-inch Floppy® guidewire and opened with a 3.0mm Passage® balloon.
(d, e) A 3.5mm, 18mm long Microstent™ was implanted.
(f) This gave a good angiographic result. There was almost immediate improvement of left ventricular function.

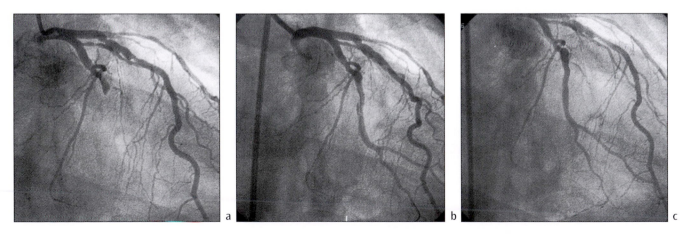

Figure 5.20

A 51-year-old man presented with acute myocardial infarction. (a) Emergency cardiac catheterization revealed a chronically occluded RCA, an acutely occluded LCx and a significant stenosis in the LAD. (b) The LCx was recanalized with a 0.014-inch Floppy® guidewire and a 3.0mm Cruiser® balloon but local coronary artery dissection was evident. (c) The dissection was successfully repaired with a Palmaz-Schatz™ 153 stent. The patient made a good recovery but he returned 18 months later with anterior ischaemia. The LCx site had remained free of significant disease but the LAD lesion had become very severe. This was treated successfully by PTCA and stenting.

Courtesy of Dr LDR Smith, Royal Devon and Exeter Hospital, Exeter, UK.

Rescue PTCA and stent implantation in acute myocardial infarction

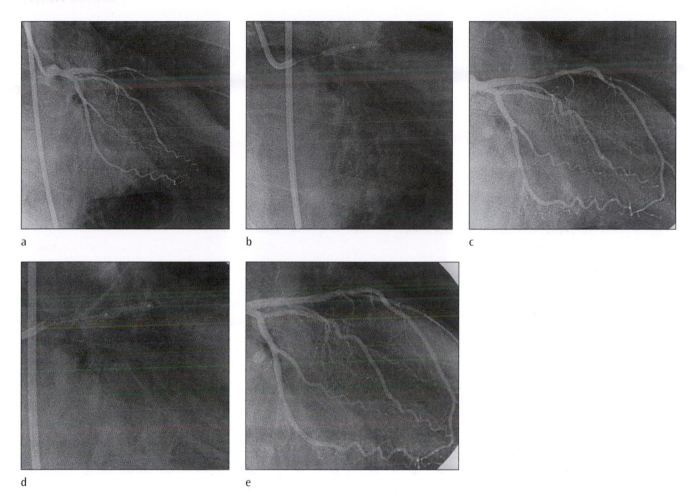

a   b   c

d   e

Figure 5.21

A 50-year-old sales manager had uncontrolled angina after receiving rtPA twice for an acute anterior myocardial infarction. His ECG showed persisting ST-segment elevation and T-wave inversion in the anterior leads. (a) Angiography showed subtotal occlusion of the proximal LAD with TIMI I flow.

(b) The lesion was crossed with a 0.014-inch guidewire and dilated with a 3.0mm Passage® balloon.

(c) This re-established flow, although there was a residual stenosis, and (d) a 3.0mm, 15mm long Palmaz-Schatz Powergrip™ stent was implanted with a good angiographic result (e).

Intravenous heparin was continued for 24 hours. The procedure was complicated by a retroperitoneal haemorrhage, and the patient required a blood transfusion, although there were no further cardiac problems.

PTCA and stent implantation after thrombolytic therapy (requiring intravenous heparin, oral antiplatelet agents and glycoprotein IIb-IIIa inhibitors such as abciximab) are likely to be associated with a greater frequency of bleeding complications and increased morbidity than primary PTCA and stenting after acute myocardial infarction.

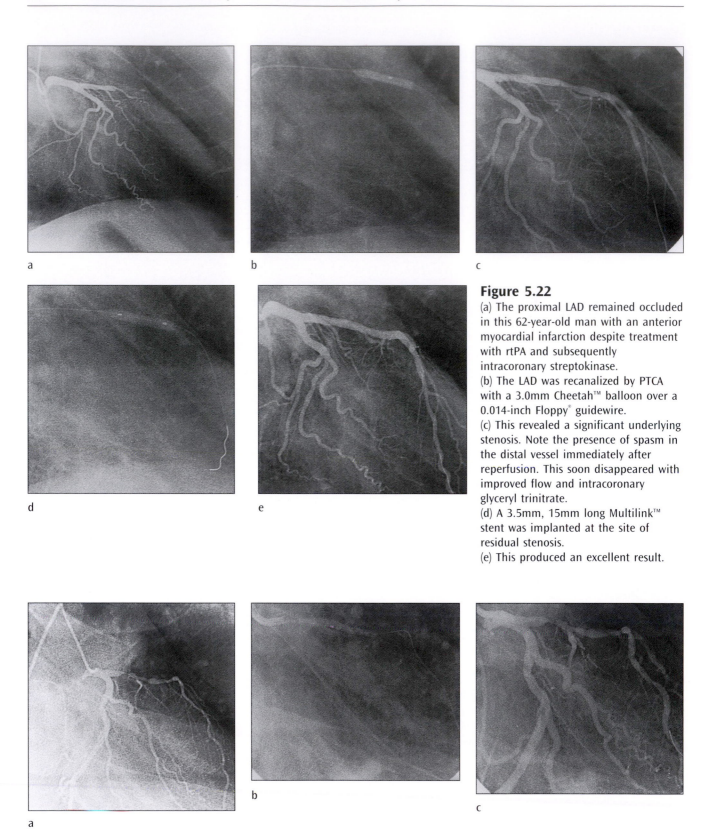

Figure 5.22
(a) The proximal LAD remained occluded in this 62-year-old man with an anterior myocardial infarction despite treatment with rtPA and subsequently intracoronary streptokinase.
(b) The LAD was recanalized by PTCA with a 3.0mm Cheetah™ balloon over a 0.014-inch Floppy® guidewire.
(c) This revealed a significant underlying stenosis. Note the presence of spasm in the distal vessel immediately after reperfusion. This soon disappeared with improved flow and intracoronary glyceryl trinitrate.
(d) A 3.5mm, 15mm long Multilink™ stent was implanted at the site of residual stenosis.
(e) This produced an excellent result.

Figure 5.23
A 61-year-old retired plumber had unstable angina after rtPA had been given for an acute anterior myocardial infarction.
Angiography showed a severe stenosis in the RCA and (a) severe stenoses in the proximal LAD.
The LAD stenoses were first dilated with (b) a 3.0mm Elipse™ balloon.
(c) A residual stenosis was evident.

continued

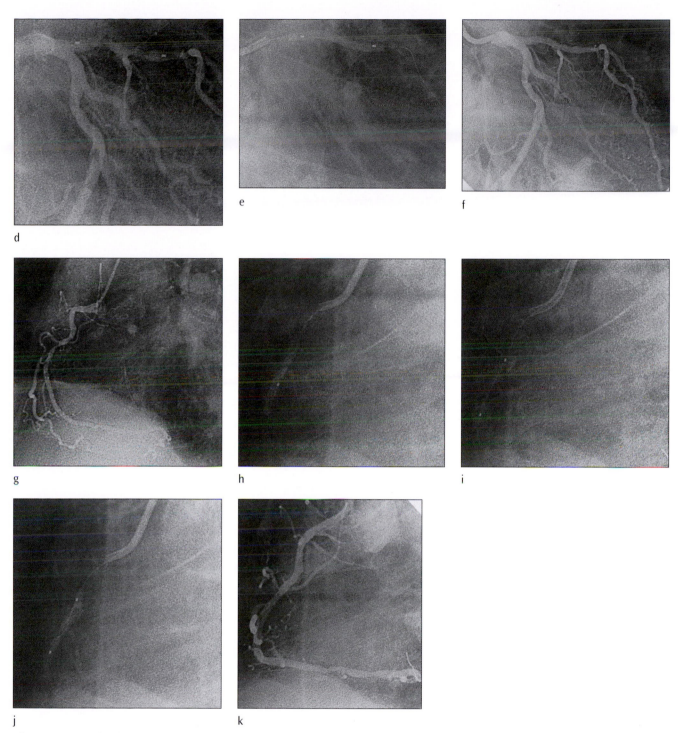

Figure 5.23 *continued*

(d, e) A 3.0mm, 25mm long Multilink™ stent was then deployed.

(f) This produced a good result.

(g) The RCA stenosis was then dilated with a 2.5mm Elipse™ balloon without success before balloon rupture.

(h) A 2.5mm Worldpass™ balloon dilated the lesion at 17 atmospheres.

(i, j) A 2.5mm, 18mm long Microstent II™ was then deployed.

(k) This gave a satisfactory result.

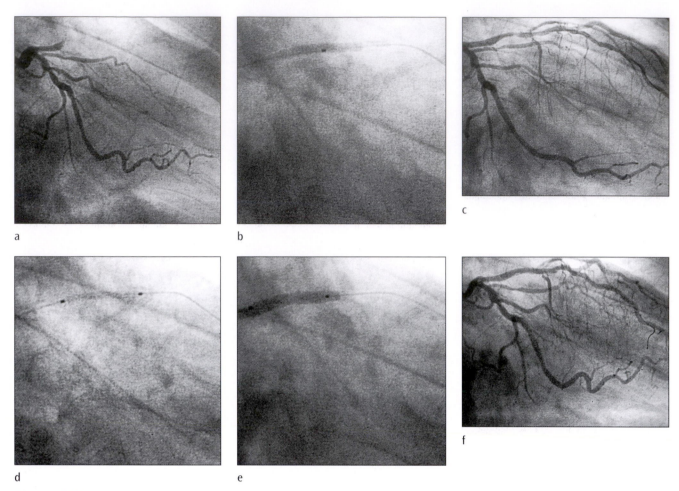

a

b

c

d

e

f

Figure 5.24

A 69-year-old retired docker with severe angina was found to have a subtotal occlusion of the proximal LAD at diagnostic angiography. He developed severe chest pain after returning to the ward and became sweaty and hypotensive. He returned immediately to the catheter laboratory with extensive anterior ST-segment elevation on his ECG. (a) Repeat angiography confirmed LAD occlusion.

(b, c) The occlusion was crossed with a 0.014-inch Floppy® guidewire and dilated with a 3.0mm Passage® balloon.

(d, e) A 3.0mm, 18mm long Microstent™ was then implanted.

(f) This produced an excellent result.

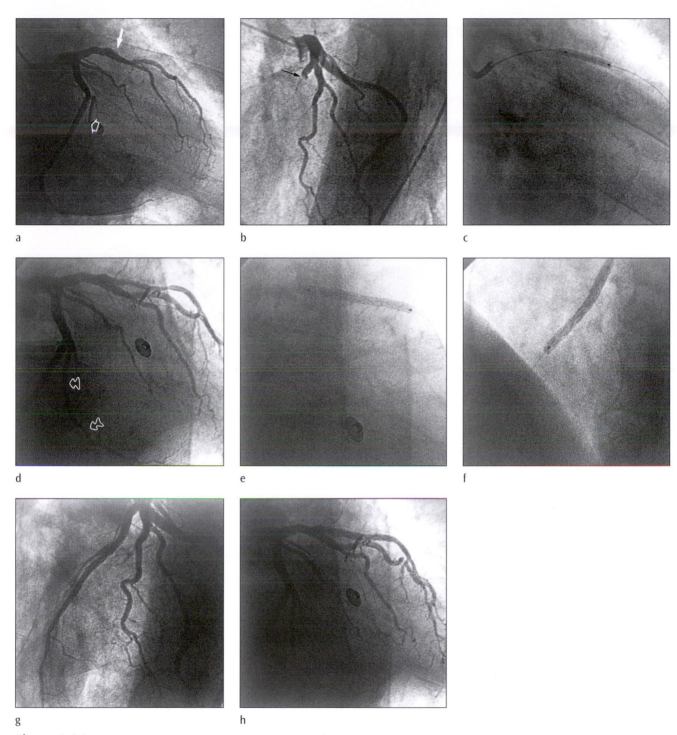

Figure 5.25

(a) A 62-year-old man with severe chest pain and atrial fibrillation was found to have proximal occlusion (arrow) of the LAD and first obtuse marginal (open arrowhead) coronary arteries. He was not receiving anticoagulant therapy.

(b) The proximal occlusion (arrow) in the LAD can be seen in the LAO cranial view.

(c) The LAD was crossed with a 0.014-inch Floppy® guidewire and reopened with a 3.0mm Worldpass™ balloon.
   Thrombus was clearly visible in the LAD and this was treated with 5mg boluses of rtPA up to a total of 25mg.
   Because of residual stenosis in the proximal LAD (d), a 30mm, 39mm long Microstent™ was deployed (e, f).

(g, h) This gave an excellent final result.

   In (d), note that after rtPA, the OMCx reappeared (open arrows). No stenosis was seen. It was assumed that the thrombus occluding the OMCx had been lysed by the thrombolytic agent.

Rescue PTCA and stenting for acute left main stem occlusion

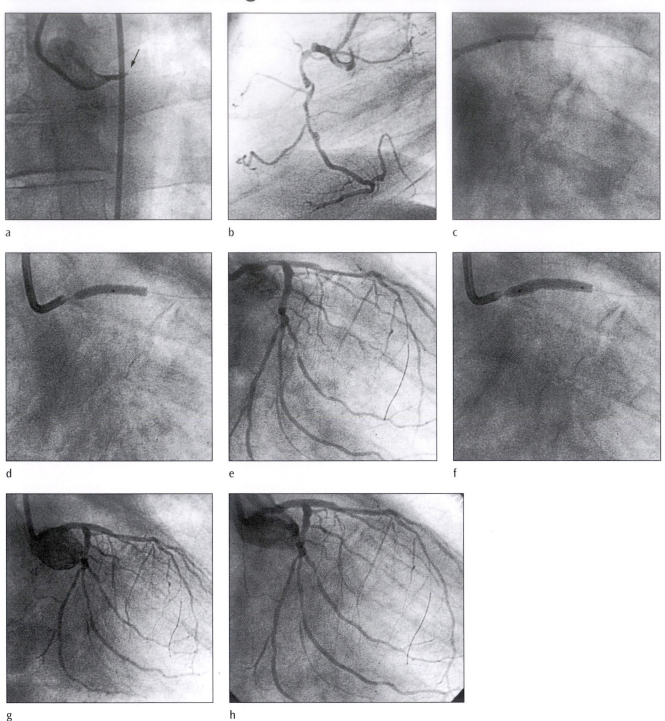

Figure 5.26

A 70-year-old man who had a strongly positive exercise test was transferred with severe unstable angina and marked ST-segment depression in leads V1-V6 on his ECG. He developed cardiogenic shock and pulmonary oedema during transfer to the cardiac catheterization laboratory. Coronary arteriography showed (a) left main stem occlusion and (b) severe disease in the right coronary artery. The patient was quickly intubated and ventilated and the left coronary artery was opened by rapidly crossing it with a 0.014-inch Intermediate® guidewire and dilatating with (c) a 2.0mm Worldpass™ balloon and then (d) a 3.0mm Worldpass™ balloon. The systolic blood pressure immediately rose from 50mm Hg to 140mm Hg as (e) the whole of the left coronary artery reopened. (f) The left main coronary artery was stented with a 3.0mm, 18mm long Microstent™ as a 'bridge to surgery' in this case. (g) An excellent angiographic result was achieved, and emergency CABG surgery was successfully performed. (h) Magnified view of the left coronary artery. Interestingly, within 5 minutes of establishing TIMI III flow and normotension, hypotension recurred acutely despite a fully patent vessel. It was presumed that this was due to reperfusion injury; the patient responded sufficiently well to intravenous adrenaline to enable him to be transferred to theatre for surgical revascularization.

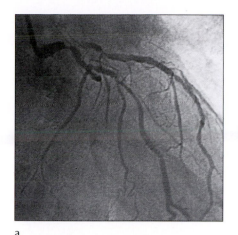

a

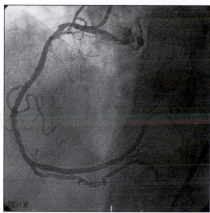

b

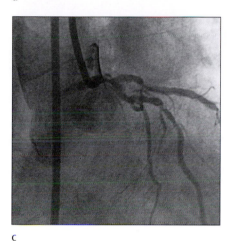

c

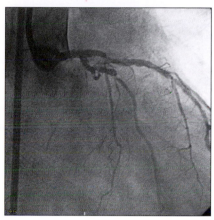

d

Figure 5.27
A 76-year-old man had acute widespread myocardial ischaemia and cardiogenic shock. Intra-aortic balloon counterpulsation was commenced and coronary arteriography was performed. (a) The left main coronary artery was found to be subtotally occluded and the ostium of the LAD was critically stenosed. The LCx was occluded after the OMCx branch. (b) The RCA showed only mild disease.

Emergency PTCA was performed to the left main artery using a 0.014-inch Scimed guidewire and a 3.0mm Viva™ balloon.

(c) An inadequate result was obtained with local dissection.

(d) Therefore, a 3.5mm, 9mm long NIR™ stent (Scimed/Boston Scientific) was deployed at 14 atmospheres, with a good angiographic result.

Courtesy of Dr LDR Smith, Royal Devon and Exeter Hospital, Exeter, UK.

Although systemic pressure and oxygenation often improve immediately after such a rescue procedure, this should only be used as a 'bridge' to emergency CABG surgery. Reperfusion arrhythmias, left ventricular stunning and sustained hypotension despite an open artery are not infrequent in this situation, and a period of bypass and reliable revascularization are probably more effective than high doses of inotropes.

Primary PTCA in patients after coronary artery bypass graft surgery

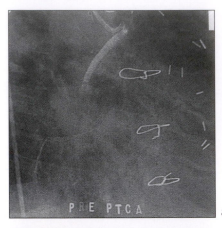

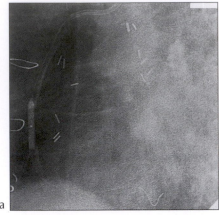

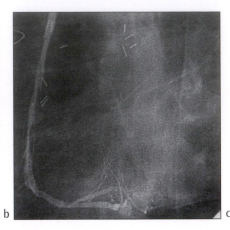

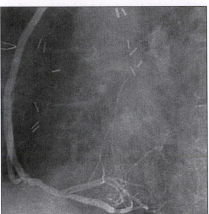

Figure 5.28

Acute occlusion of an SVG can be particularly troublesome. (a) This occluded 8-year-old vein graft to the RCA caused inferior myocardial infarction. Thrombus is clearly visible blocking the proximal third of the RCA.

(b) The SVG was easily traversed with a 0.014-inch Floppy® guidewire and the occlusion was reopened by serial inflations along the length of the SVG using a 3.0mm balloon catheter.

(c) Much thrombus is visible once flow is established down the SVG.

(d) However, the angiographic appearance is significantly improved by intragraft streptokinase infusion and further (more prolonged) inflations along the graft.

The end result was satisfactory without complication, although distal embolization is not uncommon in such a situation.

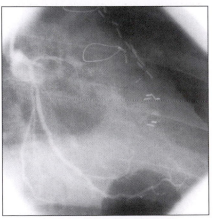

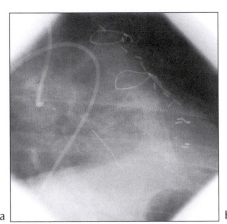

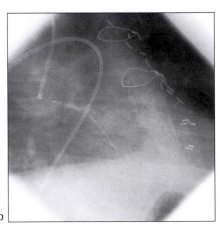

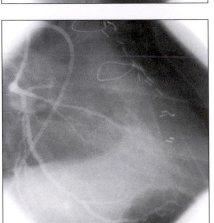

Figure 5.29

Acute occlusion of a native vessel may be responsible for acute myocardial infarction in some patients after CABG surgery. (a) This acutely occluded intermediate artery caused a 47-year-old boilermaker to present with an acute anterolateral myocardial infarction.

(b) The occlusion was crossed with a 2.5mm fixed-wire Compass™ balloon catheter (Datascope).

(c) The underlying lesion was evident on initial balloon inflation.

(d) The result after PTCA produced immediate pain relief and normalization of the ECG.

Angiojet thrombectomy

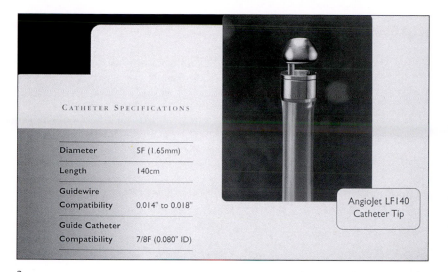

CATHETER SPECIFICATIONS

Diameter	5F (1.65mm)
Length	140cm
Guidewire Compatibility	0.014" to 0.018"
Guide Catheter Compatibility	7/8F (0.080" ID)

AngioJet LF140 Catheter Tip

a

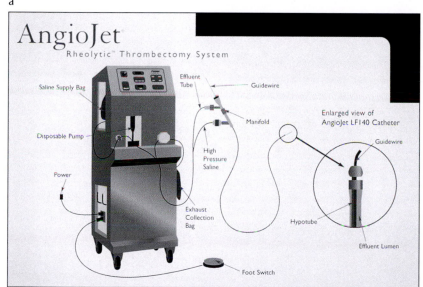

b

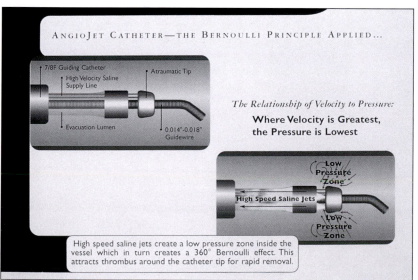

c

Figure 5.30

The Possis Angiojet® is a rheolytic thrombectomy catheter designed for the percutaneous disruption and removal of unorganized thrombus from native coronary arteries and bypass grafts using high velocity saline. It consists of a 5F double-lumen catheter that is 140cm long and it accepts a guidewire of between 0.014 and 0.018 inches and is compatible with an 8F guiding catheter (a).

The smaller lumen of the catheter is used to supply the catheter tip with saline jets. The saline jets that emerge at the tip of the catheter are generated by an external drive unit with a positive displacement pump that generates 6-8 atmospheres pressure (b). The saline jets exit at the tip of the catheter through five radially oriented holes each 25-50μm in diameter. These jets aid in the formation of a recirculation pattern that fragments the thrombotic material.

An additional three saline jets are directed retrogradely into the larger exhaust lumen of the catheter. These jets create a 'Venturi effect' that aids in evacuation of the macerated thrombotic material (c).

The exhaust of the catheter is controlled by a roller pump so that the entire catheter operates in an isovolumic mode. It has flexible tracking for deep distal thrombus in vessels with a diameter of 2.0mm or more.

The safety and efficacy of the Angiojet® rheolytic coronary thrombectomy device were demonstrated in the VEGAS I and the Euro ART studies. The VEGAS II study is a randomized trial comparing the safety and effectiveness of the Angiojet® device followed by definitive treatment with that of prolonged intracoronary urokinase followed by definitive treatment in native and SVGs that have angiographic evidence of thrombus.

Angiojet thrombectomy and stent implantation

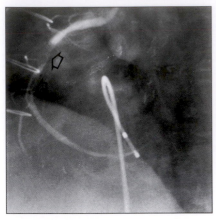

a

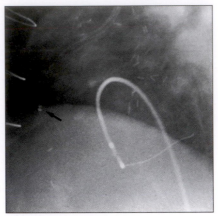

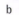

b

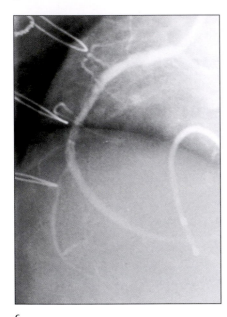

c

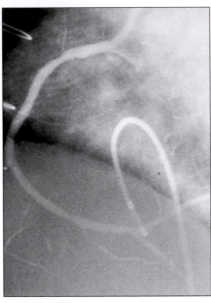

d

Figure 5.31

A 32-year-old man with diabetes mellitus presented with an acute inferior myocardial infarction. His ECG showed hyperacute ST-segment elevation in leads II, III and avF and ST-segment depression in leads V4-V6, I and avL. He had undergone CABG surgery to the LAD and OMCx 1 year earlier. (a) Coronary arteriography revealed 70% stenosis in the mid-RCA with TIMI II flow. Thrombus (open arrows) filled the mid-RCA. The SVGs were patent.

The RCA was intubated with an 8F JR 3.5 guiding catheter and the lesion was crossed with a 0.014-inch ExtraSupport™ guidewire (Guidant).

(b) The Possis Angiojet® catheter was advanced over the wire (arrow). The lesion was debulked after three passes.

(c) There was significant reduction in thrombus burden and a residual stenosis of 50% with luminal irregularity and brisk TIMI III flow was achieved.

(d) A 3.5mm, 32mm long NIR™ stent was deployed at 14 atmospheres with no significant residual stenosis.

The patient received aspirin, low-molecular-weight heparin for 3 days and ticlopidine for 1 month. There were no complications and the patient remained asymptomatic at 6 months' follow-up.

Courtesy of Drs A Seth and R Salwan, Escorts Heart Institute and Research Centre, New Delhi, India.

The Possis Angiojet® removes thrombus via the Venturi effect. The device is not bulky and can be activated rapidly. It selectively acts on unorganized thrombus and the atherosclerotic plaque is left unaltered.

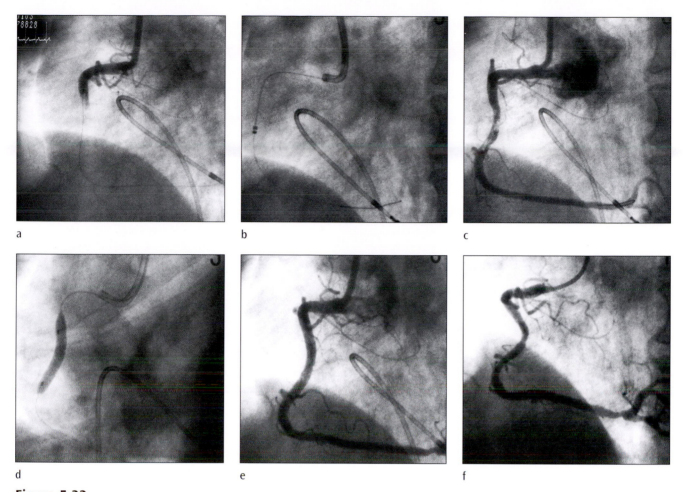

a   b   c

d   e   f

Figure 5.32

A 62-year-old man with a 12-hour history of acute inferior myocardial infarction and persistent ST-elevation in leads II, III and AVF was found to have (a) occlusion of the proximal RCA.

There appeared to be a large amount of thrombus and so AngioJet® thrombectomy was indicated. Aspirin was given before angiography.

(b) An 8F JR4 guiding catheter was positioned in the ostium of the RCA and the occlusion crossed with a 0.014-inch Floppy® guidewire. The AngioJet® LF140 thrombectomy catheter was prepared and advanced slowly with antegrade operation.

Two passes were made, resulting in removal of much thrombus and restoration of TIMI III flow.

(c) An ulcerated residual stenosis was evident.

The AngioJet® catheter was exchanged for a 3.5mm balloon, which was inflated to 10 atmospheres for 1 minute.

(d) A 3.5mm, 15mm long Multilink™ stent was then implanted.

The stent was post-dilated to 18 atmospheres with an excellent angiographic and clinical result. (e)

Neither distal embolization nor no-reflow were observed. Intravenous heparin was continued for 48 hours and the patient was prescribed ticlopidine.

(f) Follow-up angiography at 5 months did not show restenosis.

Courtesy of Drs Y Nakagawa and M Nobuyoshi, Kokura Hospital, Kitakyushu, Japan.

The use of abciximab after primary PTCA

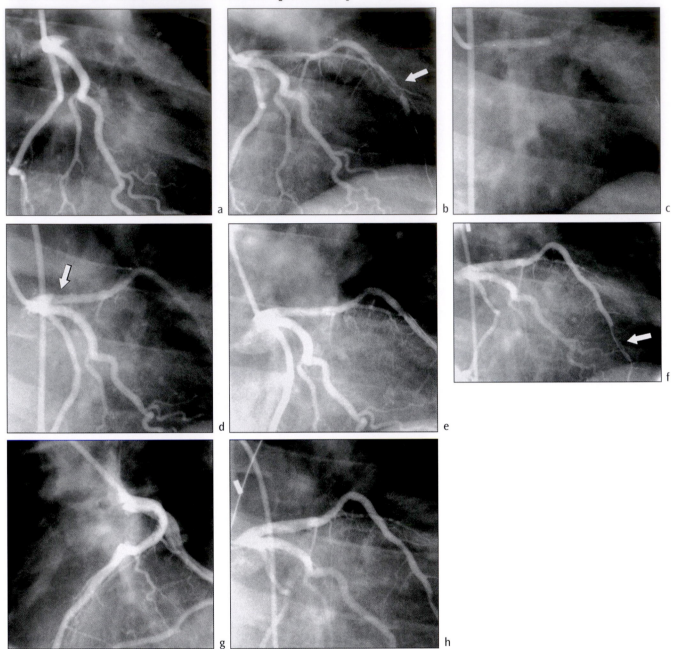

Figure 5.33

A 36-year-old man with chronic renal failure presented with a 3-hour history of extensive anterior myocardial infarction. (a) Coronary arteriography showed a proximal occlusion of the LAD. The occlusion was crossed with a 0.014-inch Clyde™ guidewire (Schneider) and PTCA was performed with a 3.0mm Samba™ balloon. (b) After the vessel had been reopened, several filling defects (arrow), presumed to be thrombus, were visible in the proximal LAD, but there was TIMI II flow. After multiple inflations in the proximal LAD, coronary flow deteriorated. (c) A 3.5mm, 18mm long GFX™ stent (AVE/Medtronic) was therefore implanted proximally, which improved the flow. (d) However a mass (arrow) protruded into the proximal part of the stent. (e) Inflation at high pressure (18 atmospheres) with a 3.5mm, 9mm long Chubby™ balloon (Schneider) significantly improved the appearance.

(f) However, there appeared to be evidence of distal embolization (arrow). An intra-aortic balloon pump was therefore inserted and the glycoprotein IIb-IIIa receptor antagonist abciximab was given to reduce intracoronary thrombus formation and embolization and to reduce the likelihood of stent thrombosis. There were no further problems. (g) After 48 hours, repeat angiography showed TIMI III flow and no evidence of the mass that had originally been seen in the proximal LAD. (h) A magnified view shows an excellent appearance of the stented segment. Residual thrombus was seen in the distal LAD, but flow was not compromised. The patient was continued on intravenous heparin for 5 days without further events.

Courtesy of Dr MJ de Boer, Hospital de Weezenlanden, Zwolle, The Netherlands.

The RAPPORT randomized trial showed that abciximab reduced the risk of acute vessel closure in patients undergoing primary PTCA for acute myocardial infarction. In particular, it reduced the risk of early mortality, reinfarction and target-vessel revascularization.

The CADILLAC randomized trial suggests that adding abciximab to primary PTCA or primary stenting in acute myocardial infarction results in a beneficial reduction in recurrent ischaemia.

Reading

Antoniucci D, Santoro GM, Bolognese L, et al. A clinical trial comparing primary stenting of the infarct-related artery with optimal primary angioplasty for acute myocardial infarction. Results from the Florence Randomized Elective Stenting in Acute Coronary Occlusions (FRESCO) trial. J Am Coll Cardiol 1998;31:1234-9.

Antoniucci D, Valenti R, Santoro GM, et al. Systematic direct angioplasty and stent-supported direct angioplasty therapy for cardiogenic shock complicating acute myocardial infarction: in-hospital and long-term survival. J Am Coll Cardiol 1998;31:294-300.

Bauters C, Lablanche J-M, Van Belle E, et al. Effects of coronary stenting on restenosis and occlusion after angioplasty of the culprit vessel in patients with recent myocardial infarction. Circulation 1997;96:2854-8.

Brener SJ, Barr LA, Burchenal JEB, et al on behalf of the ReoPro, Primary PTCA Organization and Randomized Trial (RAPPORT) Investigators. Randomized, placebo-controlled trial of platelet glycoprotein IIb/IIIa blockade with primary angioplasty for acute myocardial infarction. Circulation 1998;98:734-741.

Christiaens L, Coisne D, Allal J, Barraine R. Emergency stenting for complete thrombosis of an unprotected left main coronary artery in evolving myocardial infarction. J Invas Cardiol 1997;9:435-7.

de Boer MJ, Suryapranata H, Hoorntje JCA et al. Limitation of infarct size and preservation of left ventricular function after primary coronary angioplasty compared with intravenous streptokinase in acute myocardial infarction. Circulation 1994;90:753-61.

Grines C, Browne K, Marco J, et al. A comparison of immediate angioplasty with thrombolytic therapy for acute myocardial infarction. N Engl J Med 1993;328:673-79.

Hammerman H. Thrombolytic vs interventional treatment in acute myocardial infarction. In: Beyar R, Keren G, Leon MB, Serruys PW. Frontiers in Interventional Cardiology. London: Martin Dunitz; 1997:41-5.

Hibbard MD, Holmes DR Jr, Bailey KR, et al. Percutaneous transluminal coronary angioplasty in patients with cardiogenic shock. J Am Coll Cardiol 1992;19:639-46.

Hochman JS, Sleeper LA, Godfrey E et al. for the SHOCK Trial Study Group. SHould we emergently revascularize Occluded Coronaries for cardiogenic shocK: an international randomized trial of emergency PTCA/CABG – trial design. Am Heart J 1999;137:313-21.

Hochman JS, Sleeper LA, Webb JG et al. for the SHOCK Investigators. Early revascularization in acute myocardial infarction complicated by cardiogenic shock. N Engl J Med 1999;341:625-34.

Kahn JK, Rutherford BD, McConahay DR, et al. Results of primary angioplasty for acute myocardial infarction in patients with multivessel disease. J Am Coll Cardiol 1990;16:1089-96.

Kahn JK, Rutherford BD, McConahay DR, et al. Usefulness of angioplasty during acute myocardial infarction in patients with prior coronary artery bypass grafting. Am J Cardiol 1990;65:698-702.

Kornowski R, et al. Procedural results and long term outcomes following stenting in perimyocardial infarction syndromes. Am J Cardiol 1998;82:1163-7.

Mahdi NA, Lopez J, Leon M, et al. Primary stenting vs PTCA with bailout stenting for acute myocardial infarction. Am J Cardiol 1998;81:957-63.

Nishida Y, Nonaka H, Ueda K, et al. In-hospital outcome of primary stenting for acute myocardial infarction using Wiktor coil stent: results from a multicenter randomized PRISAM study. Circulation 1997;96(Suppl I):I-397.

Nunn CM, O'Neill WW, Rothbaum D, et al for the Primary Angioplasty in Myocardial Infarction I Study Group. Long-term outcome after primary angioplasty: report from the Primary Angioplasty in Myocardial Infarction (PAMI-I) trial. J Am Coll Cardiol 1999;33:640-6.

O'Neill WW, Brodie BR, Ivanhoe R, et al. Primary coronary angioplasty for acute myocardial infarction (the Primary Angioplasty Registry). Am J Cardiol 1994;73:627-34.

Rodriguez AE, Bernardi VH, Santaera OA, et al. on behalf of the GRAMI Investigators. Coronary stents improve outcome in acute myocardial infarction: immediate and long-term results of the GRAMI trial. Am J Cardiol 1998;81:1286-91.

Saito S, Hosokawa G. Primary Palmaz-Schatz stent implantation for acute myocardial infarction: the results of Japanese PASTA (Primary Angioplasty vs Stent Implantation in AMI in Japan) trial. Circulation 1997;96: I-595.

Smyth DW, Richards M, Elliott JM. Direct angioplasty for myocardial infarction: one-year experience in a centre with surgical backup 220 miles away. J Invas Cardiol 1997;9:324-32.

Stauffer JC, Urban P, Bleed D, et al. Result of the 'SWISS' multicenter evaluation of early angioplasty for shock following myocardial infarction. Circulation 1997;96(Suppl I):I-206.

Stone G, Brodie BR, Griffin JJ, et al. for the Primary Angioplasty In Myocardial Infarction (PAMI) Stent Pilot Trial Investigators. Prospective, multicenter study of the safety and feasibility of primary stenting in acute myocardial infarction: in-hospital and 30-day results of the PAMI Stent Pilot Trial. J Am Coll Cardiol 1998;31:23-30.

Stone GW, Brodie BR, Griffin JJ, et al for the PAMI Stent Pilot Trial Investigators. Clinical and angiographic follow-up after primary stenting in acute myocardial infarction. The Primary Angioplasty in Myocardial Infarction (PAMI) Stent Pilot Trial. Circulation 1999;99:1548-54.

Stone GW, Grines CL, Topol EJ. Update on percutaneous transluminal coronary angioplasty for acute myocardial infarction. In: Topol EJ, Serruys PW, eds. Current Review of Interventional Cardiology, 2nd ed. Philadelphia: Current Medicine; 1995:1-56.

Stone GW, Marsalese D, Brodie BR, et al. on behalf of the second Primary Angioplasty in Myocardial Infarction (PAMI-II) Trial Investigators. A prospective, randomized evaluation of prophylactic intraaortic balloon counterpulsation in high risk patients with acute myocardial infarction treated with primary angioplasty. J Am Coll Cardiol 1997;29:1459-67.

Stone GW, Rutherford BD, McConahay DR, et al. Direct coronary angioplasty in acute myocardial infarction: outcome in patients with single vessel disease. J Am Coll Cardiol 1990;15:534-43.

Suryapranata H, van't Hof AWJ, Hoorntje JCA, et al. Randomized comparison of coronary stenting with balloon angioplasty in selected patients with acute myocardial infarction. Circulation 1998;97:2502-5.

Sweeney J, Whisenant BK, Ports TA. Stenting of an unprotected ulcerated left main coronary artery in the setting of acute myocardial infarction. J Invas Cardiol 1997;9:479-81.

Ueda K, Nishida Y, Iwase T, et al. Quantitative angiographic restenosis of primary stenting using Wiktor coil stent for acute myocardial infarction: results from a multicenter randomized PRISAM study. Circulation 1997;96(Suppl I):I-531.

Waldecker B, Waas W, Haberbosch W, et al. Long-term follow-up after direct percutaneous transluminal coronary angioplasty for acute myocardial infarction. J Am Coll Cardiol 1998;32:1320-5.

Zijlstra F, de Boer MJ, Hoorntje C, et al. A comparison of immediate coronary angioplasty with intravenous streptokinase in acute myocardial infarction. N Engl J Med 1993;328:680-4.

6

Directional coronary atherectomy

DCA involves the selective excision and retrieval of atherosclerotic material from diseased coronary arteries. The Simpson coronary atherectomy device (Atherocath®) is a coaxial over-the-wire catheter for use with a steerable 0.014-inch guidewire. The distal portion of the device consists of a non-flexible, gold-plated, stainless steel biopsy housing in which lies a cup-shaped cutter. This portion has a longitudinal window of a 120° arc and a support balloon on its opposite side. Immediately distal to the housing is a tapered, flexible, stainless steel, braided nose cone that functions as a specimen collection chamber. Once the lesion is captured within the housing by inflation of the balloon, the material is collected by advancing the cutter, which spins at 2000 rpm, driven by a special motor drive unit.

DCA is indicated in large vessels (over 3mm in diameter) for bulky, non-calcified, concentric or eccentric lesions when the lesion is discrete. Bifurcation lesions, ostial lesions, discrete SVG lesions and balloon-resistant lesions are also suitable for DCA.

Specific training in this technique is necessary, since the guiding catheter and atherectomy device have specific handling characteristics and because their large size and rigid nature make them potentially traumatic. Maximum safe debulking is likely to be necessary if restenosis rates are to be minimized by DCA alone.

The OARS and BOAT studies showed that optimal atherectomy produced better long-term results than PTCA alone, in contrast to the earlier CAVEAT I and CCAT trials, in which DCA was probably used suboptimally.

The ABACAS study showed that, with IVUS guidance, adjunctive PTCA after aggressive DCA produces a larger lumen than after DCA alone. Although the long-term angiographic results were similar in the two groups, restenosis rates were very low with such optimal DCA (17% versus 16%).

The START trial showed that aggressive DCA of native coronary lesions is associated with a larger lumen diameter and less restenosis than stenting.

DCA may prove to be a useful debulking manoeuvre prior to effective coronary stent deployment, and the AMIGO study will compare the long-term restenosis rates in patients undergoing stent implantation with or without adjunctive DCA.

Finally, many of the recent advances in the understanding of coronary pathology have come from the study of histological specimens retrieved by the device.

However, DCA adds significantly to the expense of PTCA and the procedure is contraindicated in tortuous vessels, small vessels, degenerated SVGs and calcified lesions and for extensive or spiral dissections.

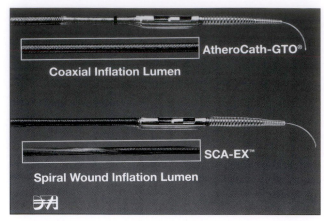

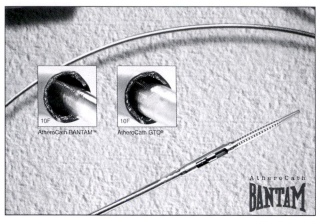

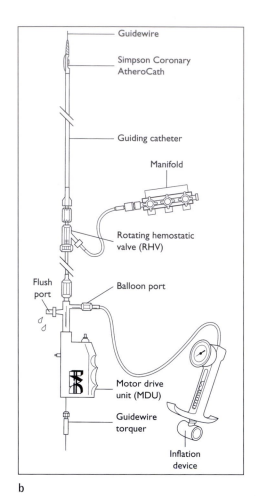

a

b

c

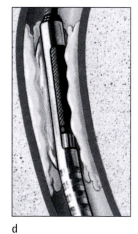

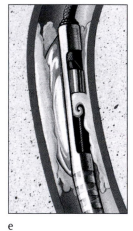

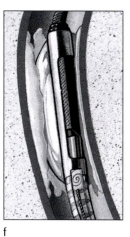

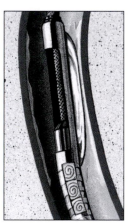

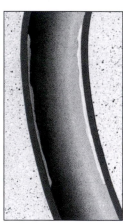

d   e   f   g   h

Figure 6.1

(a) Atherocath-GTO® and SCA-EX™ devices available from DVI/Guidant.

(b) Schematic representation of the equipment required for DCA.

(c) The Bantam™ (DVI/Guidant) has a 'downsized' shaft that allows a 7F device to be used within a 9F Tourguide™ guiding catheter (DVI/Guidant) that has an internal lumen of 0.101 inches.

(d) The schematic diagram shows how the housing is pushed into the plaque by the balloon.

This allows the cutter to slice off small pieces of tissue (e) and push them into the nose-cone of the device (f).

The atherectomy device is then reoriented towards more plaque and the cutting manoeuvre is repeated.

The additional specimens are collected in the nose cone (g) until a satisfactory angiographic result is obtained (h).

DCA in native vessels

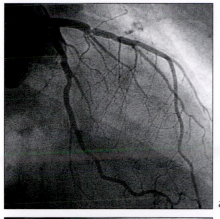

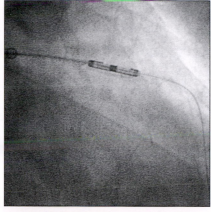

b

Figure 6.2
A 68-year-old man. (a) A short, discrete, slightly eccentric, balloon-resistant stenosis in the proximal LAD before DCA.
(b) During DCA with a 7F Simpson Atherocath®, the cutter has travelled half-way along the housing.
(c) Result after DCA shows an excellent appearance after removal of 6 pieces of tissue.
(d) Histology showed heavily calcified, fibrous plaque.

a

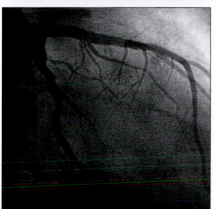

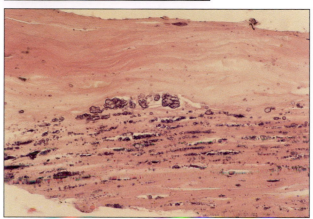

c

d

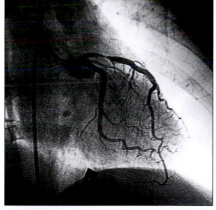

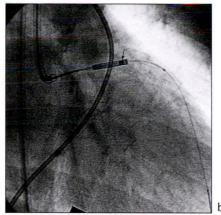

Figure 6.3
(a) Severe eccentric stenosis in the proximal LAD in a 41-year-old woman with severe unstable angina.
A 7F Atherocath was used for DCA.
(b) The cutter has reached the distal end of the housing (arrow).
(c) Result after DCA with a 7F SCA-1® device.
Six small specimens were retrieved.
(d) One of these specimens showed thrombus on an ulcerated fibrous plaque.

a

b

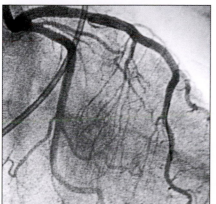

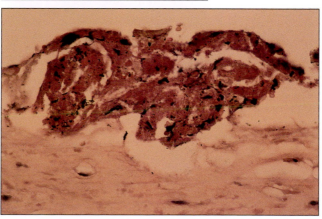

c

d

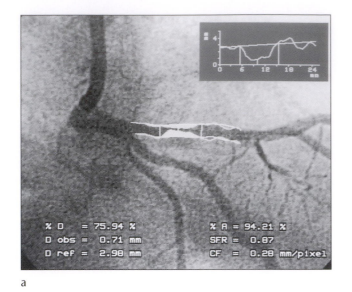
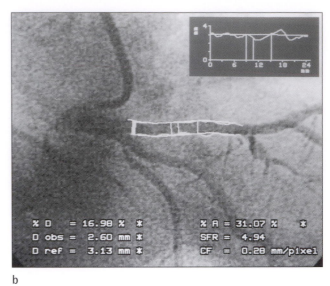

a

b

Figure 6.4
Severe, eccentric stenosis in proximal LAD (a) before and (b) after DCA in a 50-year-old man with a recent onset of unstable angina.

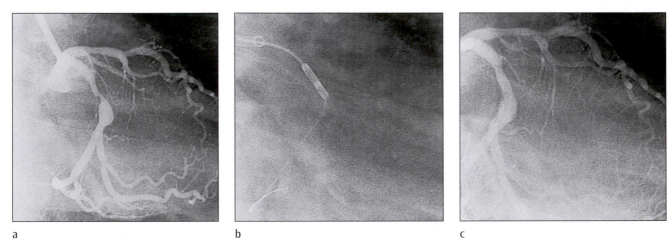

a

b

c

Figure 6.5
(a) Severe eccentric and somewhat bulky stenosis in the proximal LCx in a 57-year-old woman with moderately severe angina. A short left main stem and the shallow angle of take-off of the LCx make this a suitable case for DCA.
(b) A 7F SCA-EX™ device was placed across the lesion and the cutter advanced slowly during one of 15 cuts in circumferential fashion.
(c) The result after DCA was acceptable, although a 15-20% residual stenosis remained. Ten specimens were retrieved.

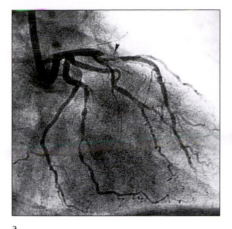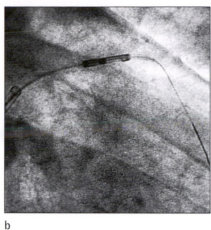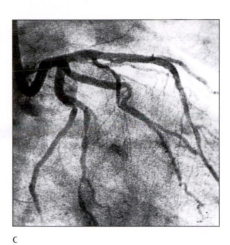

a   b   c

Figure 6.6
(a) Severe, bulky, concentric, proximal LAD stenosis (arrow) was treated by (b) DCA (7F SCA-EX™ device).
(c) The excellent result after DCA revealed no residual stenosis.

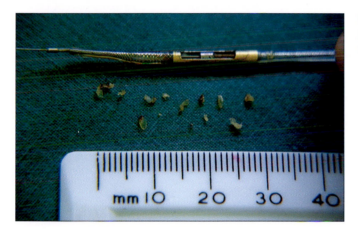

a

Figure 6.7
Macroscopic appearance of specimens retrieved from a bulky LAD stenosis using the early SCA-1® device.

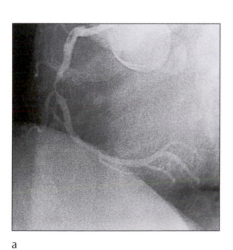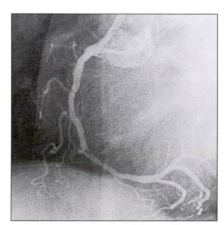

a   b

Figure 6.8
A 46-year-old woman with unstable angina. Severe eccentric stenosis in the mid-third of the RCA (a) before and (b) after DCA with a 6F SCA-EX™ device.

The START trial showed that aggressive DCA of native coronary lesions is associated with a larger lumen diameter and less restenosis than stenting.

DCA for restenosis lesions

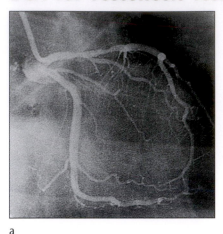

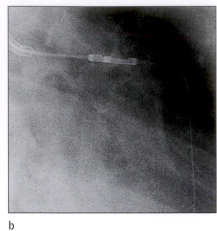

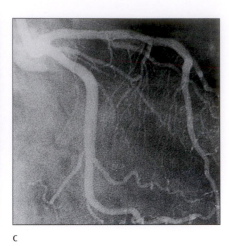

a   b   c

Figure 6.9
(a) Two angiographically insignificant restenotic lesions in proximal LAD of a 47-year-old woman with severe angina. Intracoronary ultrasound showed dense non-calcific plaque.
(b) DCA with a 7F SCA-EX™ device removed eight large specimens.
(c) There was an excellent angiographic result, and the patient had complete relief of symptoms.

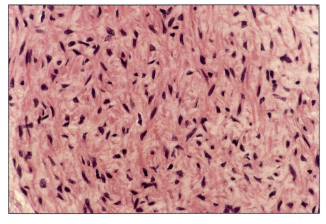

a

Figure 6.10
Tissue removed from restenotic lesions usually shows dense fibrointimal hyperplasia.

DCA of bifurcation lesions

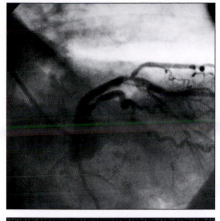

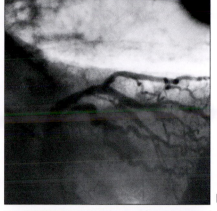

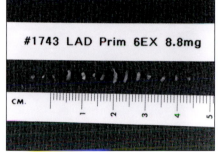

#1743 LAD Prim 6EX 8.8mg

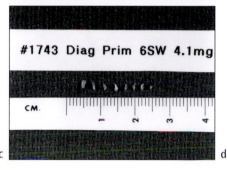

#1743 Diag Prim 6SW 4.1mg

Figure 6.11
A 45-year-old male cardiologist with hypercholesterolemia and a positive family history of ischaemic heart disease had exertional dyspnoea and a positive stress echocardiogram. (a) Diagnostic coronary angiography showed a significant stenosis affecting the LAD/first DG bifurcation.

The ostial diagonal stenosis was pre-dilated with a 2.0mm Sleek™ balloon (Cordis) and the LAD was pre-dilated with a 2.5mm Sleek™ balloon both at 60psi. DCA was then performed to the mid-LAD first using a 7F SCA-EX™ at 10psi followed by a 6F SCA-EX™ at 20psi and finally a 6F SCA-EX™ short window device at 30psi. The DG was then treated with a 6F SCA-EX™ short window device.

(b) Final angiographic result.

(c, d) The operator retrieved (c) 8.8mg of tissue from the LAD and (d) 4.1mg of tissue from the DG.

An angiogram at 7 months showed no evidence of restenosis with only 10% residual stenosis at both sites.

Courtesy of Dr G Robertson, Sequoia Hospital, Redwood City, California, USA.

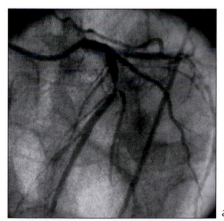

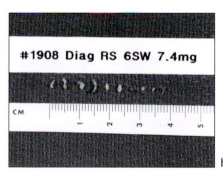

#1908 Diag RS 6SW 7.4mg

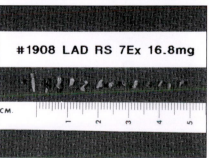

#1908 LAD RS 7Ex 16.8mg

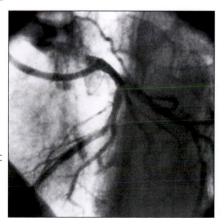

Figure 6.12
A 66-year-old man had undergone PTCA 2 months earlier to this LAD/DG bifurcation lesion after an admission to hospital with unstable angina. A recurrence of angina necessitated repeat coronary arteriography. (a) This study showed a severe restenosis involving both the LAD and the DG at the bifurcation point.

The LAD and DG lesions were pre-dilated with a 2.5mm balloon to 50psi. DCA was then performed to the ostium of the DG using a 6F SCA-EX™ short window device to a pressure of 20psi and to the LAD using a 7F SCA-EX™ device to a pressure of 20psi.

(b) A total of 7.4mg of tissue was removed from the DG and (c) 16.8mg of tissue was removed from the LAD.

(d) There was an excellent angiographic result.

Two years later the patient remained free of angina.

Courtesy of Dr T Hinohara, Sequoia Hospital, Redwood City, California, USA.

DCA in SVGs

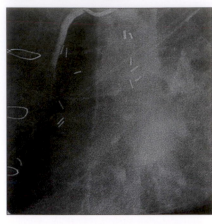

a

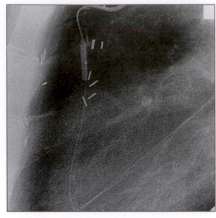

b

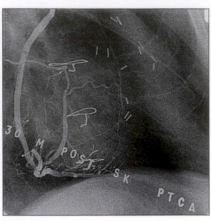

c

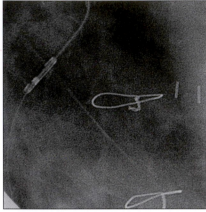

d

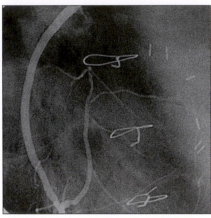

e

Figure 6.13

DCA can be useful in SVGs. (a) This 6-year-old RCA SVG in a 56-year-old newspaper proprietor was occluded for the second time. He had undergone two previous CABG operations.
(b) The SVG was reopened by PTCA with a 3.5mm Gold-Ex® balloon catheter and intragraft streptokinase was infused to lyse visible thrombus within the graft.
(c) A persistent filling defect was evident at the site of previous occlusion, which remained despite PTCA at high pressure.
(d) DCA was performed with a 7F SCA-EX™ device.
(e) An excellent angiographic result was achieved.

Three specimens were retrieved, which histologically showed organized thrombus.

The randomized CAVEAT II trial involving patients with SVG lesions demonstrated improved acute angiographic results after DCA compared with PTCA but similar restenosis rates in the two groups at 6 months.

DCA-Rotablator® synergy in calcified lesions

DCA can be combined with Rotablator® atherectomy for bulky calcified lesions (see Chapter 12).

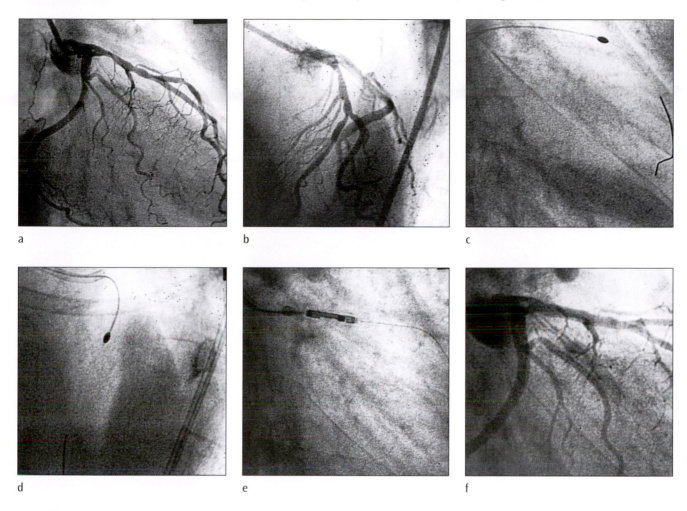

a b c

d e f

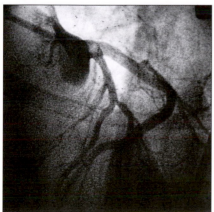

g

Figure 6.14

A 60-year old man. (a) Two bulky, eccentric, calcified lesions (one proximal and one just before the diagonal branch), together with two additional lesions (one just beyond the bifurcation and one in the middle third).

(b) The lesions are best seen in the cranial LAO projection.

They were first treated with a 1.75mm Rotablator® burr and then a 2.25mm Rotablator® burr – (c) RAO projection; (d) cranial LAO projection.

(e) A 7F SCA-EX™ device was used to remove six specimens from the more proximal three lesions.

The final angiographic result was satisfactory – (f) RAO projection; (g) cranial LAO projection.

DCA in native vessels after CABG surgery

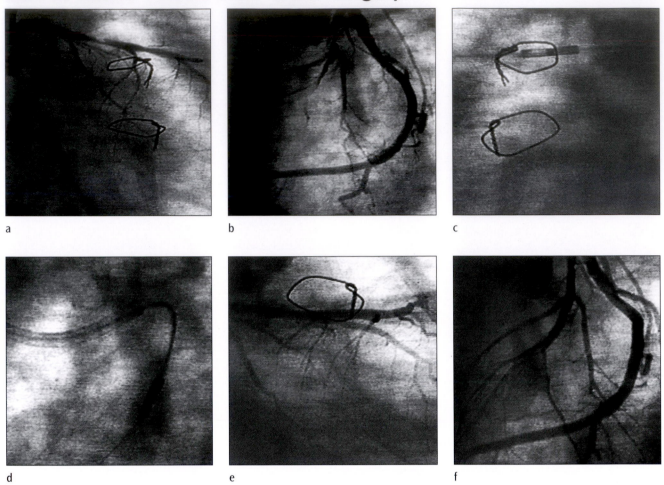

a   b   c

d   e   f

Figure 6.15

DCA can be used in native coronary arteries after CABG surgery. A 60-year-old man had severe stable angina and an occluded LAD SVG, but the LAD was still patent although severely stenosed – (a) RAO; (b) cranial LAO projection.

DCA was performed using a 7F SCA-EX™ device – (c) RAO projection; (d) cranial LAO projection.

This produced an excellent angiographic result – (e) RAO projection; (f) cranial LAO projection – and an excellent clinical result.

Primary atherostenting

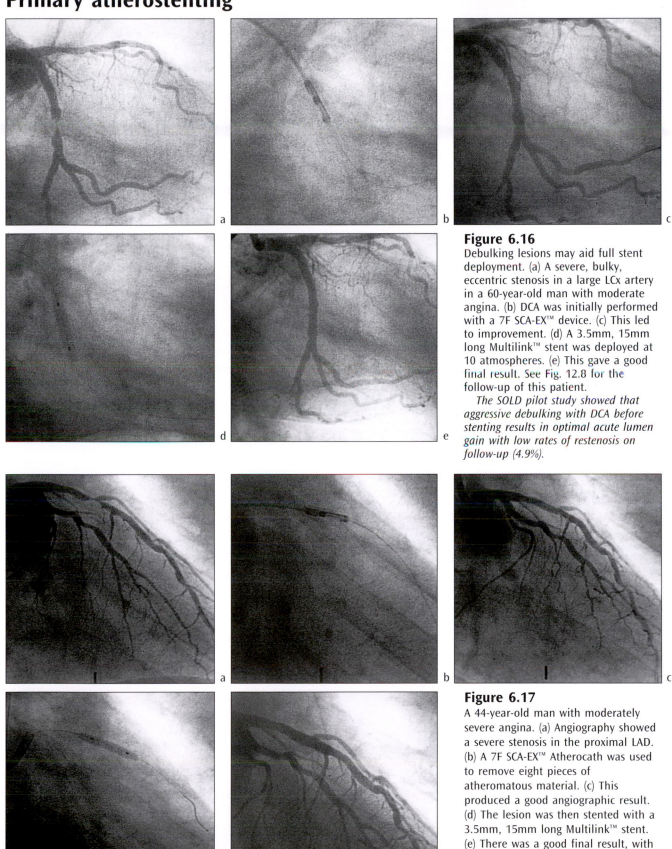

a   b   c

Figure 6.16
Debulking lesions may aid full stent deployment. (a) A severe, bulky, eccentric stenosis in a large LCx artery in a 60-year-old man with moderate angina. (b) DCA was initially performed with a 7F SCA-EX™ device. (c) This led to improvement. (d) A 3.5mm, 15mm long Multilink™ stent was deployed at 10 atmospheres. (e) This gave a good final result. See Fig. 12.8 for the follow-up of this patient.
The SOLD pilot study showed that aggressive debulking with DCA before stenting results in optimal acute lumen gain with low rates of restenosis on follow-up (4.9%).

d   e

Figure 6.17
A 44-year-old man with moderately severe angina. (a) Angiography showed a severe stenosis in the proximal LAD. (b) A 7F SCA-EX™ Atherocath was used to remove eight pieces of atheromatous material. (c) This produced a good angiographic result. (d) The lesion was then stented with a 3.5mm, 15mm long Multilink™ stent. (e) There was a good final result, with negative residual stenosis. Quantitative coronary arteriography showed a large MLD.

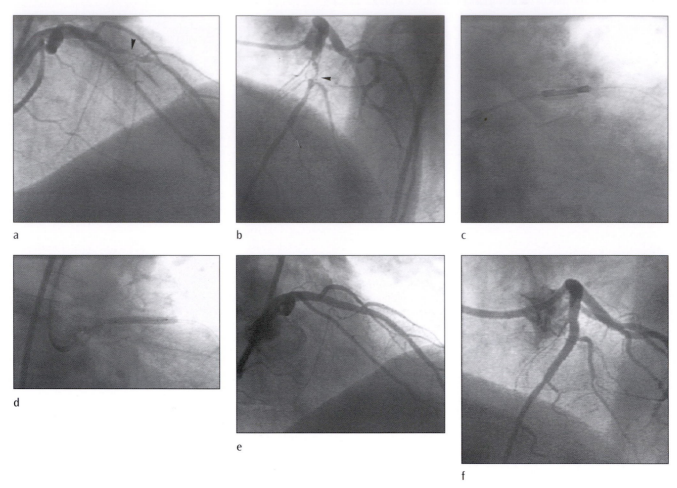

a b c

d e

f

Figure 6.18

(a, b) A 61-year-old man with hypertension and severe unstable angina was found to have mild disease in the RCA and LCx coronary arteries but a severe complex lesion in the proximal LAD (arrow).

The patient was treated with abciximab.

The LAD lesion was crossed with a 0.014-inch Floppy® guidewire and pre-dilated with a 3.5mm, 30mm long Goldie Longy™ balloon at 2 atmospheres.

(c) A 7F SCA-EX™ was then used to make 18 cuts to the lesion site.

A large amount of tissue was removed.

(d) A 3.5mm, 25mm long Multilink™ stent was then implanted.

A 3.5mm, 30mm long Goldie Longy™ balloon was used to post-dilate the stent up to 14 atmospheres.

(e, f) The final result was excellent. Moreover, there was no elevation in CPK.

Courtesy of Dr M de Belder, Cardiothoracic Unit, South Cleveland Hospital, Middlesbrough, UK.

Intracoronary ultrasound after DCA

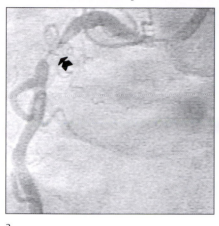

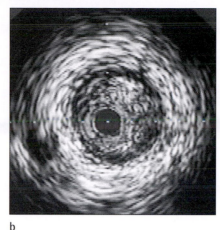

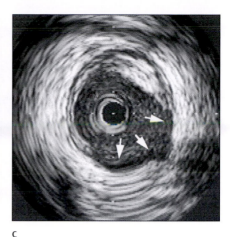

a

b

c

Figure 6.19

A 56-year-old man with severe angina had (a) a critical stenosis in the proximal RCA (arrow). (b) Intracoronary ultrasound before intervention showed dense non-calcific plaque tightly surrounding the IVUS catheter. DCA was performed with a 7F Atherocath®. (c) After three cuts, IVUS showed excellent debulking of plaque but a deep eccentric cut extending deep into the media (arrows).

A final angiogram (not shown) showed extravasation of contrast. There was no acute complication, but 6 months later the patient presented with chest pain. An angiogram at this time showed a large aneurysm at the site of the previous perforation.

Courtesy of Dr S Schwarzacher, Center for Research in Cardiovascular Interventions, Stanford University, Stanford, California, USA.

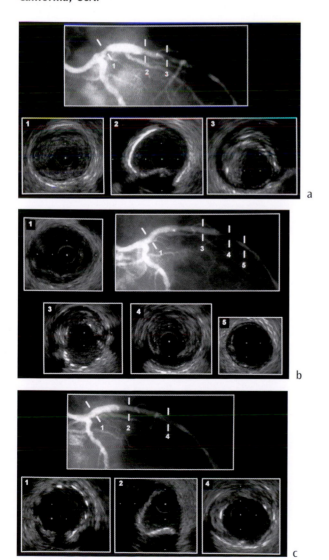

a

b

c

Combined DCA and stent implantation using intracoronary ultrasound

Figure 6.20

A 70-year-old man with diabetes, hypertension and moderately severe angina had (a) three significant lesions in the LAD. Intracoronary ultrasound showed soft plaque in the proximal lesion (1), heavy calcification (>180°) in the second lesion (2) and a more fibrotic, eccentric lesion with mild calcification in the middle third (3).

(b) The proximal lesion was treated with DCA using a 7FG SCA-EX™ Atherocath.

The typical appearance with multiple cuts can be identified in the IVUS image (1). The calcified segment was left untreated (IVUS image not shown). The middle third lesion was stented with a 16mm long 9 cell NIR™ stent mounted on a 3.5mm Viva Primo™ balloon (Scimed) inflated up to 14 atmospheres. The stent showed a relatively eccentric expansion, owing to the eccentric, hard plaque that was present (3). Beyond this lesion there remained eccentric, ruptured plaque with a dissection from 4 o'clock to 8 o'clock; this can be seen in the IVUS image (4). The distal reference segment was practically free from disease (5).

(c) The proximal lesion was then stented with a 14mm long JJIS II® stent mounted on a 3.5mm Viva Primo™ balloon inflated at 16 atmospheres.

The IVUS showed a homogenous expansion with a relatively small residual plaque burden (1). The calcified segment was left untreated (2) and the most distal lesion was stented with an additional 16mm long 9 cell NIR™ stent mounted on a 3.5mm Viva Primo™ balloon inflated up to 14 atmospheres (4). The IVUS showed homogenous stent expansion (4).

The final angiographic result was satisfactory and the patient was rendered symptom-free.

Courtesy of Dr F Werner and H Mudra, Klinikum Innenstadt der LMU Medizinische Klinik, Munich, Germany.

Reading

Abdelmeguid AE, Whitlow PL. Coronary atherectomy: directional, rotational and extraction catheters. In: White CJ, Ramee SR, eds. Interventional Cardiology. New York: Marcel Dekker; 1995:175-200.

Adelman AG, Cohen EA, Kimball BP, *et al*. A comparison of directional atherectomy with balloon angioplasty for lesions of the left anterior descending coronary artery. N Engl J Med 1993;329:228-33.

Baim DS, Cutlip DE, Sharma SK, *et al*. Final results of the Balloon vs Optimal Atherectomy Trial (BOAT). Circulation 1998;97:322-31.

Baim DS, Kent KM, King SB, *et al* for the NACI Investigators. Evaluating new devices. Acute (in-hospital) results from the new approaches to coronary intervention registry. Circulation 1994;89:471-81.

Dauerman HL, Higgins PJ, Sparano AM, *et al*. Mechanical debulking versus balloon angioplasty for the treatment of true bifurcation lesions. Circulation 1998;98(Suppl I):I-350.

Ellis SG, De Cesare NB, Pinkerton CA, *et al*. Relation of stenosis morphology and clinical presentation to the procedural results of directional coronary atherectomy. Circulation 1991;84:644-53.

Garratt KN, Bell MR, Berger PB, *et al*. and the US Directional Atherectomy Study Group. Outcome of directional coronary atherectomy by new operators: comparison with experienced operators. J Am Coll Cardiol 1992;19(Suppl A):352A.

Hinohara T, Robertson GC, Selmon MR, *et al*. Directional coronary atherectomy. J Invas Cardiol 1990;2:217-26.

Hinohara T, Selmon MR, Robertson GC, *et al*. Directional atherectomy: new approaches for treatment of obstructive coronary and peripheral vascular disease. Circulation 1990;81(Suppl IV):79-91.

Hinohara T, Selmon MR, Robertson GC, *et al*. Directional coronary atherectomy. In: Holmes DR, Garratt KN, eds. Atherectomy. Boston: Blackwell Scientific; 1992:18-42.

Holmes DR Jr, Topol EJ, Califf RM *et al* and the CAVEAT-II Investigators. A multicenter, randomized trial of coronary angioplasty versus directional atherectomy for patients with saphenous vein bypass graft lesions. Circulation 1995;91:1966–74.

Hosokawa H, Kato O, Tamai H, *et al*. Role of adjunctive balloon angioplasty following coronary atherectomy: a serial intravascular ultrasound analysis from the ABACAS trial. J Am Coll Cardiol 1997;29:281A.

Moussa I, Moses JW, Strain JE, *et al*. Angiographic and clinical outcome of patients undergoing 'Stenting after Optimal Lesion Debulking': the 'SOLD' pilot study. Circulation 1997;96(Suppl I):I-81.

Ramsdale DR, Grech ED. Directional coronary atherectomy. In: Grech ED, Ramsdale DR, eds. Practical Interventional Cardiology. London: Martin Dunitz; 1997:141-76.

Simonton CA, Leon MB, Baim DS, *et al*. 'Optimal' directional coronary atherectomy: final results of the Optimal Atherectomy Restenosis Study (OARS). Circulation 1998;97:332-9.

Simonton CA. Lesion-specific technique considerations in directional coronary atherectomy. Cathet Cardiovasc Diagn 1993;Suppl I:3-9.

Topol EJ, Leya F, Pinkerton CA, *et al*. for the CAVEAT study group. A comparison of directional atherectomy with coronary angioplasty in patients with coronary artery disease. N Engl J Med 1993;329:221-7.

Tsuchikane E, Sumitsuji S, Awata N, *et al*. Final results of the STent versus directional coronary Atherectomy Randomized Trial (START). J Am Coll Cardiol 1999;34:1050-7.

Tsuchikane E, Sumitsuji S, Nakamura T, *et al*. Angiographic follow-up results of STent versus Atherectomy Randomized Trial (START). J Am Coll Cardiol 1998;31:379A.

Waksman R, Popma JJ, Kennard ED, *et al*. Directional coronary atherectomy (DCA): a report from the New Approaches to Coronary Intervention (NACI) Registry. Am J Cardiol 1997;80:50K-59K.

Whitlow PL, Franco I. Indications for directional coronary atherectomy. Am J Cardiol 1993;72: 21E-29E.

7

Rotablator® coronary atherectomy

Percutaneous coronary rotational atherectomy (PTCRA) – Rotablator® coronary atherectomy – uses a diamond-studded, elliptically shaped brass burr that is 1.25-2.5mm in diameter to remove plaque while it is rotating at speeds of between 150,000 and 200,000 rpm. The drive shaft of the device is rotated by a turbine that is housed within an 'advancer unit'. The turbine is driven by compressed air. The catheter is passed over a special 325cm long, 0.009-inch diameter stainless steel guidewire (RotaWire™) in order to advance the burr through the lesion. A floppy RotaWire™ and an ExtraSupport RotaWire™ are available. The Rotawire™ Floppy Gold wire has a 12.5 cm gold-coated segment distally to enhance visibility and make guidewire bias more obvious.

Saline is infused into the sheath surrounding the drive shaft at a basal rate of 3 ml/min which increases to a rate of 12 ml/min during burr rotation. In each 500 ml bag of saline is placed 5,000 units of heparin, 5 mg GTN and 5 mg verapamil. This infusion not only reduces heat generated by the rotating burr but also helps to reduce coronary artery spasm. Rotaglide™, a lipid-based emulsion designed to further lubricate the Rotablator™ system, should soon be available. A total of 10 ml added to the infusion will further reduce friction within the system.

PTCRA has particular use for lesions that are unresponsive to PTCA, such as complex or calcified lesions, hard fibrotic lesions and restenotic lesions. Other lesions such as ostial, bifurcation, angulated and long lesions are also more attractive for PTCRA than PTCA. Currently, adjunctive PTCA at low pressure is recommended after PTCRA, and this is essential in large vessels since the largest burr is 2.5mm in diameter. A multiple step-up burr technique may be the best method of achieving a smooth, non-dissected result but the extraordinary expense of the procedure may make it difficult to justify financially. The procedure is quite different from PTCA and requires special expertise and training.

PTCRA is contraindicated in degenerated SVGs and in lesions in which there is a lot of thrombus. Other cases in which PTCRA is contraindicated include cases of diffuse disease with poor distal vessel run-off and cases in which the patient has severely impaired left ventricular function. Coronary artery spasm and bradyarrhythmias not uncommonly occur in dominant RCA or LCx procedures and temporary pacemaker insertion is indicated here.

A new 'Rotalink'™ system is now available. This enables burrs to be interchanged on the same advancer unit, reducing the cost of the procedure.

Table 7.1 shows the recommended guiding catheter (French size and internal diameter) for each burr size as well as the respective target rpm proximal to the lesion. Table 7.2 shows the most appropriate burr size for the artery in order to achieve 70-85% burr-artery ratio.

The DART trial compared the clinical and angiographic outcomes after rotational atherectomy versus PTCA in non-complex native coronary lesions.

The STRATAS trial showed that, in native coronary arteries, an aggressive Rotablator® strategy with no adjunctive PTCA or low-pressure adjunctive PTCA (burr-artery ratio 0.7-0.9 as 'stand-alone' or with adjunctive PTCA at less than 1 atmosphere) does not decrease restenosis or adverse clinical events when compared with conservative Rotablator® use with adjunctive PTCA (burr-artery ratio of 0.6-0.8 followed by routine adjunctive PTCA with balloon-artery ratio of 1.1-1.3 and balloon pressure of 3 atmospheres).

Table 7.1
The recommended Guiding Catheter (French size and internal diameter) for each burr size as well as the respective target rpm proximal to the lesion.

Burr diameter			[1]Minimum recommended guiding catheter size (French)	Recommended guiding catheter internal diameter (inches)	Target rpm (proximal to lesion)
mm	inches	French			
1.25	0.049	3.75	8.0	0.053	175,000–180,000
1.50	0.059	4.50	8.0	0.063	175,000–180,000
1.75	0.069	5.25	8.0	0.073	175,000–180,000
2.00	0.079	6.00	9.0	0.083	175,000–180,000
2.15	0.085	6.45	9.0	0.089	160,000–165,000
2.25	0.089	6.75	9.0	0.093	160,000–165,000
2.38	0.094	7.14	9.0[2]	0.098	160,000–165,000
2.50	0.098	7.50	10.0	0.102	160,000–165,000

[1]Large lumen catheter with side holes recommended (maintain at least 0.004" clearance between burr and inner diameter of guide catheter)
[2]Large lumen catheter with an inner diameter of at least 0.098"

Table 7.2
The most appropriate burr size for the artery in order to achieve 70-85% burr-artery ratio.

Artery (mm)	70% (mm)	Closest burr (mm)	85% (mm)	Closest burr (mm)
1.5	1.05	–	1.28	1.25 (83%)
1.75	1.22	1.25 (71%)	1.49	1.50 (86%)
2.00	1.40	1.50 (75%)	1.70	1.50 (75%)
2.25	1.57	1.50 (66%)	1.91	1.75 (77%)
2.50	1.75	1.75 (70%)	2.13	2.15 (86%)
2.75	1.92	2.00 (73%)	2.33	2.25 (82%)
3.00	2.10	2.15 (72%)	2.55	2.50 (83%)
3.25	2.27	2.25 (69%)	2.76	2.50 (76%)
3.50	2.45	2.50 (71%)	2.98	2.50 (71%)
4.00	2.80	2.50 (62%)	3.40	2.50 (62%)
4.50	3.15	2.50 (56%)	3.83	2.50 (56%)

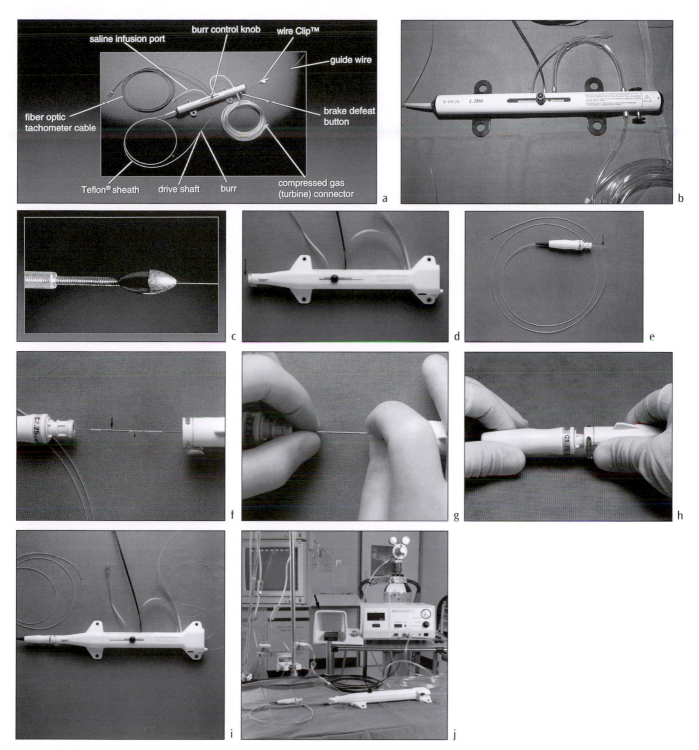

Figure 7.1

(a, b) Rotablator® catheter and advancer components. (c) Close-up view of Rotablator® catheter and burr over a guidewire.
(d) The newer Rotalink™ system has a more streamlined advancer unit, which can be attached to an individual catheter/burr by a unique locking mechanism (arrow). (e) A 2.25mm catheter/burr that is separate from its advancer unit. The brass tube (arrow) that covers the bayonet locking mechanism is shown. (f) Close-up view showing the interlocked drive shaft joining the catheter/burr (left) to the advancer unit (right). The arrow shows the brass tube which will cover the bayonet locking mechanism (arrowhead).
(g) The brass tube covers the bayonet locking mechanism, which rotates at high speed and through which the RotaWire™ passes.
(h) The catheter/burr is then locked into the advancer unit. (i) The system is ready for use. (j) The Rotalink™ system set up in the catheter laboratory. Activation of the foot pedal (arrow) allows the operator to start and stop the Rotablator®.
Courtesy of Heart Technology, Boston Scientific Ltd, USA.

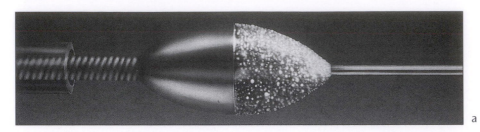

a

Figure 7.2
(a) Magnified view of diamond-studded burr.
Courtesy of Heart Technology,
Boston Scientific Ltd, USA.
(b) A floppy and an ExtraSupport RotaWire™ are available.

- Flexible, easily navigates anatomy
- Significantly increased torqueability
- 2.2 cm spring tip for distal treatment
- Minimal vessel straightening
- Reduced guidewire bias – more neutrally placed in vessel

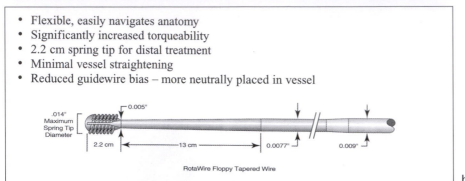

RotaWire Floppy Tapered Wire

b

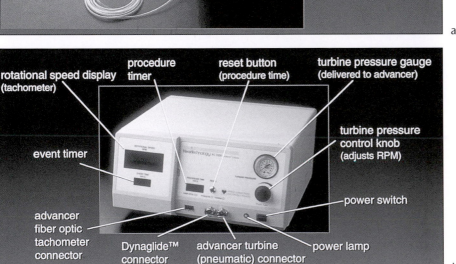

Percutaneous Transluminal Coronary Rotational Ablation (PTCRA)

System Overview

a

Figure 7.3
(a, b) System overview shows the console into which the fiberoptic tachometer cable and the compressed-air line are inserted.

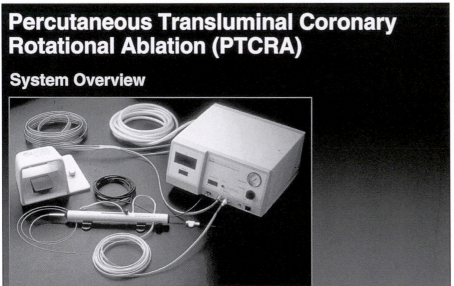

b

Complex or calcified lesions

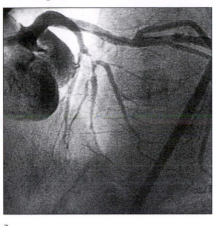
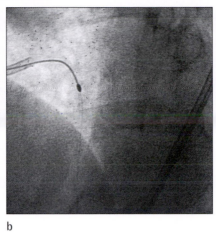
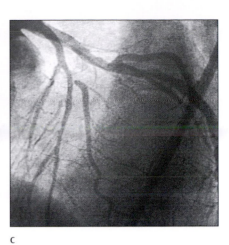

a   b   c

Figure 7.4

(a) This morphologically complex and calcified stenosis in the proximal LAD is ideal for high-speed rotational coronary atherectomy with the Rotablator® device (cranial LAO projection).

(b) A 1.5mm burr is advanced across the lesion at 190,000 rpm.

(c) Result after 2.0mm burr and adjunctive PTCA with a 3.0mm balloon catheter at a pressure of 1.5 atmospheres.

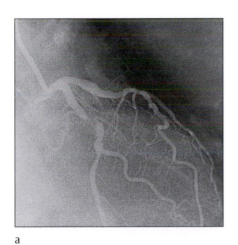
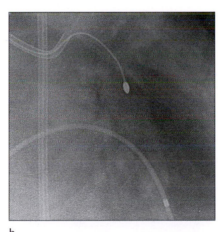

a   b

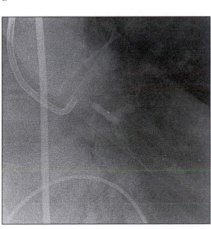
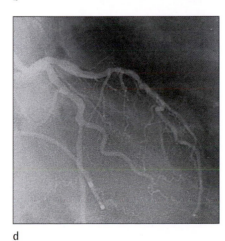

c   d

Figure 7.5

(a–c) Bulky, eccentric and calcified stenosis in LCx treated by a 1.75mm and a 2.25mm Rotablator® burr and adjunctive PTCA with a 3.0mm Goldie™ balloon.

(d) A good angiographic result was obtained.

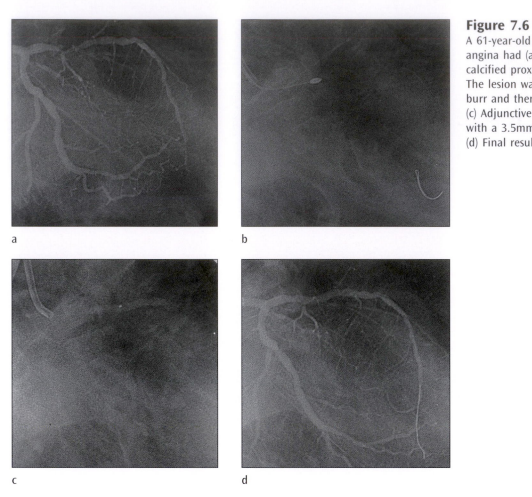

a

b

c

d

Figure 7.6
A 61-year-old care assistant with severe angina had (a) a complex, bulky and calcified proximal LAD lesion.
The lesion was ablated with a 1.5mm burr and then (b) a 2.25mm burr.
(c) Adjunctive dilatation was performed with a 3.5mm Elipse™ balloon.
(d) Final result.

Tubular lesions

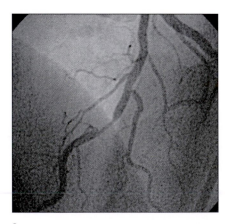

a

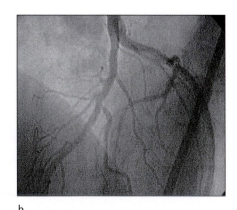

b

Figure 7.7
A 42-year-old man with uncontrolled angina. Tubular lesion in mid-third of LAD (a) before and (b) after PTCRA with a 1.75mm and 2.25mm burr and adjunctive PTCA with a 3.5mm Gold Ex® (Medtronic) balloon catheter.

Aorta-ostial lesions

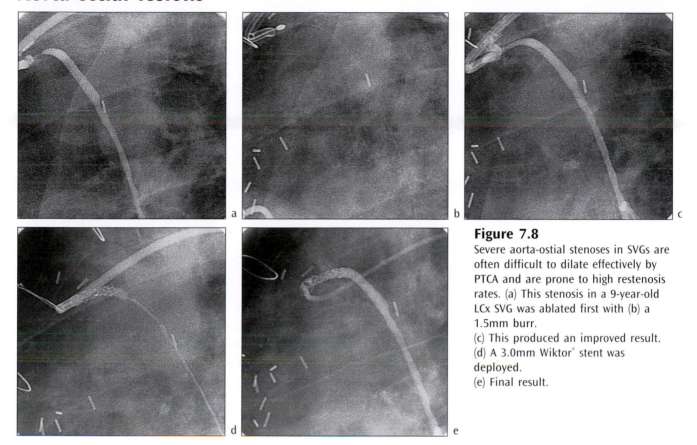

Figure 7.8
Severe aorta-ostial stenoses in SVGs are often difficult to dilate effectively by PTCA and are prone to high restenosis rates. (a) This stenosis in a 9-year-old LCx SVG was ablated first with (b) a 1.5mm burr.
(c) This produced an improved result.
(d) A 3.0mm Wiktor® stent was deployed.
(e) Final result.

Ostial or bifurcation lesions

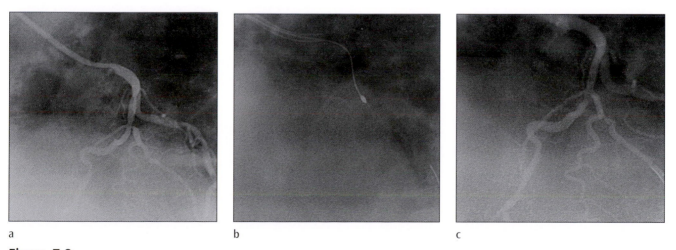

Figure 7.9
(a) A severe ostial stenosis in the first diagonal branch of the LAD.
(b) The lesion was ablated with a 1.75mm Rotablator® burr followed by a 2.25mm Rotablator® burr.
(c) The excellent final result.

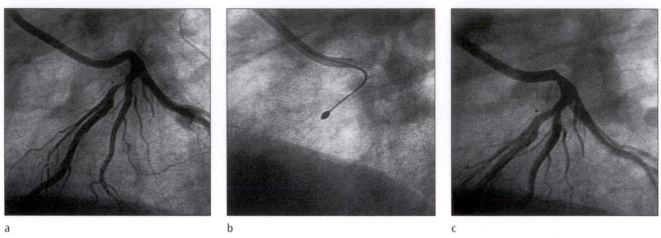

a   b   c

Figure 7.10
(a) Lesions at or just beyond bifurcations, such as this LAD stenosis, can be ablated by PTCRA.
(b) A 1.75mm burr was followed by a 2.25mm burr and adjunctive PTCA with a 3.0mm balloon at 1.5 atmospheres.
(c) This produced an acceptable result.

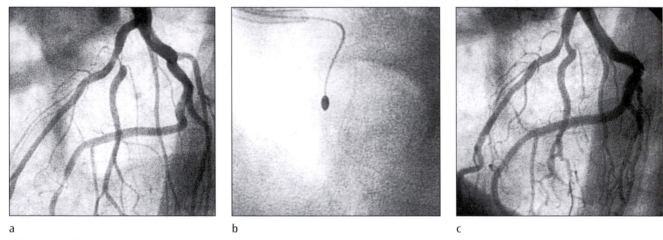

a   b   c

Figure 7.11
A 35-year-old engineer had moderate angina and (a) a severe ostial diagonal lesion.
(b) The lesion was ablated with a 1.5mm Rotablator® burr and a 2.0mm Rotablator® burr in turn.
   The lesion was post-dilated with a 3.0mm Elipse™ balloon.
(c) The angiographic result was excellent, as was the clinical result.

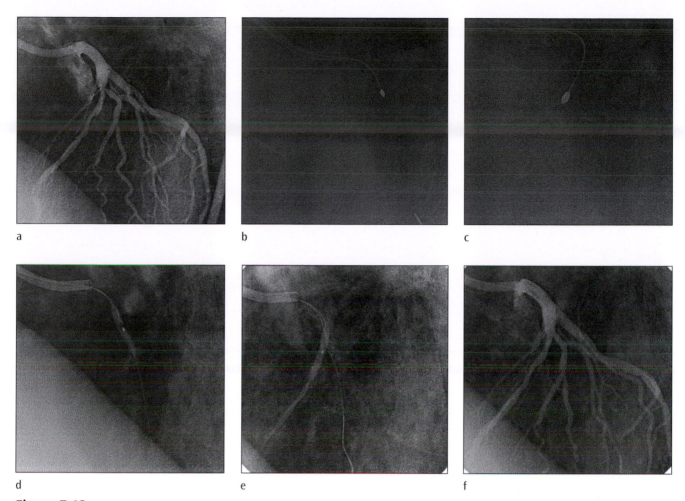

Figure 7.12
(a) A severe ostial stenosis in the first DG in a 53-year-old brewery representative was associated with significant disease in the adjacent LAD.
(b, c) Both lesions were ablated with a 1.75mm Rotablator® burr followed by a 2.25mm Rotablator® burr.
(d, e) Adjunctive PTCA was performed with a 3.0mm Elipse™ balloon in the DG (d) and LAD (e).
(f) Final result.

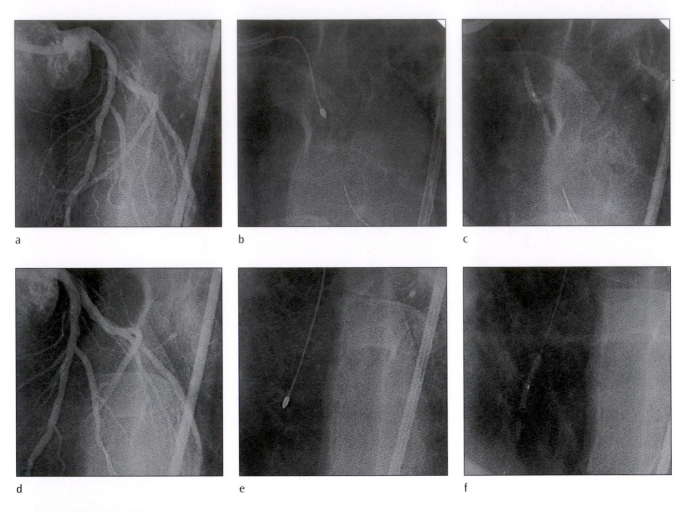

a

b

c

d

e

f

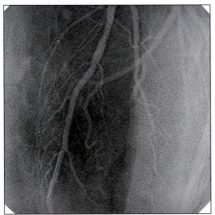

g

Figure 7.13

(a) Severe ostial stenosis in the first DG in a 47-year-old gastroenterologist who had moderate angina.

(b) The stenosis was ablated with a 1.75mm burr and a 2.25mm burr.

(c) This was followed by adjunctive dilatation by PTCA with a 3.0mm Express Supra™ balloon with an excellent result (d).

   A distal LAD lesion was also treated with (e) a 1.75mm burr and (f) a 3.0mm Express Supra™ balloon.

(g) This produced a similar good angiographic result and a satisfactory clinical outcome.

True bifurcation lesions

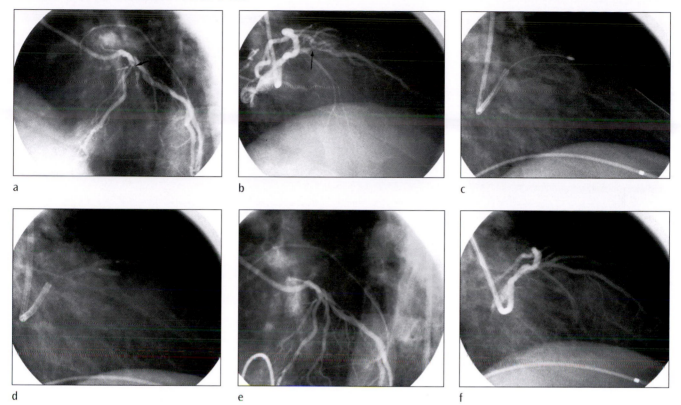

a b c

d e f

Figure 7.14

A 51-year-old man had severe angina on exertion and rest angina. His ECG showed ST-segment depression in leads V3-V6. Coronary arteriography showed a severe and calcified bifurcation stenosis (arrow) involving the LAD and the first DG – (a) LAO cranial projection; (b) RAO cranial projection.

PTCA and primary stenting was considered to be potentially difficult because of the degree of calcification and the bifurcation anatomy. The degree of calcification and the vessel size made DCA and ELCA unattractive options.

Five days later the patient was brought back for bifurcation rotational atherectomy and adjunctive administration of abciximab. The origin of the DG had progressed to occlusion. A 9FL guiding catheter was chosen to accommodate a wide range of burr sizes and provide good support.

(c) The LAD lesion was crossed with a floppy C-wire™ and ablated with sequential 1.5mm and 1.75mm Rotablator® burrs (RAO projection).

After removing the guidewire from the LAD and placing it down the DG branch, the DG was then similarly treated with the 1.5mm and 1.75mm burrs.

(d) Adjunctive PTCA was then performed with two 3.0mm balloon catheters.

(e, f) This resulted in an excellent angiographic appearance.

There were no complications and the patient was allowed home the next day.

Courtesy of Dr CS Rihal, Cardiovascular Diseases and Internal Medicine, Mayo Clinic, Minnesota, USA.

Angulated lesions

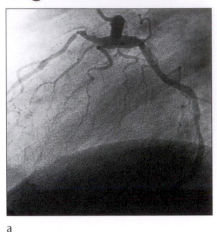
a

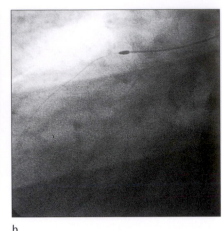
b

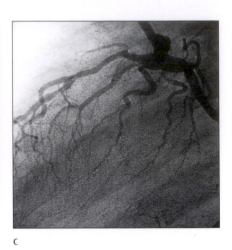
c

Figure 7.15
Severe stenoses in sharply angulated segments are prone to dissection by PTCA. (a) This stenosis in the proximal LAD was ablated with a 1.5mm burr and then a 2.0mm burr (b).
(c) The lesion was gently dilated by PTCA with a 2.5mm balloon catheter at low pressure.

Long lesions

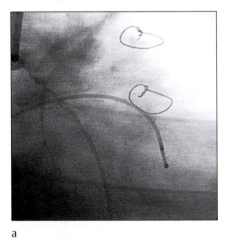
a

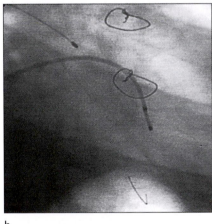
b

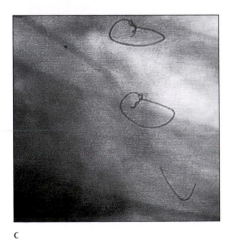
c

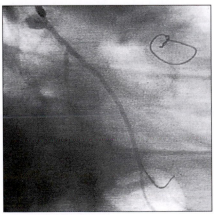
d

Figure 7.16
PTCRA can be used effectively to produce smooth, non-dissected results in very long lesions. (a) This stenosis, in a 56-year-old man with previous CABG surgery and a patent SVG to the LAD, extended from the left main coronary artery down the LCx and along its obtuse marginal branch.

A step-up technique is ideal. This was carried out with (b) a 1.5mm followed by a 2.0mm burr and (c) adjunctive PTCA with a 3.0mm, 30mm long Elipse™ balloon catheter.

(d) This produced a good angiographic result.

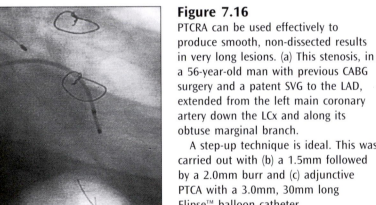

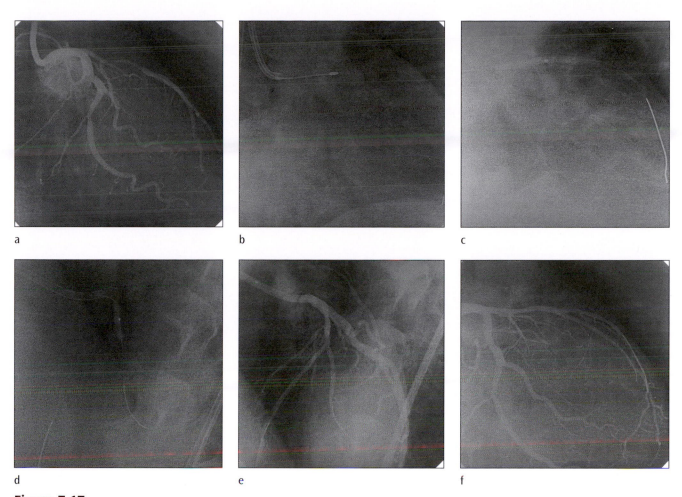

a   b   c

d   e   f

Figure 7.17

A 57-year-old postman with severe angina and recent rest pain had (a) a long and severe stenosis in the proximal LAD.
(b) A 1.5mm burr and a 2.25mm burr were passed across the stenosis in turn.
(c) The lesion was post-dilated with a 3.0mm, 40mm long Elipse™ balloon catheter.
(d) The ostium of the diagonal branch required dilatation.
(e, f) A good angiographic result was obtained in both vessels.

Diffuse disease and multiple lesions

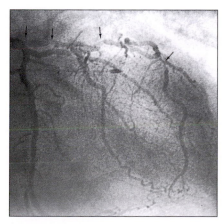

a

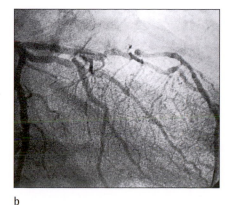

b

Figure 7.18

A 65-year-old inventor with hypertension, hypercholesterolemia and severe angina was found to have (a) significant three-vessel disease, including diffuse disease along the length of the LAD (arrows).

The series of LAD lesions were ablated with a 1.5mm followed by a 1.75mm Rotablator® burr and then post-dilated with a 2.0mm Supercrosse® (Progressive Angioplasty Systems) balloon and subsequently a 2.5mm Express™ balloon.

(b) The angiographic result was acceptable.

The lesions in the OMCx and the RCA were dilated during the same procedure.

Balloon-resistant lesions

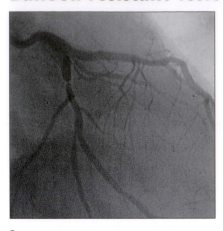

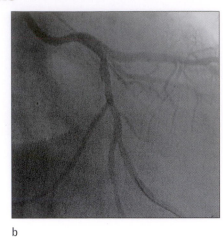

a

b

Figure 7.19
(a) A discrete, hard, balloon-resistant stenosis in the proximal LCx (RAO projection).
(b) The stenosis was ablated by a single 2.25mm burr.

Short lesions such as this may be treated by single burr unless they are extremely severe or in a large vessel, when a step-up technique should be preferred. Unfortunately the latter approach is significantly more expensive.

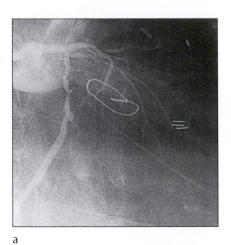

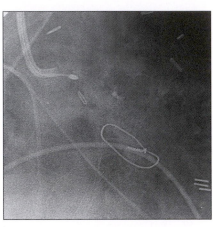

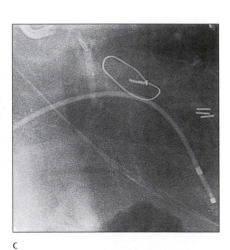

a

b

c

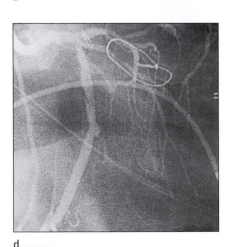

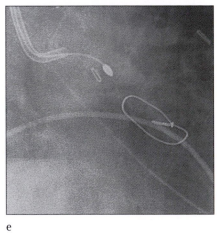

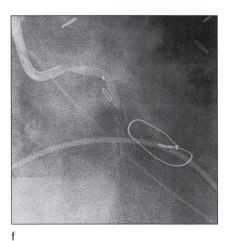

d

e

f

Figure 7.20
A 70-year-old man who had undergone previous CABG surgery and who had severe angina had (a) a long segment of severe disease in the proximal LCx.

The lesion could not be crossed with a low-profile balloon catheter. IVUS demonstrated heavy calcification that extended from the distal left main stem and into the most severe part of the stenosis, although the IVUS probe would not cross the stenosis either.

A 1.75mm burr (b) was followed by a 3.0mm Elipse™ balloon (c) and a 3.5mm Passage® balloon.

(d) This produced an improved result but local dissection.

continued

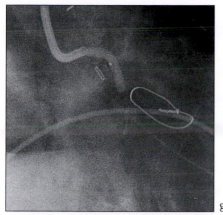

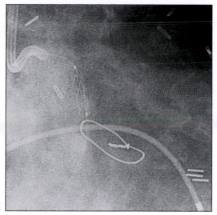

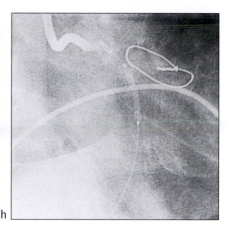

g   h   i

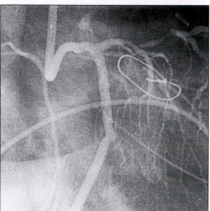

Figure 7.20 *continued*

Initially it proved impossible to pass a 3.5mm, 18mm long Microstent II™ around the ostium of the LCx owing to residual calcification; balloon dilatation did not help.

After Rotablator® atherectomy with a 2.25mm burr (e) and adjunctive PTCA with a 3.5mm balloon (f, g), it was possible to (h) deliver and then deploy the stent (i).

(j) This gave a good angiographic result.

j

Branch vessels

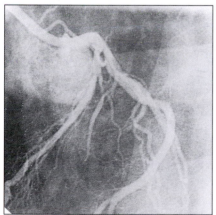

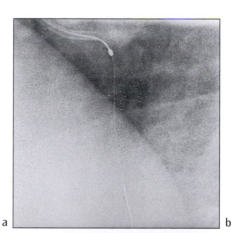

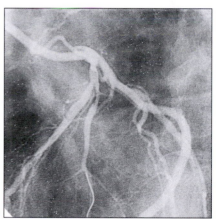

a   b   c

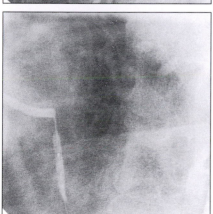

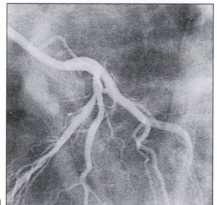

Figure 7.21

A 46-year-old solicitor with moderate angina. (a) A severe stenosis in a diagonal branch of LAD (LAO cranial projection).

(b) The stenosis was ablated by a 1.5mm burr.

(c) This produced an improved result.

(d, e) The result was further improved by a low pressure inflation with a 3.0mm Passage® balloon.

(e) Final result.

d   e

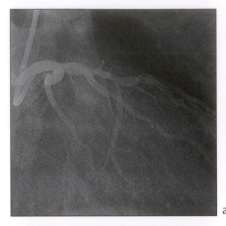

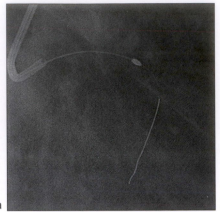

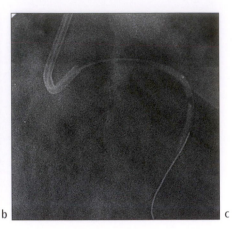

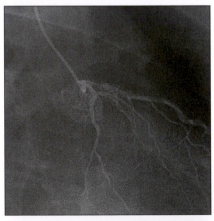

Figure 7.22
A 57-year-old car worker with moderate angina had (a) a significant stenosis in the proximal part of a large first septal artery.
(b) The lesion was easily crossed with a 0.009-inch C-wire™ and ablated with a 1.75mm Rotablator® burr.
(c) After adjunctive PTCA with a 3.0mm balloon, no residual stenosis was visible (d).

In-stent restenosis

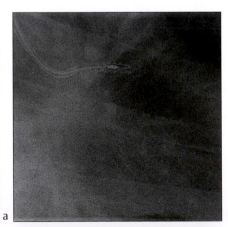

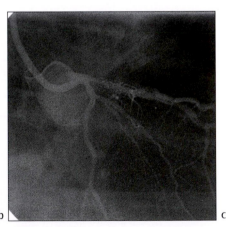

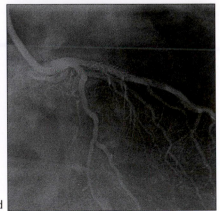

Figure 7.23
A 44-year-old man (the same patient as in Figs 12.7, 15.43 and 15.48) developed (a) a second restenosis proximal to and within two coronary stents (Microstent® and Wiktor®).
(b) The lesion was ablated with a 1.5mm burr and a 2.0mm burr.
(c) This produced an improvement.
(d) The lesion was post-dilated with a 3.0mm Samba™ balloon.
(e) Final result.

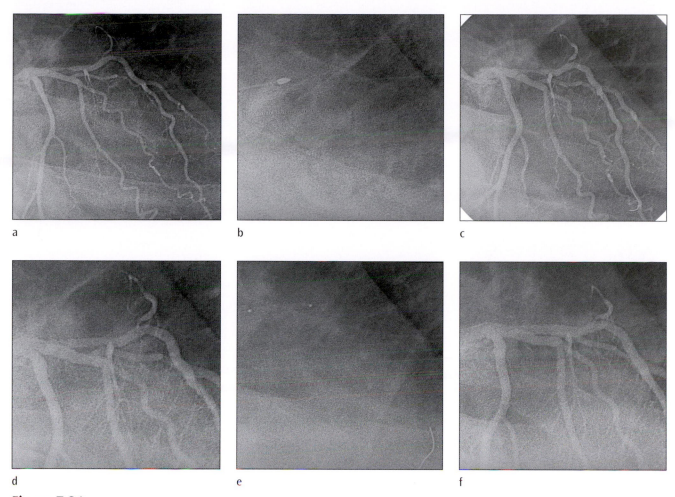

Figure 7.24

A 57-year-old bricklayer developed recurrent angina of effort that was caused by a second restenosis inside (a) this Palmaz-Schatz™ stent in the proximal LAD that had been implanted 9 months earlier.

(b) The lesion was ablated with a 1.75mm Rotablator® burr.

(c) This produced some improvement.

(d) It was then dilated with a 3.0mm Passage® balloon.

(e) A 3.0mm, 18mm long Microstent II™ was deployed at the lesion site and inside the original Palmaz-Schatz™ stent.

(f) The final result was good.

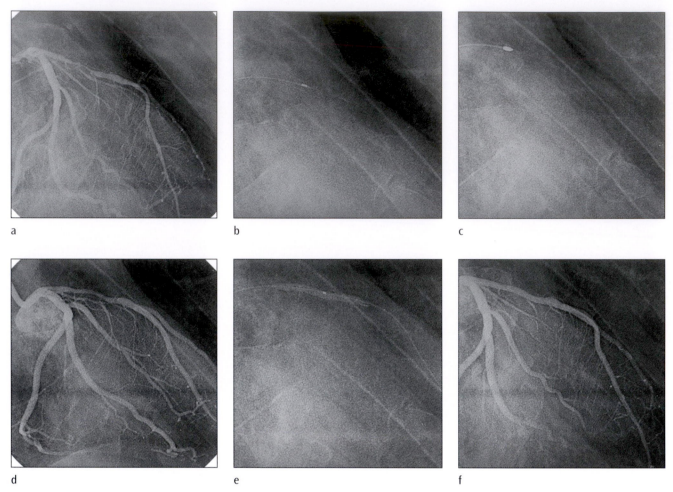

a   b   c

d   e   f

Figure 7.25

A 73-year-old man developed recurrent angina that was caused by a restenosis inside (a) this Multilink™ stent, 6 months after implantation in the LAD.

The lesion was ablated by (b) a 1.75mm Rotablator® burr and a 2.0mm Rotablator® burr (c).

(d) This produced a marked improvement.

(e) The lesion was then post-dilated with a 3.0mm, 30mm long Elipse™ balloon.

(f) The final result was excellent.

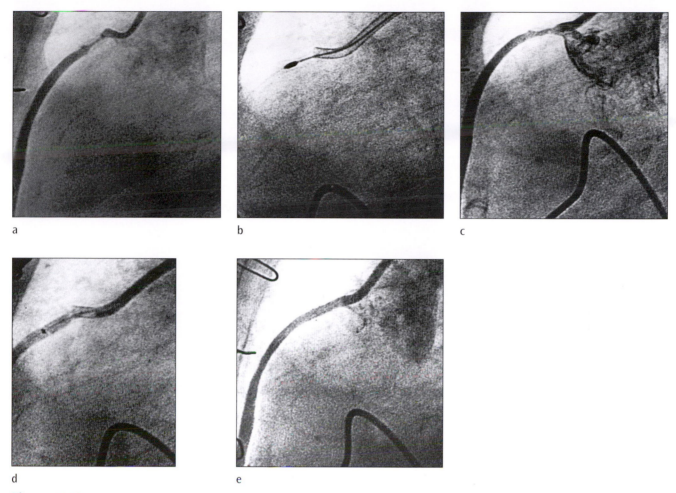

a   b   c

d   e

Figure 7.26

A 58-year-old lady developed recurrent angina 5 months after PTCRA and NIR™ stenting ('rotastenting') to the aorta-ostial segment of her 6-year-old RCA SVG.

(a) Angiography showed a severe restenosis within the stent.
IVUS showed full stent deployment.

(b) Rotablator® atherectomy was performed using a 1.5mm and then a 2.0mm Rotablator® burr with improvement (c).

(d) The lesion was post-dilated with a 3.0mm, 10mm long Finale™ balloon.

(e) This produced a good final result.

   The BARASTER Registry compared the acute procedural results after stand-alone rotational atherectomy versus rotational atherectomy and adjunctive PTCA versus PTCA alone for the treatment of in-stent restenosis. Whether rotational atherectomy reduces the frequency of recurrent in-stent restenosis was investigated by the ARTIST and ROSTER randomized trials.

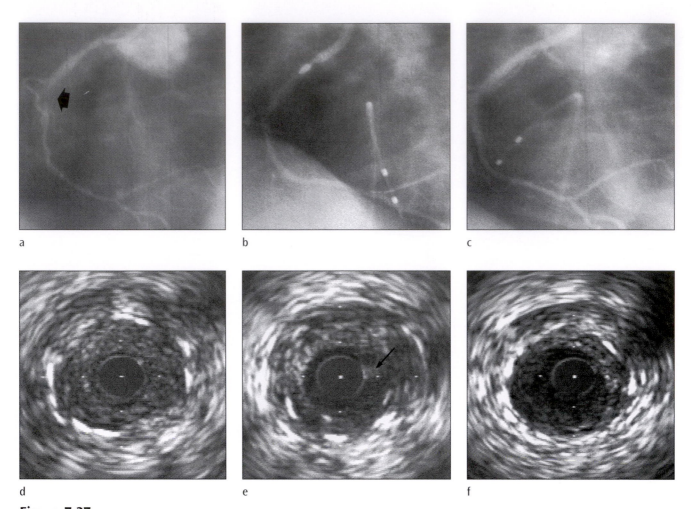

Figure 7.27

(a) This RCA had severe in-stent restenosis (arrow).

A 2.38mm Rotablator® burr was advanced via a 10F JR guiding catheter. Several passes were made along the entire stented segment.

(b) This produced angiographic improvement.

(c) The final result after PTCA with a 4.0mm non-compliant balloon at 14 atmospheres is satisfactory.

(d) Before treatment, IVUS using the CVIS 30MHz 3.2F MicroRail® ultrasound catheter (Boston Scientific) shows dense homogeneous material with low echogenicity occluding the vessel lumen around the IVUS catheter. The lumen area measures $1.1mm^2$ and the stent area $9.6mm^2$.

(e) After multiple passes with a 2.38mm Rotablator® burr, a regular circular lumen is re-established with a lumen area that is smaller than the burr area ($3.7mm^2$ vs $4.4mm^2$). Guidewire artefact is visible at 3 o'clock (arrow).

(f) Final result after PTCA with the 4.0mm balloon shows further lumen enlargement from $3.7mm^2$ to $6.9mm^2$, which is the combined effect of stent expansion (stent area increased from $9.8mm^2$ to $11.8mm^2$) and plaque extrusion through the struts.

Note that a thin rim of in-stent hyperplasia remains between 12 and 6 o'clock.

Courtesy of Drs C Di Mario, O Kovalenko, R Albiero and A Colombo, EMO-Centro-Cuore, Columbus Hospital, Milan, Italy.

Primary rotastenting

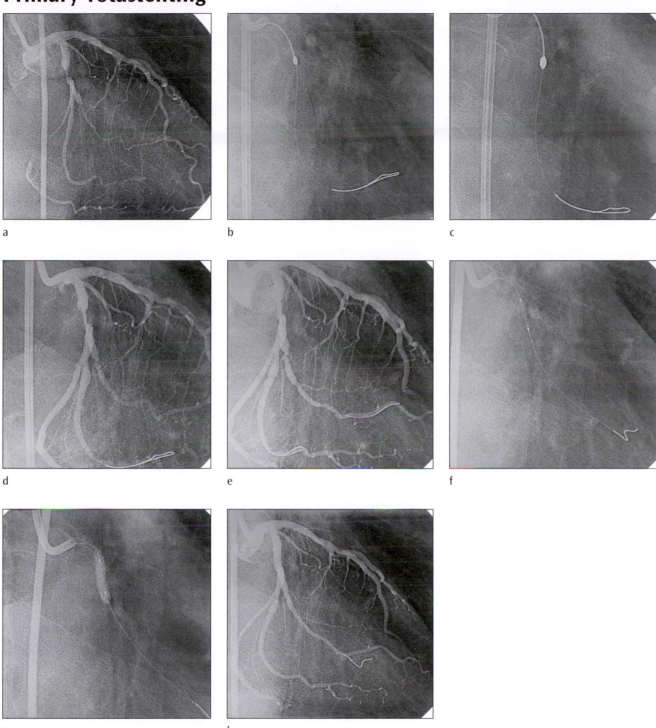

a

b

c

d

e

f

g

h

Figure 7.28

A 70-year-old man with severe angina was found to have (a) a severe bulky stenosis in the proximal LCx, just above a trifurcation point. Flow was very sluggish down the true LCx and the first OMCx.

(b, c) The proximal LCx lesion was first ablated with a 1.75mm and then a 2.25mm Rotablator® burr.

(d) This produced a marked improvement.

(e) Two stenoses were then identified in the first OMCx; these were crossed with a 0.014-inch Floppy® guidewire. PTCA with a 3.0mm Samba™ balloon produced a satisfactory result (see h below).

(f, g) The proximal LCx lesion was then stented with a 3.5mm, 15mm long Multilink™ stent.

(h) This gave an excellent angiographic result.

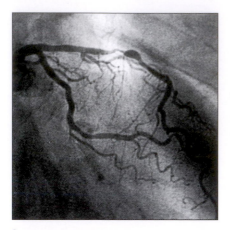

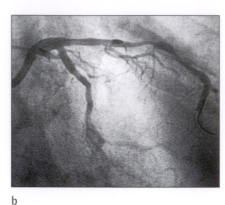

b

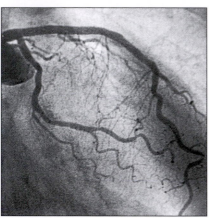

a

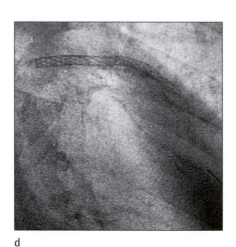

c

d

Figure 7.29
A 70-year-old man with severe angina was found to have severe calcification in the proximal half of the LAD on fluoroscopy. (a) It proved impossible to dilate the most severe lesion even at high pressure in order to deliver a stent.
(b) Rotational atherectomy was performed using a 1.75mm Rotablator® burr and then a 2.25mm Rotablator® burr.
The segment was post-dilated with a 3.0mm, 30mm long Worldpass™ balloon. The LAD was then stented with a 3.0mm, 16mm long NIRoyal™ stent (Scimed/Boston Scientific), placed distally, a 3.0mm, 32mm long NIRoyal™ stent placed proximal to this, and a 3.0mm, 16mm long NIRoyal™ stent, placed more proximally towards the ostium of the LAD. The stents were overlapped and post-dilated to 14 atmospheres and an excellent result was obtained (c). (d) The stents are very radio-opaque.
   The SPORT trial is currently investigating whether rotastenting provides better short- and long-term results than PTCA and NIR® stenting alone.

Reading

Abdelmeguid AE, Whitlow PL. Coronary atherectomy: directional, rotational and extraction catheters. In: White CJ, Ramee SR, eds. Interventional Cardiology. New York: Marcel Dekker; 1995:175-200.

Brown DL, George CJ, Steenkiste AR, *et al*. High-speed rotational atherectomy of human coronary stenoses: acute and one-year outcomes from the New Approaches to Coronary Intervention (NACI) Registry. Am J Cardiol 1997;80:60K-67K.

Casterella PJ, Teirstein PS. Rotational coronary atherectomy. In: Grech ED, Ramsdale DR, eds. Practical Interventional Cardiology. London: Martin Dunitz; 1997:189-204.

Goldberg SL, Shawl F, Buchbinder M, *et al*. Rotational atherectomy for in-stent restenosis: The BARASTER Registry. Circulation 1997;96(Suppl I):I-80.

Moses JW, Whitlow PL, Kuntz RE, *et al*. Myocardial infarction after rotational atherectomy: predictors and influence on late outcome in the STRATAS trial. J Am Coll Cardiol 1998;31:455A.

O'Neill WW, Niazi KA. Rotational coronary atherectomy using the Rotablator atherectomy device. In: Holmes DR, Garratt KN, eds. Atherectomy. Boston: Blackwell Scientific; 1992:43-60.

Reifart N, Vandormael M, Krajcar M, *et al*. Randomized comparison of angioplasty of complex coronary lesions at a single center. Excimer laser, Rotational atherectomy and Balloon angioplasty Comparison (ERBAC) Study. Circulation 1997;96:91-8.

Reisman M. Guide to rotational atherectomy. Birmingham, Michigan, USA: Physician's Press; 1997.

Schechtmann NS, Rosenblum J, Stertzer SH, *et al*. Rotational ablation of chronic coronary occlusions. Cathet Cardiovasc Diagn 1991;24:295-9.

Sharma SK, Kini A, Duvvuri S, *et al*. Randomized trial of ROtational atherectomy vs balloon angioplasty for in-STEnt Restenosis (ROSTER). J Am Coll Cardiol 1998;40:142A.

Warth DC, Leon MB, O'Neill W, *et al*. Rotational Atherectomy Multicenter Registry: acute results, complications and 6-month angiographic follow-up in 709 patients. J Am Coll Cardiol 1994;24:641-8.

8

Transluminal extraction catheter coronary atherectomy

TEC® coronary atherectomy uses an over-the-wire, 5.5-7.5F catheter that possesses two rotating cutting blades at its tip. As the device is slowly advanced over the guidewire, the blades are rotated at 750 rpm by a drive shaft that is powered by a battery pack. Plaque and debris are aspirated into a vacuum collection chamber at the distal end of the catheter. A special guidewire with an enlarged olive-shaped tip and a special guide catheter are necessary.

TEC® atherectomy is therefore useful in diseased vein grafts that contain diffuse grumous, atherosclerotic material or voluminous thrombus and in native vessels that contain much thrombus. The procedure is limited by the rigidity and small size of the catheter. Adjunctive PTCA and stenting is usually necessary.

TEC® atherectomy is contraindicated in heavily calcified lesions, severely angulated stenoses, small vessels, bifurcation lesions and dissections.

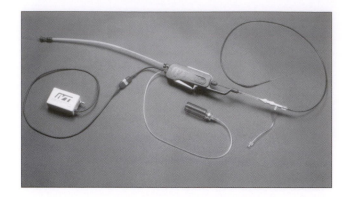

Figure 8.1
TEC® atherectomy catheter over a TEC® guidewire, placed through TEC® guide catheter. The hand-held drive and the advancer unit are connected to the battery pack and vacuum collection chamber.
Courtesy of Interventional Technologies Ltd, San Diego, California, USA.

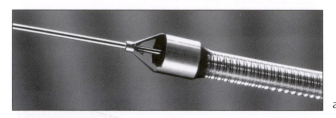

a

Figure 8.2
(a) Close-up view of conical-shaped cutting head of a TEC® atherectomy catheter.
(b) Its two rotating cutting blades cut plaque, which is aspirated down the hollow shaft of the device and into the vacuum bottle.

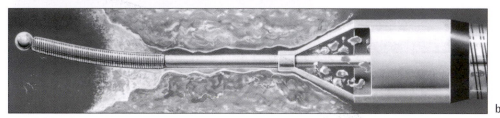

b

Lesions in native coronary arteries

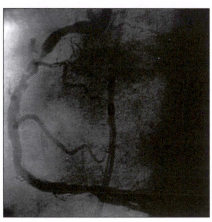
a

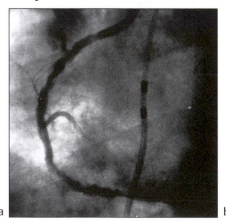
b

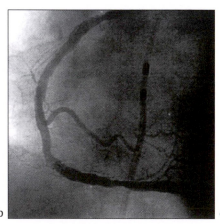
c

Figure 8.3
A 65-year-old man with angina and congestive cardiac failure had severe three-vessel coronary artery disease and a left ventricular ejection fraction of 16%. A staged procedure was planned. (a) The large dominant RCA had diffuse disease of the entire vessel and 90% stenosis at its tightest segment.

A 10F TEC® guide catheter was placed in the ostium of the RCA and a 7F (2.33mm) TEC® catheter was advanced slowly through the stenosis while maintaining continuous rotation and aspiration.

(b) A post-procedure angiogram demonstrated a residual stenosis of 50%.

A 3.5mm, 40mm long balloon was used for adjunctive PTCA.

(c) Final result shows a residual stenosis of less than 30%.

Courtesy of Drs BG Denys and MR Izzo, Presbyterian University Hospital, Pittsburgh, Pennsylvania, USA.

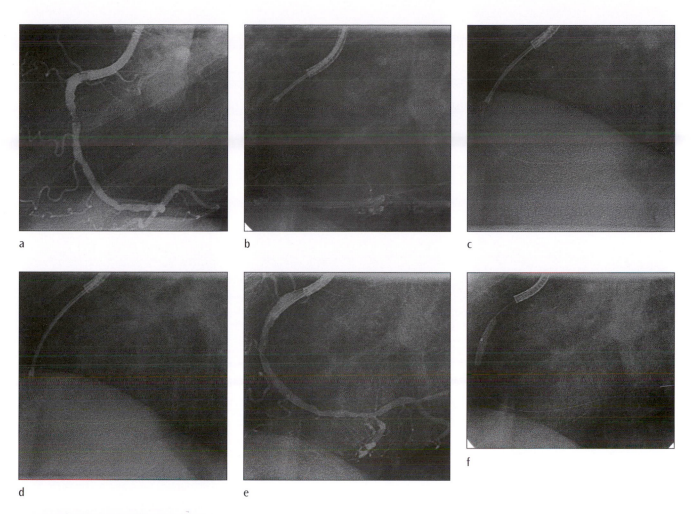

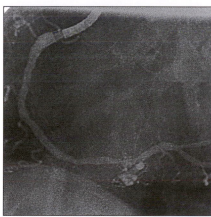

Figure 8.4

A 67-year-old retired theatre technician underwent angiography 11 days after presenting with chest pain and inferolateral ECG abnormalities. The patient had not received thrombolytic therapy. (a) The RCA had a significant mid-third stenosis and much intracoronary thrombus.

(b-d) A 6.5F TEC® device aspirated thrombus as it was slowly advanced through the lesion.

(e) Result after TEC® atherectomy.

(f) A 15mm Palmaz-Schatz™ stent was then deployed over the ulcerated plaque with a 3.5mm/4.0mm CAT™ balloon (Cardiovascular Dynamics).

(g) Final result.

Courtesy of Drs M Chester and R Perry, Cardiothoracic Centre, Liverpool, UK.

The TOPIT trial compared the clinical and angiographic outcomes after TEC atherectomy or PTCA for thrombus-containing lesions in native vessels.

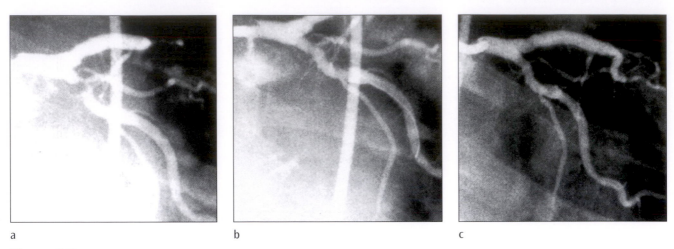

a   b   c

Figure 8.5

A 72-year-old man with acute chest pain developed ventricular tachycardia and ventricular fibrillation. (a) Coronary arteriography performed after resuscitation showed a 95% stenosis with thrombus in the proximal LCx.

Through a 10F TEC® guide catheter and over a 0.014-inch, 300cm long TEC® guidewire, a 5.5F (1.83mm) TEC® catheter was advanced through the stenosis while continuous rotation and aspiration was maintained.

(b) A 7.5F (2.5mm) TEC® device was then advanced through the lesion to remove more thrombotic material.

A 4.0mm balloon was used for adjunctive PTCA.

(c) The final result is satisfactory.

Courtesy of Drs MH Bowles and R Kipperman, HCA Wesley Medical Center, Wichita, Kansas, USA.

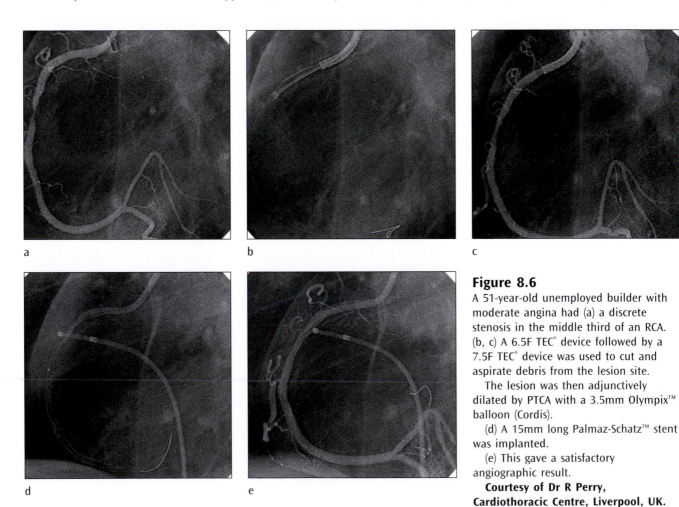

a   b   c

d   e

Figure 8.6

A 51-year-old unemployed builder with moderate angina had (a) a discrete stenosis in the middle third of an RCA. (b, c) A 6.5F TEC® device followed by a 7.5F TEC® device was used to cut and aspirate debris from the lesion site.

The lesion was then adjunctively dilated by PTCA with a 3.5mm Olympix™ balloon (Cordis).

(d) A 15mm long Palmaz-Schatz™ stent was implanted.

(e) This gave a satisfactory angiographic result.

Courtesy of Dr R Perry, Cardiothoracic Centre, Liverpool, UK.

Totally occluded native vessels

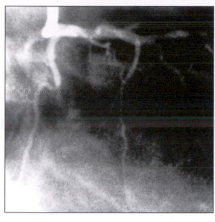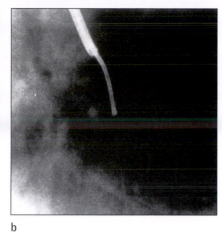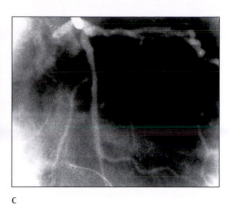

a   b

c

Figure 8.7

A 48-year-old lady had had an inferolateral myocardial infarct treated with thrombolysis 7 weeks earlier. Angiography initially showed a severe stenosis of the LCx with thrombus, but (a) by 7 weeks the vessel was totally occluded.
(b) A 6.5F (2.17mm) TEC® catheter was advanced across the lesion over a 0.014-inch TEC® guidewire.
(c) Post-procedure angiography demonstrated a good result.
   Adjunctive PTCA was performed with a 3.0mm balloon.
   Courtesy of Dr JM McClure, St. Luke's Hospital, Saginaw, Michigan, USA.

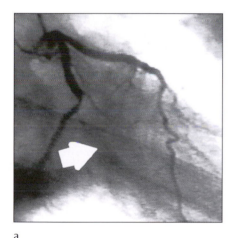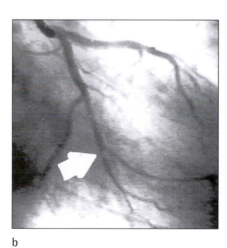

a   b

Figure 8.8

A 73-year-old man presented with acute inferolateral myocardial infarction. (a) Coronary angiography demonstrated total occlusion of the OMCx.

A 6.5F (2.17mm) TEC® catheter was advanced over a TEC® guidewire passed through the totally occluded OMCx. Six slow passes were performed, resulting in extraction of considerable amounts of thrombus and atheromatous material and (b) a good angiographic result.

A 2.5mm balloon was used for adjunctive PTCA.

Courtesy of Dr A Spring, Washoe Medical Center, Reno, Nevada, USA.

TEC atherectomy in SVGs

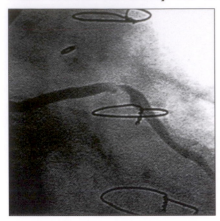

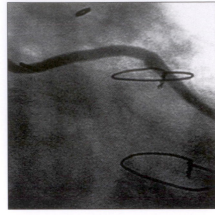

a

b

Figure 8.9
A 68-year-old diabetic man with unstable angina had undergone CABG surgery 11 years previously. (a) This ulcerated lesion in the OMCx SVG appears to be associated with intraluminal thrombus.
(b) It was satisfactorily treated by TEC® atherectomy using a 7.5F (2.5mm) TEC® device and adjunctive PTCA with a 3.5mm balloon.
Courtesy of Drs TC Trageser amd CM Furr, Hamot Medical Center, Erie, Pennsylvania, USA.

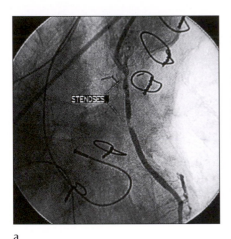

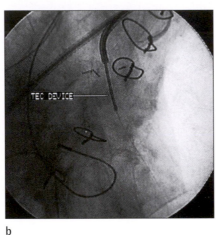

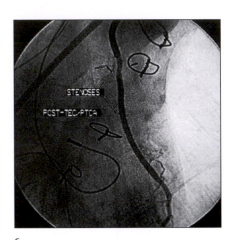

a

b

c

Figure 8.10
A 70-year-old man had undergone CABG surgery 10 years previously. A 2-month history of angina was associated with two stenoses in the SVG to the LAD.
(a) The mid-third lesion was accompanied by a filling defect.
(b) A 7.5F (2.5mm) TEC® catheter was used.
This was followed by adjunctive PTCA with a 4.0mm balloon.
(c) The final result was satisfactory.
Courtesy of Dr RS Gottleib, The Graduate Hospital, Philadelphia, Pennsylvania, USA.

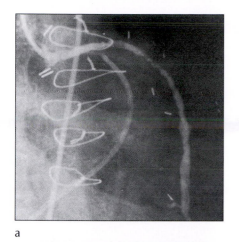
a

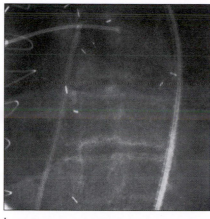
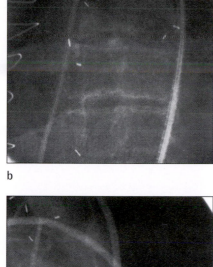
b

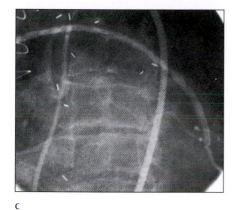
c

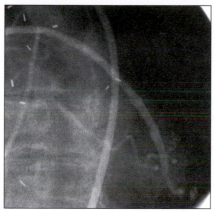
d

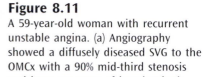

Figure 8.11

A 59-year-old woman with recurrent unstable angina. (a) Angiography showed a diffusely diseased SVG to the OMCx with a 90% mid-third stenosis and large amounts of intraluminal filling defects.

(b) A 7.5F (2.5mm) TEC® catheter was used to extract large amounts of thrombus and debris.

(c) This produced marked improvement.

The SVG was then dilated with a long 3.5mm PTCA balloon.

(d) This gave an excellent angiographic result.

Long-term anticoagulation with warfarin is appropriate in a case such as this.

Courtesy of Dr R Safian, William Beaumont Hospital, Royal Oak, Michigan. USA.

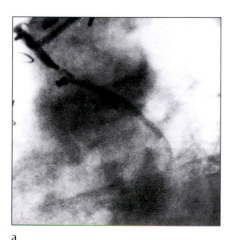
a

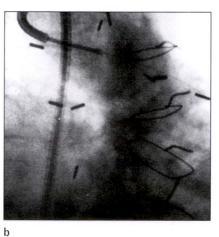
b

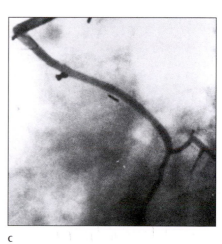
c

Figure 8.12

A 61-year-old male had undergone CABG surgery 14 years earlier. He presented with acute onset of chest pain and ECG changes of acute injury. Thrombolytic therapy was given and, although the pain initially resolved, symptoms recurred that day. (a) Emergency angiography showed subtotal occlusion of the SVG to the LAD with extensive intraluminal thrombus.

(b) Multiple slow passes with a 6F (2.0mm) TEC device over a 0.014-inch TEC® guidewire aspirated much thrombus.

(c) Final result.

Courtesy of Drs T LaLonde and V Abiragi, St John's Hospital, Detroit, Michigan. USA.

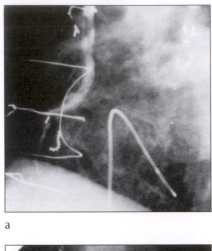
a

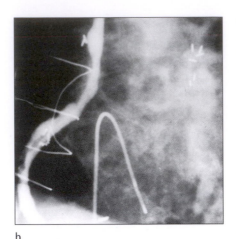
b

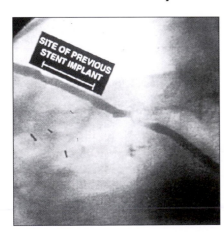
c

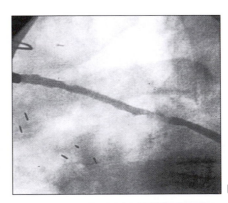
d

Figure 8.13
A 61-year-old man had undergone CABG surgery 3 years earlier. He was admitted with an acute inferior myocardial infarction.
(a) Emergency angiography showed an SVG to the RCA to be occluded in its middle third, and there were filling defects that were consistent with thrombus. The patient was given an overnight infusion of 250,000U of urokinase directly into the SVG.

However, intraluminal thrombus persisted (b). Multiple passes with a 2.5mm (7.5F) TEC° catheter were made along the SVG and into the posterior descending artery.

(c) A post-TEC° angiogram showed a residual stenosis in the middle third and at the anastomosis site.

Adjunctive PTCA was performed with a 2.5mm balloon along the length of the SVG and at the anastomosis site and a 3.0mm balloon in the proximal graft stenosis.

(d) This produced a good angiographic result.
Courtesy of Drs R Cain, J Work and JA Fleisher, Encino-Tarzana Medical Center, Encino, California. USA.
The TECBEST I study compared the incidence of cardiac enzyme elevation after debulking using TEC° atherectomy versus PTCA before elective stenting in low-risk SVGs. The TECBEST II study is comparing TEC° before elective stenting with and without abciximab in high-risk SVG lesions.

TEC atherectomy for thrombus in an SVG stent

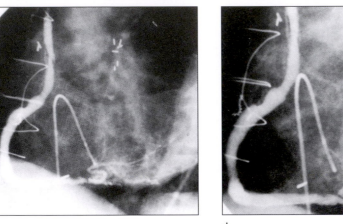

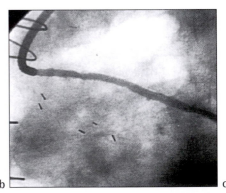
a   b   c

Figure 8.14
(a) This SVG to an OMCx had a 95% stenosis distal to a stent that had been implanted 5 months earlier. The eccentric lesion had an irregular contour and appeared to be associated with thrombus.

Three slow passes with a 2.0mm TEC® catheter left a significant residual stenosis (b).

The residual stenosis was dilated with a 3.5mm perfusion balloon.

(c) Final result.
Courtesy of Dr JM Parks, University of Alabama, Birmingham, Alabama, USA.

Reading

Abdelmeguid AE, Whitlow PL. Coronary atherectomy: directional, rotational and extraction catheters. In: White CJ, Ramee SR, eds. Interventional Cardiology. New York: Marcel Dekker; 1995:175-200.

Hara K, Ikari Y, Tamura T, *et al*. Transluminal extraction atherectomy for restenosis following Palmaz-Schatz stent implantation. Am J Cardiol 1997;79:801-2.

Matthews RV. Extraction atherectomy vs PTCA in treating saphenous vein graft disease: focus on embolization. J Invas Cardiol 1996;8(Suppl C):16C-21C.

Mehta S, Margolis J, Moore L. Transluminal extraction atherectomy. In: Grech ED, Ramsdale DR, eds. Practical Interventional Cardiology. London: Martin Dunitz; 1997:177-88.

Sketch MH, Davidson CJ, Yeh W *et al*. Predictors of acute and long-term outcome with transluminal extraction atherectomy: the New Approaches to Coronary Intervention (NACI) Registry. Am J Cardiol 1997;80:68K-77K.

Sketch MH, Stack RS. The transluminal extraction-endarterectomy catheter (TEC) device. In: Holmes DR, Garratt KN, eds. Atherectomy. Boston: Blackwell Scientific; 1992:61-80.

TEC extraction atherectomy advanced operators workshop. J Invas Cardiol 1995;7(Suppl D):3D-24D.

9

Excimer laser coronary atherectomy

Excimer laser coronary atherectomy (ELCA) uses laser light with a frequency of 308nm of xenon chloride to ablate plaque by delivering nanosecond pulses of energy at various repetition rates. The device is ideal for:

- balloon-resistant lesions;
- aorta-ostial stenoses;
- moderately calcified lesions;
- long lesions (over 10-20mm in length);
- total occlusions that can be crossed by a guidewire;
- SVG lesions; and
- diffuse disease.

However, its use is limited by the size of the device and the expense of the equipment. Special expertise is necessary and although the catheter is now more flexible than previously, ELCA is difficult or, indeed, may be impossible in tortuous vessels. Because the catheters are still small, adjunctive PTCA is usually necessary. Perforation remains an important complication, and bifurcation lesions are potentially still a problem. Adjunctive stenting may reduce restenosis rates.

ELCA catheters

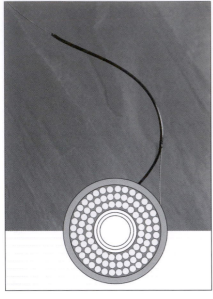

a

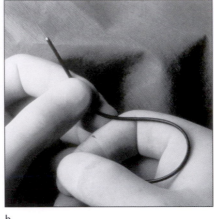

b

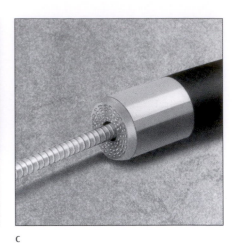

c

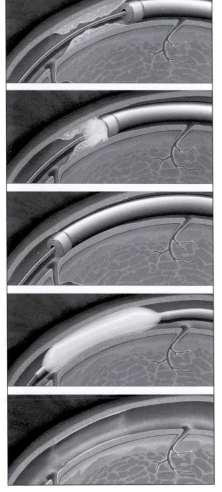

d

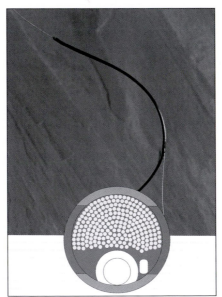

e

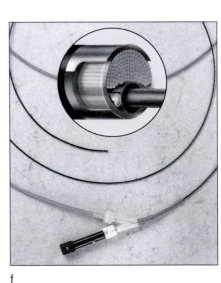

f

Figure 9.1

(a) The Spectranetics Vitesse®-C concentric excimer laser catheter is currently available in 1.4mm, 1.7mm and 2.0mm diameters. These catheters require 7F, 8F and 9F guide catheters, respectively. The laser catheters are rapid-exchange catheters and are compatible with a 0.018-inch guidewire, although a 1.4mm device is available that is compatible with a 0.014-inch wire. The fibres (of which there are between 80 and 250) are 61μm in diameter and the catheters have a radio-opaque metal ring tip for improved visibility and precise lesion contact.

(b) The catheter is reasonably flexible.

(c) Close-up of the catheter-tip.

(d) Schematic representation of debulking a lesion with ELCA using a Vitesse®-C device.

(e) The Spectranetics Vitesse®-E eccentric excimer rapid-exchange laser catheter is available as a 1.7mm and a 2.0mm device. It has a torque knob to allow laser-lesion alignment in eccentric or bulky lesions and bifurcation lesions when the laser energy needs to directed away from the carina. The 220 fibres are each 45μm in diameter.

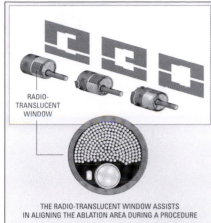

RADIO-TRANSLUCENT WINDOW

THE RADIO-TRANSLUCENT WINDOW ASSISTS IN ALIGNING THE ABLATION AREA DURING A PROCEDURE

g

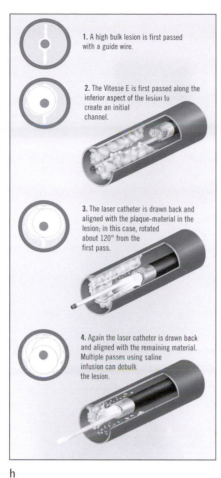

1. A high bulk lesion is first passed with a guide wire.

2. The Vitesse E is first passed along the inferior aspect of the lesion to create an initial channel.

3. The laser catheter is drawn back and aligned with the plaque-material in the lesion; in this case, rotated about 120° from the first pass.

4. Again the laser catheter is drawn back and aligned with the remaining material. Multiple passes using saline infusion can debulk the lesion.

h

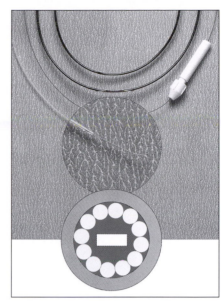

i

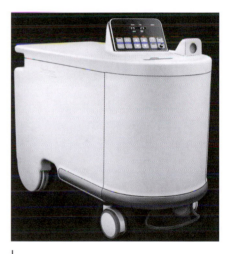

l

j

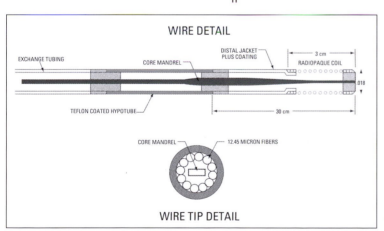

WIRE DETAIL

EXCHANGE TUBING   CORE MANDREL   DISTAL JACKET PLUS COATING   3 cm   RADIOPAQUE COIL

.018

TEFLON COATED HYPOTUBE   30 cm

CORE MANDREL   12.45 MICRON FIBERS

WIRE TIP DETAIL

k

The catheter is compatible with a 0.014-inch guidewire and an 8F guide catheter.

(f) Close-up view of the distal end of a Vitesse®-E catheter. The torque knob enables lesion alignment (g), which can be further assisted by observing the radiolucent window at the tip of the catheter on fluoroscopy.

(h) Schematic diagram of debulking a lesion using the eccentric catheter.

(i) The Spectranetics Prima™ laser wire has an 0.018-inch diameter and possesses twelve fibres, each with a diameter of 45μm. It has a lubricious coating, a 3cm shapeable radio-opaque tip and a torque knob for steerability. A support catheter provides additional back-up and a conduit for exchanging guidewires. Its primary use is the recanalization of chronic total occlusions.

(j) Close-up view of a Prima™ laser wire.

(k) Internal structure of a Prima™ laser wire.

(l) The Spectranetics CVX-300® unit produces a long-pulse, ultraviolet laser beam at a wavelength of 308 nm for plaque ablation. It has a catheter output fluence of 30-60mJ/mm², a maximum repetition rate of 40 pulses per second and a pulse width of 125-200ns. It measures 49 inches in length, 35 inches in height and 24 inches in width, and it weighs 295kg.

ELCA and stenting for totally occluded native vessels

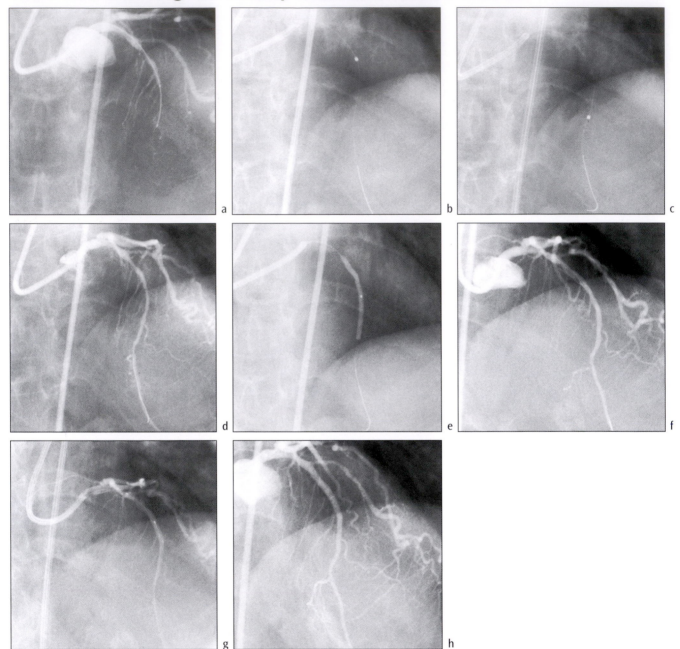

Figure 9.2

A 52-year-old Caucasian male had sustained an anterior myocardial infarction 8 months previously, and he continued to experience exertional angina. Angiography showed 80% and 100% lesions in the mid-LAD. (a) The lesions were crossed with a 0.014-inch Intermediate® guidewire supported by a Transit® catheter (Cordis).

(b) A Spectranetics 1.4mm Vitesse®-C concentric laser catheter was then advanced through the 80% stenosis to the level of the total occlusion.

(c) The total occlusion was ablated at a fluence of 45mJ/mm² and a repetition rate of 25 pulses per second. The total time of laser therapy that was used to cross through the 3cm of plaque was 65 seconds.

(d) The laser catheter was removed and restoration of antegrade flow was documented. The channel created was approximately 1.5mm in diameter.

(e) A 2.75mm, 4cm long Bandit™ balloon (Scimed) was used to dilate the artery after laser ablation.

Balloon dilatation improved the luminal diameter of the lased section but resulted in (f) a linear dissection at the proximal 80% stenosis.

(g) Three 3.0mm Palmaz-Schatz™ coronary stents were implanted, covering the proximal lesion through the area of total occlusion.

(h) Final result after high pressure balloon inflation.

Courtesy of Dr JE Tcheng, Duke Medical Center, Durham, North Carolina, USA.

The EXACTO randomized trial is comparing the outcome of ELCA plus PTCA (debulking strategy) with PTCA alone in chronic total occlusions that have been crossed with a conventional guidewire.

ELCA and stenting for left main disease

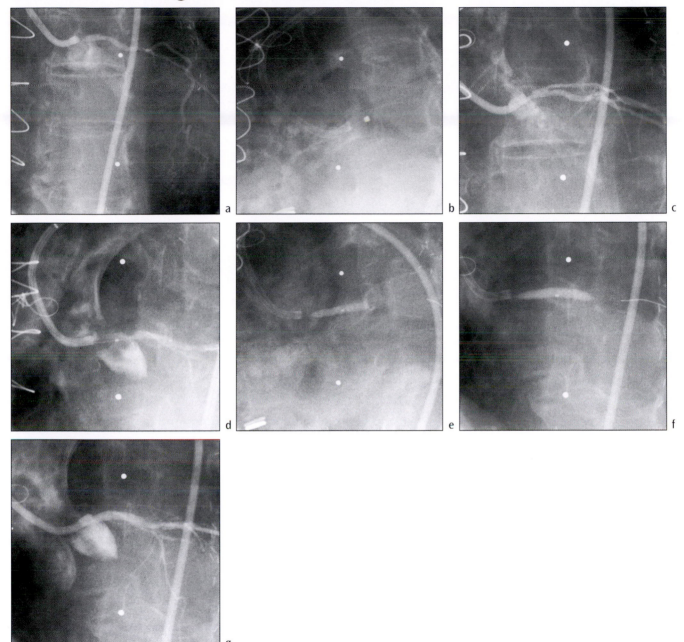

Figure 9.3

A 63-year-old woman with hypertension and diabetes had previously undergone CABG surgery and presented now with recurrence of angina. (a) Angiography demonstrated occlusion of the SVG in the OMCx and a 99% stenosis of the left main coronary artery.
(b) Ablation of the left main ostial stenosis was performed with a Spectranetics 2.0mm Excimer laser over a 0.014-inch ExtraSupport™ guidewire via a 9.0FL4 guide catheter.
(c) Ablation was performed at a fluence of 50mJ/mm^2 and a repetition rate of 25 pulses per second. The total ablation time was 7 seconds.
(c) After laser ablation, a channel of approximately 2.0mm diameter was established.
(d, e) A 3.0mm Palmaz-Schatz™ coronary stent was then implanted. Care was taken to ensure adequate coverage of the entire ostium with the stent, and approximately 1mm of stent was left outside the ostium in the aorta.
(f, g) Final result after high-pressure (20 atmospheres) balloon dilation with a 3.0mm NC Bandit™ balloon catheter.
Courtesy of Dr JE Tcheng, Duke Medical Center, Durham, North Carolina, USA.

ELCA in eccentric lesions

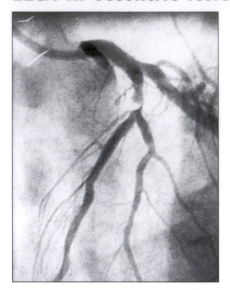

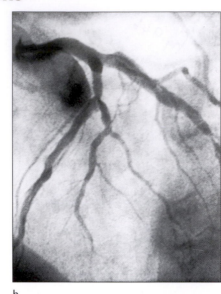

a   b

Figure 9.4
(a) A severe eccentric stenosis in the LAD just above a large first DG in a 53-year-old man with easily provoked angina.
(b) Three passes with a 1.7mm eccentric Spectranetics Laser catheter (with a saline flush technique) achieved a satisfactory result.
Courtesy of Dr CW Hamm, University of Hamburg, Hamburg, Germany.

ELCA in concentric lesions

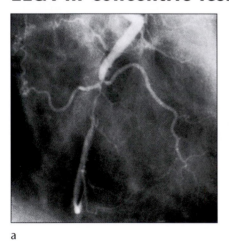

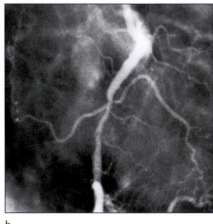

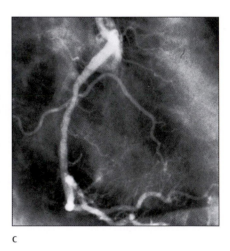

a   b   c

Figure 9.5
This 64-year-old woman with Canadian Cardiovascular Society class III angina had (a) a long stenosis in the mid-third of an RCA.

(b) A 1.6mm Laser catheter (Advanced Interventional Systems Inc®) was used to ablate the lesion with a single pass using energy densities of 60mJ/mm², a pulse duration of 219ns and a repetition rate of 20Hz.

The lesion was post-dilated with a 2.5mm balloon catheter.

(c) Final result.

The patient was free of symptoms at 6 months' follow-up.

Courtesy of Drs YEA Appelman and JJ Piek, Department of Cardiology, Academic Medical Centre, Amsterdam, The Netherlands.

The AMRO trial failed to demonstrate any significant acute or long-term clinical or angiographic benefit of ELCA alone over PTCA alone in patients with diffuse native vessel or SVG lesions.

ELCA for in-stent restenosis

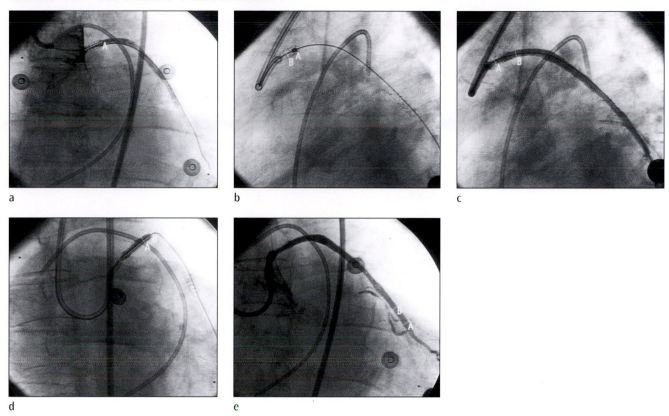

a   b   c

d   e

Figure 9.6

A 72-year-old man had undergone CABG surgery in 1982. He developed early recurrence of angina. This was due to progressive native disease, including occlusion of the native RCA. In February 1994, he was restudied because of uncontrolled angina. The SVG to the PLCx had developed a 60% ostial stenosis and a 70% mid-shaft stenosis. Wiktor® stents were implanted to both regions, and a Palmaz-Schatz™ stent was placed between them because of dissection. In November 1994, restenosis within both stents was treated successfully by PTCA.

(a) By August 1996, the ostial stent had developed further restenosis (60%).

A new restenosis (50%) was present in the graft shaft between the Palmaz-Schatz stent and the second Wiktor® stent; this extended into the proximal part of the Wiktor® stent. A new eccentric lesion had occurred in the distal graft (70%).

A 9F Amplatz Left 1 guiding catheter with side holes was used to intubate the SVG and the lesion was crossed with a 0.014-inch guidewire.

(b) The ostial restenosis was treated with three passes of a 2.0mm diameter monorail laser catheter (energy 50mJ, repetition rate 25Hz, saline flush during laser activation). Note the radio-opaque ring tip.

(c) This produced improvement.

(d) A 3.5mm Pronto Rely™ balloon (USCI) was used to post-dilate the lesion up to 20 atmospheres.

The mid-graft 50% lesion was dilated with the same balloon. The distal 70% lesion was pre-dilated with the same balloon and stented with a 3.5mm, 12mm long Microstent II™ deployed at 10 atmospheres.

(e) Final result.

The occluded RCA was then reopened and stented (not shown).

Courtesy of Dr M Webb-Peploe, St. Thomas's Hospital, London, UK.

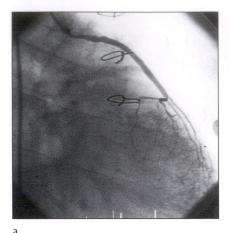
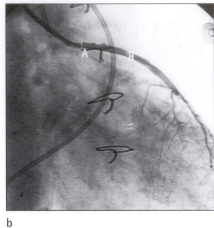
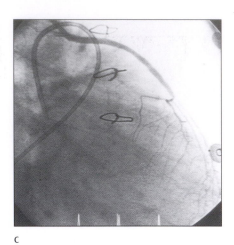

a   b   c

Figure 9.7

A 63-year-old woman had had a 3.5mm Palmaz-Schatz™ stent deployed in the ostial portion of an SVG to the LAD 12 years after CABG surgery. (a) Four months later she developed a 75% restenosis within the stent.

The SVG to the LAD was intubated with an 8F Multipurpose guide catheter with side holes and wired with a 0.014-inch guidewire. The lesion in the stent was treated with two passes of a 1.7mm diameter monorail laser catheter followed by (b) a 2.0mm device (energy 50mJ, repetition rate 25Hz, saline flush during firing).

Although an improvement was seen, a 3.5mm Pronto Rely™ balloon was then used (up to 18 atmospheres) for adjunctive PTCA.

(c) This produced a good final result.

Courtesy of Dr M Webb-Peploe, St. Thomas's Hospital, London, UK.

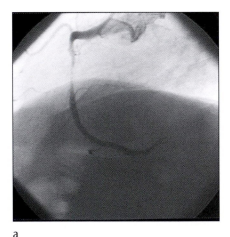
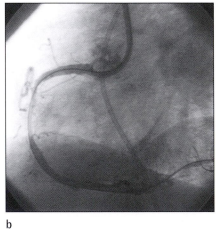
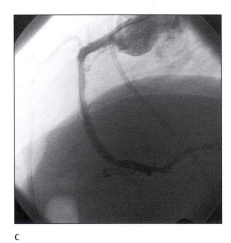

a   b   c

Figure 9.8

A 61-year-old man with severe angina had a stent implanted in the proximal third of the RCA because of dissection after PTCA 8 months earlier. (a) Angiography showed a severe within stent restenosis.

A 9F Amplatz Left 1 guiding catheter with side holes was used to intubate the RCA, which was wired with a 0.014-inch standard guidewire. The lesion was treated with 2 passes of a 1.7mm diameter monorail laser catheter (energy 50mJ, repetition rate 25Hz, saline flush during laser firing).

(b) This produced angiographic improvement.

A 3.5mm, 30mm long Goldie® balloon was used for adjunctive PTCA (10 atmospheres) in and proximal to the stent. This caused a Type A dissection, which was treated by deployment of a 4.0mm, 12mm long Microstent II™ (12 atmospheres).

(c) This gave a good final result.

Courtesy of Dr M Webb-Peploe, St. Thomas's Hospital, London, UK.

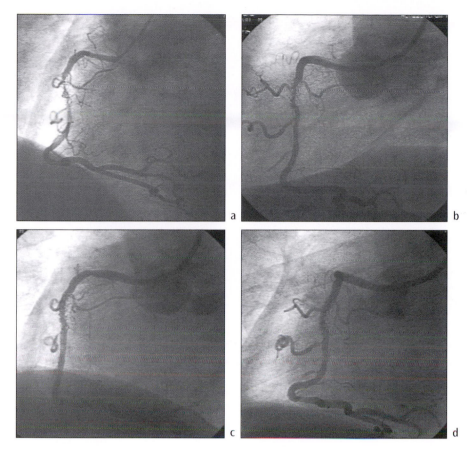

Figure 9.9
(a) In-stent restenosis within a Wiktor® stent placed in the RCA in a 65-year-old man.
(b) A 1.7mm (50mJ/mm²) laser catheter was used to ablate the lesion.
(c) Adjunctive PTCA was performed with a 3.0mm, 40mm long Speedy™ balloon (Schneider) at 8 atmospheres, with a good final result.
(d) Angiogram at 7 months showed a satisfactory appearance.
Courtesy of Drs N Reifart and N Semmler, Ambulantes Herzzentrum, Frankfurt, Germany.

The LARS European surveillance study and the LARS retrospective USA Registry reported satisfactory procedural success with ELCA and adjunctive PTCA for the treatment of in-stent restenosis. The LARS multicenter randomized study is currently comparing the acute angiographic and late clinical outcome of patients with diffuse in-stent restenosis treated with ELCA plus adjunctive PTCA with the outcome of those treated with PTCA alone.

Recanalization of chronic total occlusions by laser wire

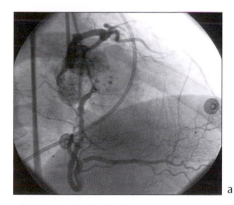
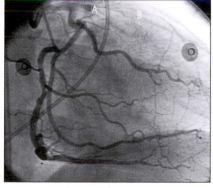
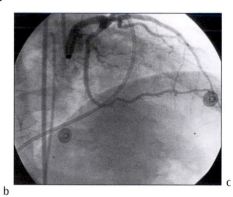

Figure 9.10
A 41-year-old seafarer was known to have had an occluded LAD artery for at least 8 months (10 months after an anterior myocardial infarction) when an attempt to reopen the vessel by PTCA failed (a).

The occlusion was approached with a 0.018-inch laser wire supported by its probing catheter. The occlusion was crossed using nine 3-second bursts of laser energy (energy 50mJ, repetition rate 25Hz), with careful reorientation of the J-tip of the laser wire between each firing as judged by simultaneous contrast injection into both the right and the left coronary arteries.

(b) The laser wire was then severed from its hub and used as a conventional exchange guidewire; the occlusion was treated with a single pass of an over-the-wire 1.4mm diameter laser catheter (energy 50mJ, repetition rate 25Hz).

The laser wire was then replaced by a conventional 0.014-inch wire, and the area of previous occlusion was dilated by a 3.0mm Europass™ balloon before a 3.0mm, 39mm long Microstent II™ was deployed at 11 atmospheres.

(c) Final result.
Courtesy of Dr M Webb-Peploe, St. Thomas's Hospital, London, UK.

The TOTAL randomized trial compared the effectiveness of the PRIMA™ Laser guidewire with that of conventional guidewires for crossing chronic total occlusions.

Reading

Deckelbaum L. Coronary laser angioplasty. In: White CJ, Ramee SR, eds. Interventional Cardiology. New York: Marcel Dekker; 1995:135-56.

Evans BH, Eigler N, Litvak F. Excimer laser coronary angioplasty. In: Faxon DP, ed. Practical Angioplasty. New York: Raven Press; 1994:197-208.

Goldberg SL, Columbo A, Akiyama T. Stent-under expansion refractory to balloon dilatation: a novel solution with excimer laser. J Invas Cardiol 1998;269-73.

Hamburger JN, Serruys PW, Seabra-Gomes R, et al. on behalf of The European TOTAL Investigators. Recanalization of total coronary occlusions using a laser guidewire (the European TOTAL surveillance study). Am J Cardiol 1997;80:1419-23.

Hamm CW, Simon R, Seabra-Gomes RJ, et al. Laser angioplasty for within stent restenosis: final results of the LARS surveillance study. J Am Coll Cardiol 1998;31:143A.

Holmes DR Jr, Mehta S, George CJ, et al. Excimer laser coronary angioplasty: the New Approaches to Coronary Intervention (NACI) experience. Am J Cardiol 1997;80:99K-105K.

Koster R, Hamm CW, Seabra-Gomes R, et al. Laser angioplasty of restenosed coronary stents: results of a multicenter surveillance trial for the Laser Angioplasty of Restenosed Stents (LARS) Investigators. J Am Coll Cardiol 1999;34:25-32.

Koster R, Hamm CW, Terres W, et al. Treatment of in-stent restenosis by excimer laser angioplasty. Am J Cardiol 1997;80:1424-8.

Litvak F, Eigler E, Margolis J, et al. Percutaneous excimer laser coronary angioplasty: results in the first consecutive 3000 patients. J Am Coll Cardiol 1994;23:323-9.

Mehran R, Mintz GS, Satler LF, et al. Treatment of in-stent restenosis with excimer laser coronary angioplasty: mechanisms and results compared with PTCA alone. Circulation 1997;96:2183-9.

Parikh A, Dev V, Litvak F. Excimer laser coronary angioplasty. In: Grech ED, Ramsdale DR. Practical Interventional Cardiology. London: Martin Dunitz; 1997;205-14.

Serruys PW, Hamburger JN, de Feyter PJ, van den Brand MJ. Recanalization of chronic total occlusions using a laser guidewire. Circulation 1994;90(Suppl I):I-331.

Serruys PW, Teunissen Y on behalf of the TOTAL Study Investigators. Randomized comparison of laser guidewire and mechanical guidewires for recanalization of chronic total coronary occlusions: the TOTAL trial, final result and follow-up at 30 days. J Am Coll Cardiol 1998;31:81A.

10

Intracoronary stenting I

Intracoronary stents are useful for preventing abrupt closure after PTCA when local dissection threatens to occlude the artery. Unacceptable angiographic results after PTCA can be improved, and restenosis rates in native vessels and SVGs may be reduced by stent implantation.

A wide range of more than 50 stents is now available. Most of these stents are balloon-expandable (e.g. NIR™ (Fig. 10.1a), Microstent GFX™ and Multilink™), although some are self-expanding (e.g. Wallstent™ (Fig. 10.1b)). Generally stents are now presented ready mounted on a balloon of appropriate length and diameter (see Fig. 10.1a) (e.g. Multilink Duet™, NIR™, Microstent GFX™ and bare or unmounted stents such as the original Palmaz-Schatz™ 153 (see Fig. 10.1c)); bare stents are used infrequently now. The structure varies from a tubular design (e.g. Multilink™ (see Fig. 10.1d), Palmaz-Schatz™ (see Fig. 10.1e)) to a coil (e.g. Wiktor® (Fig. 10.1f)) or a multicellular design (e.g. divYsio™, NIR™ (see Fig. 10.1g)). The Microstent II™ has a series of U-shaped hoops that are arranged end-to-end (see Fig. 10.1h). Some stents are specifically designed for placement on side branches or at bifurcations (e.g. JoStent®-S and JoStent®-B stents), and others have special coatings (e.g. phosphorylcholine (divYsio™) or silicon-carbide (a–SiC:H) (Tenax®)) in order to reduce the risk of thrombosis.

The radio-opacity of a stent varies according to the nature of the metal that it is made of. Stainless steel stents are difficult to visualize but those made of tantalum are easy to see on fluoroscopy. The NIRoyal™ stent is very radio-opaque because of its gold coating. The Radius™ stent is made of nitinol (see Fig. 10.1i,j). Other stents, such as BeStent™ , have small radio-opaque markers at each end of the stent.

Stents are now available in various lengths for specific anatomical problems (see Fig. 10.1a), and biliary stents can be used for large vessels and vein grafts. PTFE-covered stents are also available and may be useful for sealing coronary artery perforations and coronary artery aneurysms after intervention and for lesions in SVGs. Characteristics of stents that are currently available or have been recently available are shown in Table 10.1.

Special training is required in correct case selection and deployment techniques if complications such as failure to deliver or stent embolization are to be avoided. Pre-dilatation of the stenosis is generally recommended before stent deployment. Relative contraindications to stent implantation include:

- extremely tortuous vessels;
- heavily calcified vessels;
- poor guiding catheter support; and
- vessels under 2.5mm in diameter.

Stents are currently expensive, costing between £UK 350 and £UK 700 (about US$ 550–1100) each. However, stented patients are less likely to be rehospitalized, undergo repeat revascularization or have angina within the first year of the procedure compared with those undergoing PTCA alone, so reducing cumulative health-care costs.

Optimal stent deployment may require debulking of the atheromatous plaque burden by atherectomy, which will prolong the procedure and add to its expense. Inadequate deployment is associated with an increased risk of subacute thrombosis, and high pressure balloon inflation within the stent is advisable. IVUS may be used to confirm that the stent struts are fully deployed against the wall of the artery.

The best antithrombotic regimen for stent implantation remains to be defined, although currently most interventional cardiologists use a combination of antiplatelet agents (e.g. aspirin 150mg per day and clopidogrel 75mg per day). Clopidogrel is currently given for 4 weeks after the procedure. It has replaced ticlopidine, which had a 2% incidence of leukopenia. A loading dose of 300mg clopidogrel given at the time of stenting appears to accelerate platelet inhibition.

Progress is being made in the geometric design of stents (Fig. 10.1j–p) and in the development of coated stents (e.g. heparin, phosphorylcholine, a-SiC:H and diamond-like carbon coatings (a-C:H)) and eluting stents to attempt to prevent subacute thrombosis and restenosis, which are still significant problems, especially in smaller vessels.

Table 10.1
Characteristics of stents that are currently or have been recently available

Stent	Manu-facturer	Structure	Material	Strut thickness (mm)	Metal artery (%)	Recoil (%)	Radio opacity	Markers	Available lengths (mm)	Available diameters (mm)	Other Features
Multilink	Guidant	Multirings + links	Steel	0.06	7–15	<5	Low	No	15, 25, 35	2.5; 3.0; 3.5; 4.0	Fexc; BE; PM; BPd; UM; T;
Duet	Guidant	"	Steel	0.12	7–15	<5	Low	No	8, 13, 18, 23, 28, 38	2.5; 3.0; 3.5; 4.0	Fexc; BE; PM: Bpd; UM; T;
*Tristar	Guidant	"	Steel	0.14	15	2	Low	No	8, 13, 18, 23, 28, 33, 38	2.5; 2.75; 3.0; 3.5; 4.0	Fexc; BE; PM; Bpd; T;
*Tetra	Guidant	Multilink, corru-gated ring pattern	Steel	0.09–0.12	14	2	Low	No	8, 13, 18, 23, 28, 33, 38	2.5; 2.75; 3.0; 3.5; 4.0	Fexc; BE; PM; Bpd; T; VTS
*Ultra	Guidant	"	Steel	0.13	13–19	2	Mod	No	13, 18, 28, 38	3.5; 4.0; 4.5; 5.0	Fmod; BE; PM; Bpd; T;
Cordis stent	J&J/Cordis	Helical coil	Tantalum	0.127	15	<10	High	No	18	3.0; 3.5; 4.0	Fexc; BE; PM; Bc; C;
Crown	J&J/Cordis	Continuous sine wave/ slotted tube	Steel	0.07	17–20	2	Low	No	15, 19, 31	3.0; 3.5; 4.0	Fexc; BE; PM; Bpd; T;
Crossflex	J&J/Cordis	Weave	Steel	0.15	22	–	Mod	No	15	3.0; 3.5; 4.0	Fexc; BE; PM; Bc; T;
Crossflex LC	J&J/Cordis	Laser cut slotted tube. Continuous design & bridges Helical wrap	Steel	0.14	13–15	<2	Low	No	12, 18, 22, 27	3.0; 3.5; 4.0	Fexc; BE; PM; Bpd; T;
*Bx Velocity	J&J/Cordis	Radial rings of closed cells with connecting bridges	Steel	0.14	12–15	2	Low	No	8, 13, 18, 23, 28, 33	2.25; 2.5; 2.75; 3.0 3.5; 4.0; 4.5; 5.0	Fexc; BE; PM; Bpd; T;
MiniCrown	J&J/Cordis	Laser cut slotted tube closed cell sinusoidal wave	Steel	0.06	20	<7.5	Low	No	11, 15, 26	2.25; 2.5; 2.75; 3.0; 3.25	Fmod; BE; PM; Bpd; T;
Palmaz–Schatz 153	J&J	Slotted tube central articulation	Steel	0.07	20	5	Low	No	8, 9, 14, 18	3.0–5.0	Flow, BE; UM; T;
Palmaz-Schatz Power Grip	J&J/Cordis	Slotted tube Spiral articulation	Steel	0.07	20	5	Low	No	15	3.0; 3.5; 4.0	Flow; BE; PM; T; Bpd
Microstent II/IIXL	AVE/Medtronic	Sinusoidal 3mm crowns	Steel	0.15–0.2	8	8	Mod	No	6, 9, 12, 18, 24, 30, 39	2.5; 3.0; 3.5; 4.0	Fexc; BE; PM; Bpd; R;
Microstent GFX	"	"	Steel	0.13	21	4	Mod	No	8, 12, 18, 24, 30, 40	2.5; 3.0; 3.5; 4.0	Fexc; BE; PM; Bpd; R;
*GFXII	"	2mm sinusoidal elements (6 crown, 12 stent)	Steel				Mod	No	8, 12, 18, 24, 30, 40	2.5; 3.0; 3.5; 4.0	Fexc; BE; PM; Bpd; R;
*be Stent	"	Serpentine mesh	Steel	0.075	12–18	<4	Low	Yes	8, 15, 25, 35	2.5; 3.0; 3.5; 4.0 4.5; 5.0	Fexc; BE; PM; Bpd; T; Gold markers at end of stent
Wiktor i	"	Coil; semi-helical dense weave	Tantalum	0.13	8–9.5	9	High	No	10, 15, 20, 30	2.5; 3.0; 3.5; 4.0	Fexc; BE; PM; Bpd; C; Heparin coated available
Wiktor GX	"	Coil; semi-helical loose weave	Tantalum	0.13	7–9	9	High	No	16	3.0; 3.5; 4.0; 4.5	Fexc; BE; PM; Bpd: C;
Cardiocoil	Medtronic	Coil released by handle	Nitinol	–	14	–	Mod	No	10; 15; 20; 25	3.0; 3.5; 4.0; 4.5; 5.0	Fexc; SE; PM; Bpd; C;
Angiostent	Angio-dynamics	Helical wire Coil design Longitudinal spiral	Platinum 90% iridium 10%	0.127	9.4–12.5	7	High	No	15; 25; 35	3.0; 3.5; 4.0	Fexc; BE; PM; Bc; C;
Freedom	Global Thera-peutics	Zigzag Fishscale	Steel	0.18	10.7–15.4	5–9	Low	No	12, 16, 20, (PM) 24, 30, 40 12, 16, 22, 26, 32, 36 (UM)	3.0; 3.5 (PM) 2.5–4.5 (UM)	Fexc; BE; PM; UM; C, Bpd
*Carbostent	Sorin	Multicellular	Steel carbon coated	0.07	12–15	0	Low	Yes	9, 15, 25	2.5; 3.0; 3.5; 4.0	Fexc; BE; PM; Bpd; T; 2 platinum markers at each end
*Diamond AS	Phytis	Repeated sinusoidal ring-bridges	Steel carbon coated (DLC)	0.06	–	4	Low	No	9, 16	2.5–5.0	Fmod; BE; PM; T;
*Diamond AS Flex	"			0.08	–	4	Low	No	16, 25	2.5–5.0	Fmod; BE; PM; T;
Paragon	Vascular Therapies	Multidiamond shaped cells	Nitinol	0.15	20%	5–10	Mod	No	9, 16, 26, 36	2.75; 3.0; 3.5; 4.0	Fexc; BE; PM; Bpd; T;
X-trode (XT)	BARD	Zig-Zag modules on flex spine	Steel	0.15	13–20	5	High	No	6, 11, 15, 19, 24, 30, 37	2.5; 3.0; 3.5; 4.0; 4.5	Fexc; BE; PM; Bpd; R; Radiopaque spine
*Biodivysio	Biocom-patibles	Multicellular P.C. coated slotted tube	Steel	0.075	14	1–2	Low	No	11, 15, 18, 28, 40	3.0; 3.5; 4.0; 4.5	Fexc; BE; PM; T;

Table 10.1 *continued*
Characteristics of stents that are currently or have been recently available

Stent	Manu-facturer	Structure	Material	Strut thickness (mm)	Metal artery (%)	Recoil (%)	Radio opacity	Markers	Available lengths (mm)	Available diameters (mm)	Other Features
*Biodivysio SV	"	Interlocking arrowhead design	Steel	0.06	10–15	1	Low	No	10, 18	2.0; 2.5	Fexc; BE; PM; T;
Gianturco Roubin II	Cook	Longitudinal with spine (clamshell design)	Steel	0.076	15–20	9–11	Low	Yes	10, 20, 40	2.5; 3.0; 3.5; 4.0;4.5; 5.0	Fexc; BE; PM; Bpd; C; Gold markers at end of stent
V Flex	Cook	Flex V and	Steel	0.08	13	<1	Low	No	8, 12, 16, 20, 24	2.5; 3.0; 3.5	Fexc; BE; PM; Bpd; T;
*V Flex plus	Cook	tie bar design	Steel	0.08	13	<1	Low	No	8, 12, 16, 20, 24	2.5; 3.0; 3.5	Fexc; BE; PM; Bpd; T;
ACT-1	PAS	Slotted tube articulated	Nitinol	0.18	23		Mod	No	8, 17	3.0; 3.5; 4.0	Fmod; BE; UM; T;
Tensum	Biotronik	Slotted tube design	a-SiC:H coated	0.08	14	<3	High	No	9, 13, 18	2.5; 3.0; 3.5; 4.0	Fmod; BE; PM; Bpd; T; UM;
*Tenax	"	"	Steel	0.08	14	<5	Low	Yes	10, 15, 20, 25, 30, 35	2.5; 3.0; 3.5; 4.0; 4.5	Fexc; BE; PM; UM; T; Bpd; 2 tanta-lum markers at ends
Iris II	Unicath	Cellular design Inverted C-Flex joints with diagonal struts	Steel		16	0	Mod	No	17, 27	2.5; 3.0; 3.5; 4.0	Fmod; BE; PM; UM; T; Bpd;
*Spiral Force	"	C flex joints with spiral struts	Steel		12	–	Low	No	9, 17, 27	2.5; 3.0; 3.5; 4.0	Fexc; BE; PM; UM; T;
*Magic Wallstent	Schneider/ Boston Scientific	Mesh	Cobalt + Platinum core	0.10	20	0	High	No	17–47	3.0; 3.5; 4.0; 4.5; 5.0	Fexc; SE; PM; Bpd; M; Sheath tip marker Shortens on deploy-ment*
*Seaquence	Nycomed	Tubular, linked rings, repeating 's' shapes	Steel	0.13	11–17	<5	Low	No	8, 12, 18, 28, 38	2.5; 3.0; 3.5; 4.0	Fexc; BE; PM; Bpd; T;
*Joflex	Jomed	Multicell 'M' design	Steel	0.09	14–19	<3	Low	No	9, 12, 16, 19, 26, 32	2.5; 3.0; 3.5; 4.0	Fmod; BE; PM; Bpd; T;
*Jomed S	"	Sidebranch design	Steel	0.09	10–16	<3	Low	No	17, 28	2.5; 3.0; 3.5; 4.0	Fmod; BE; PM/UM; Bpd; T; Heparin coated available
*Jomed B	"	Bifurcation design	Steel	0.09	10–16	<3	Low	No	19, 26	2.5; 3.0; 3.5; 4.0	Fmod; BE; PM/UM; Bpd; T; Heparin-coated avail-able
*Jomed Stent Graft	"	M cell design PTFE sandwiched between 2 stents	Steel PTFE				Low	No	9, 12, 16, 19, 26	2.5–5.0	Fpoor; BE; PM/UM; T;
*NIR Primo	Scimed/ Boston Scientific	Multicell 'M' design 7 or 9 cells	Steel	0.10	11–18	<1	Low	No	9, 16, 25, 32	2.5; 3.0; 3.5; 4.0	Fmod; BE; PM; M;
*Niroyal	"	"	Steel, gold-plated	0.10	11–18	<1	High	No	9, 12, 15, 18, 25, 31	2.5; 3.0; 3.5; 4.0 4.5; 5.0	Fmod; BE; PM; Bpd; T; UM
*Radius	Scimed	Slotted tube Multisegment	Nitinol	0.11	20	0	Mod	No	14, 20, 31	3.0; 3.5; 4.0	Fmod; SE; PM; Bpd; T;
*Inflow Gold stent	Inflow Dynamics	Slotted tube interconnected sinusoidal waves with oval struts	Steel, gold-plated	0.08/ 0.155	18	<5	High	No	7, 9, 11, 15, 23	2.5; 3.0; 3.5; 4.0; 4.5; 5.0	Fmod; BE; PM; Bpd; T;
*S540	Medtronic/ Ave	Rings, sinusoidal elements,	Steel	oval 0.127/	17–23	<2	Mod	No	8, 12, 16, 18, 24	2.5	Fexc; BE; PM; Bpd; R;
*S670	"	7 Crowns 14 struts per element		0.178			Mod	No	9, 12, 15, 18, 24, 30	3.0; 3.5; 4.0	Fexc; BE; PM; Bpd; R;

Key
F = flexibility; BE = Balloon expandable; SE = Self expanding; PM = Premounted; UM = Unmounted; Bpd = Proximal and distal balloon marker; Bc = Central balloon marker; Exc = Excellent; Mod = Moderate; M = Mesh design; T = Tubular design; C = Coil design; R = Ring design; VTS = variable thickness strut
*Currently available in UK

Recently available coronary stents

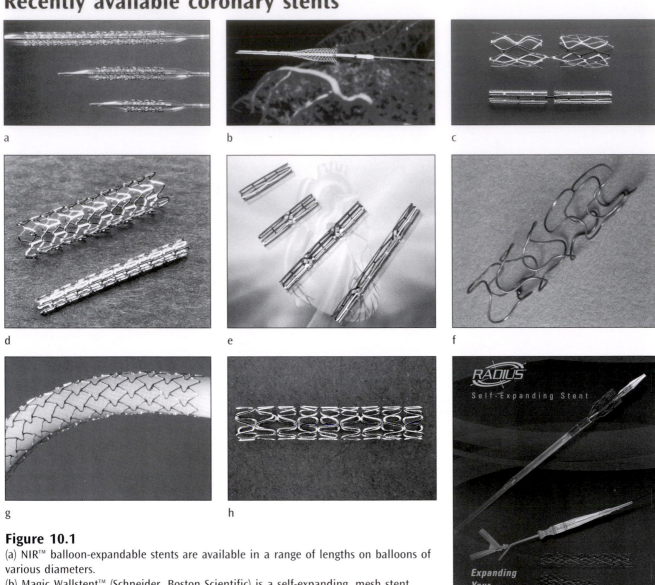

Figure 10.1

(a) NIR™ balloon-expandable stents are available in a range of lengths on balloons of various diameters.

(b) Magic Wallstent™ (Schneider, Boston Scientific) is a self-expanding, mesh stent protected by a retractable protective sheath. This shows the sheath partially withdrawn.

(c) Close-up view of a Palmaz-Schatz PS 153™ , one of the early bare or unmounted stents.

(d) Multilink™ stent unexpanded and expanded.

(e) Palmaz-Schatz Powergrip™ (8mm, 9mm, 15mm, 18mm).

(f) Wiktor® stent is a coil stent made of tantalum wire.

(g) NIR™ stent has a multicellular design.

(h) Microstent II™ has a series of U-shaped hoops that are arranged end to end.

(i) Radius™ self-expanding stent (Scimed, Boston Scientific).

(j) Close-up view of Radius™ self-expanding stent.

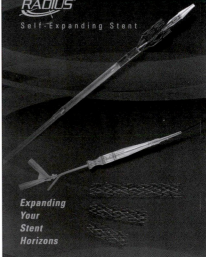

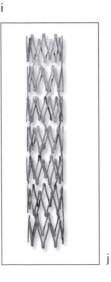

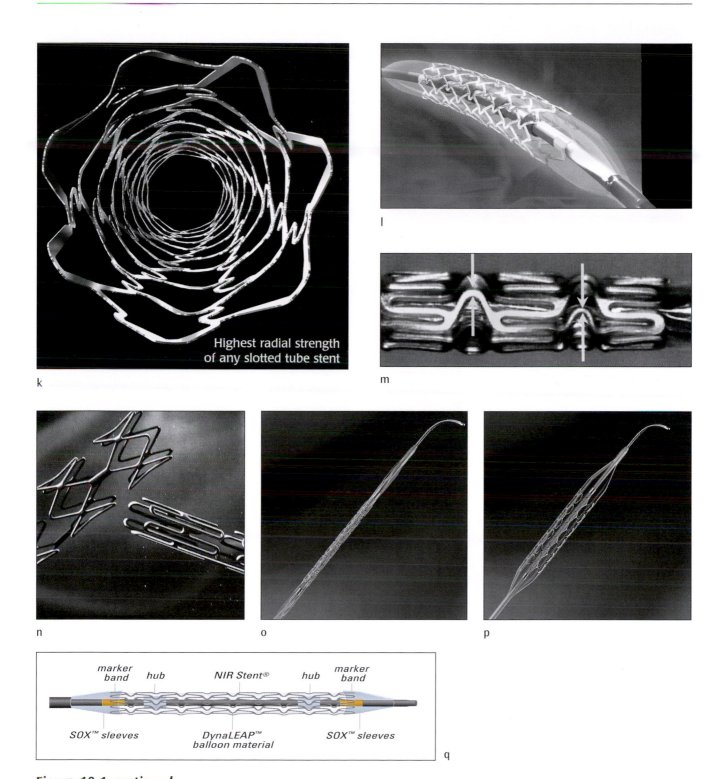

Highest radial strength
of any slotted tube stent

k

l

m

marker
band   hub   NIR Stent®   hub   marker
band

SOX™ sleeves   DynaLEAP™
balloon material   SOX™ sleeves

n

o

p

q

Figure 10.1 *continued*

(k) Spiral Force™ (Uni-Cath Inc) has a spiral arrangement of its struts.

(l) NIRoyal™ has a number of features to improve conformability and crossability, to reduce edge tears and to improve radio-opacity. These features include shortened stent end struts, (m) thinned-out longitudinal struts at the proximal and distal cell row (arrows), and gold plating.

(n) The Tensum™ stent (Biotronik) was an a-SiC:H-coated tantulum tubular stent, but it has been replaced by (o, p) the Tenax™ tubular, stainless steel stent, which is also coated with antithrombogenic a-SiC:H.

(q) Novel design features such as SOX™ technology (Boston Scientific/SCIMED) protects the leading and trailing edge of the NIR™ stent (NIR™ w/SOX™ Monorail™) for improved crossability and retractability. It also aids 'centre-out deployment' to eliminate 'dog-boning' during deployment and maximises MLD by focusing balloon pressure at the centre of the stent.

Stents to native vessels

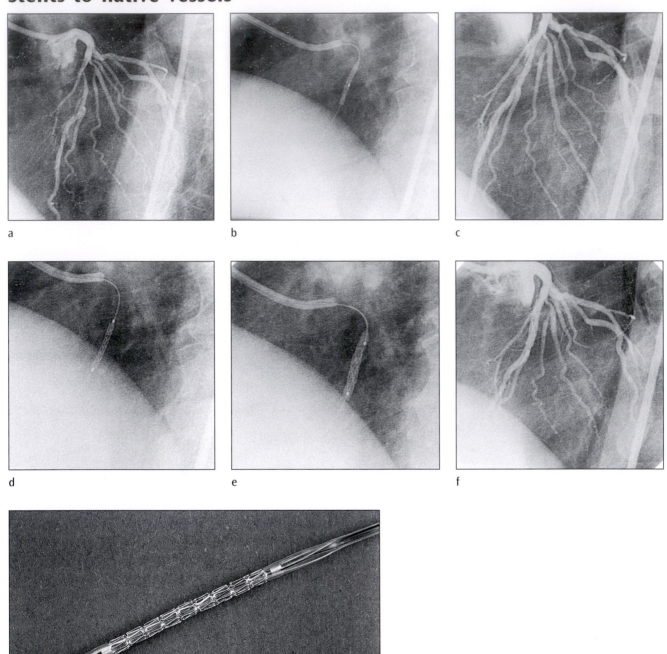

Figure 10.2

A 50-year-old clerk working for a petroleum company developed (a) a severe restenosis in the proximal LAD 4 months after PTCA (LAO cranial projection).

(b) The lesion was dilated by a 2.5mm Elipse™ balloon (LAO cranial projection).

(c) This resulted in a local dissection and a suboptimal result (LAO cranial projection).

(d) A 3.0mm, 18mm long Microstent™ was positioned and deployed successfully (e).

(f) This produced an excellent angiographic result and complete relief of symptoms.

The Microstent™ (g) was renowned for its flexibility and for being the first stent to provide ease of passage through an already deployed stent.

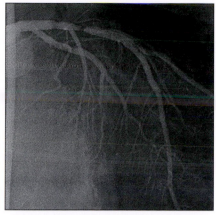

a

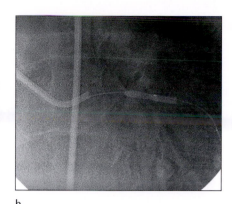

b

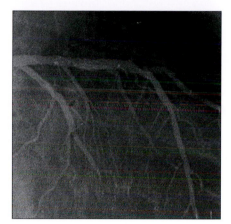

c

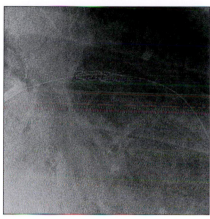

d

Figure 10.3
(a) A severe bulky lesion in the proximal LAD of a 56-year-old taxi driver with severe unstable angina.
(b) The lesion was pre-dilated with a 3.0mm Cheetah™ balloon.
(c) A 3.5mm, long Microstent II™ was implanted with good effect.
(d) The stent is clearly visible on fluoroscopy.

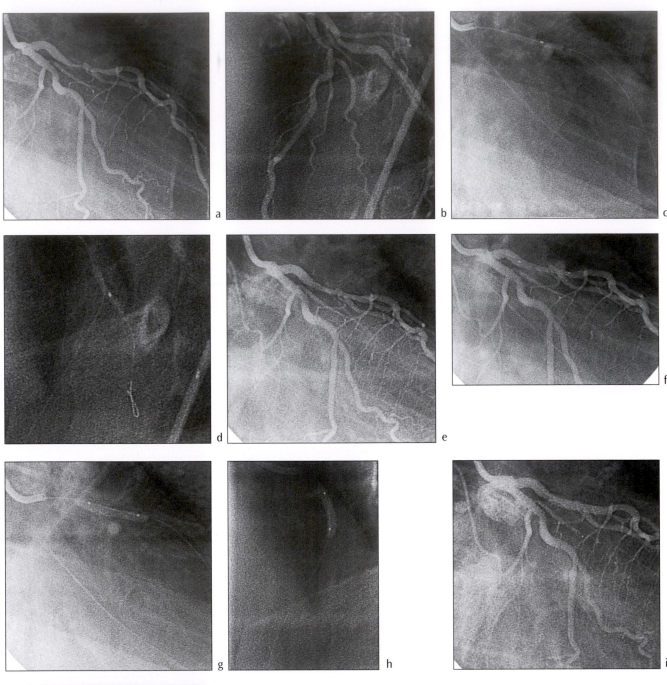

Figure 10.4

This 47-year-old professional fish farmer with recent onset unstable angina had (a) a severe proximal LAD stenosis that was approximately 16mm long.

(b) The DG had a severe ostial stenosis.

(c) The LAD stenosis was pre-dilatated with a 3.0mm Express™ balloon.

(d) The stenosis in the DG was then dilated with a 2.5mm Express™ balloon. Note that there is a guidewire down each branch.

(e) Because there was residual stenosis in the LAD, a 3.5mm, 18mm long Microstent II™ was placed in the proximal LAD (f-h).

(i, j) This produced a good angiographic result.

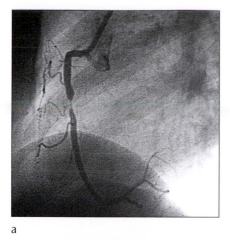

a

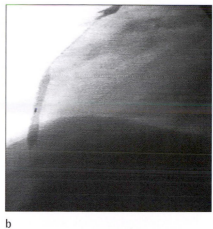

b

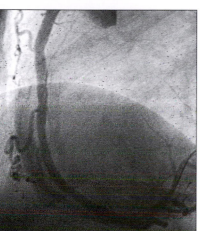

c

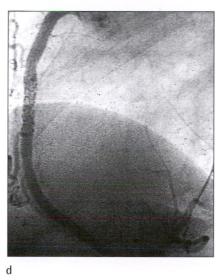

d

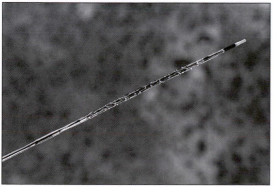

e

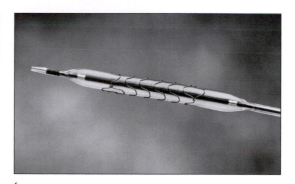

f

Figure 10.5

A 49-year-old sales manageress with unstable angina. Severe stenosis in the middle third of large dominant RCA (a) before, (b) during and (c) after PTCA with a 3.0mm Elipse™ and a 3.5mm Goldie™ balloon.

A local dissection is visible on the inner wall of the RCA.

(d) The lesion was therefore stented with a 3.5mm Wiktor® stent.

(e) The Wiktor-i™ stent is made of tantalum wire wound in a coil design and crimped on to a rapid-exchange balloon catheter. When the stent is deployed, the metal-artery ratio is low (f), which makes side branch preservation more likely and access easier.

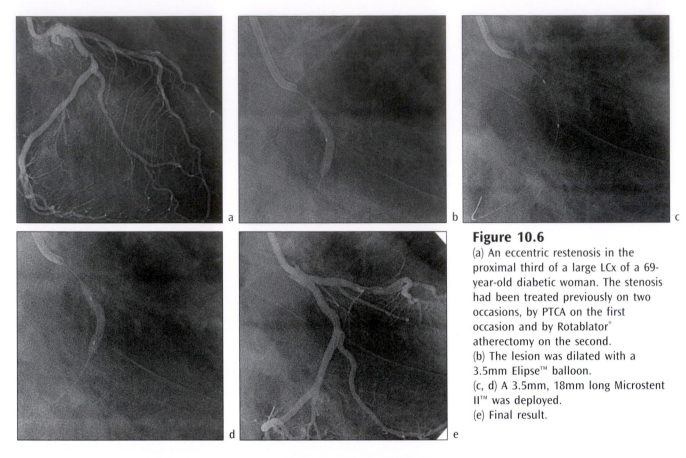

Figure 10.6
(a) An eccentric restenosis in the proximal third of a large LCx of a 69-year-old diabetic woman. The stenosis had been treated previously on two occasions, by PTCA on the first occasion and by Rotablator® atherectomy on the second.
(b) The lesion was dilated with a 3.5mm Elipse™ balloon.
(c, d) A 3.5mm, 18mm long Microstent II™ was deployed.
(e) Final result.

Stenting for poor angiographic result or local dissection

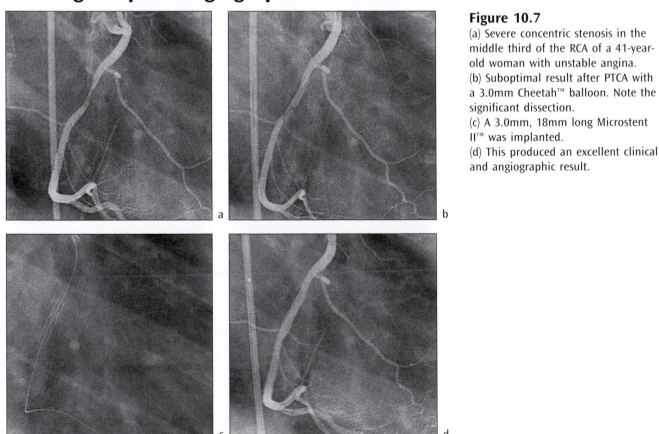

Figure 10.7
(a) Severe concentric stenosis in the middle third of the RCA of a 41-year-old woman with unstable angina.
(b) Suboptimal result after PTCA with a 3.0mm Cheetah™ balloon. Note the significant dissection.
(c) A 3.0mm, 18mm long Microstent II™ was implanted.
(d) This produced an excellent clinical and angiographic result.

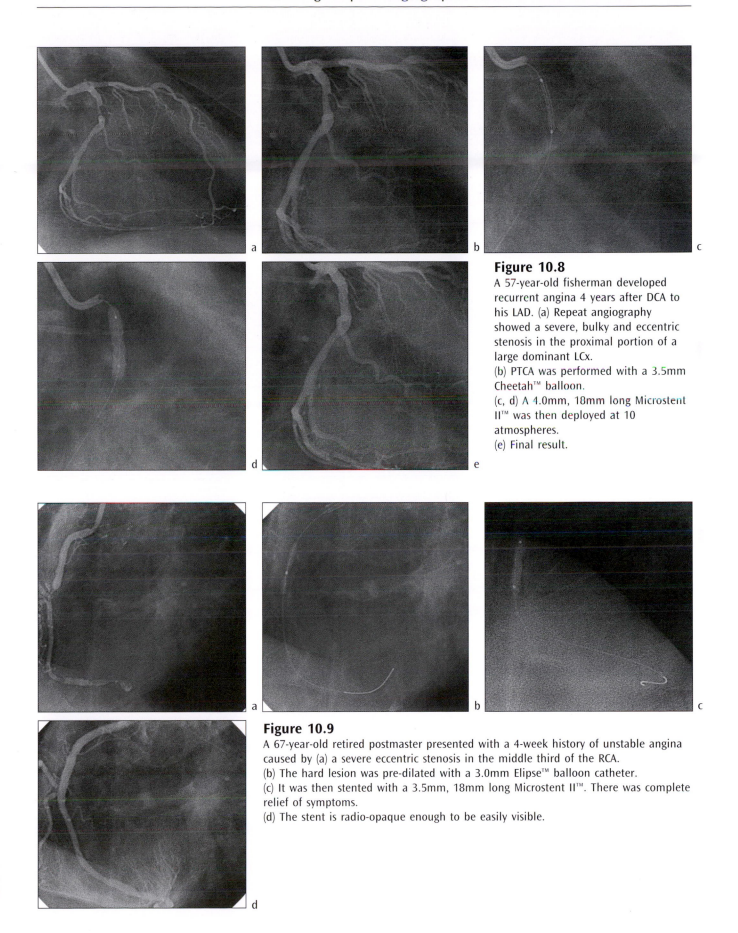

Figure 10.8

A 57-year-old fisherman developed recurrent angina 4 years after DCA to his LAD. (a) Repeat angiography showed a severe, bulky and eccentric stenosis in the proximal portion of a large dominant LCx.
(b) PTCA was performed with a 3.5mm Cheetah™ balloon.
(c, d) A 4.0mm, 18mm long Microstent II™ was then deployed at 10 atmospheres.
(e) Final result.

Figure 10.9

A 67-year-old retired postmaster presented with a 4-week history of unstable angina caused by (a) a severe eccentric stenosis in the middle third of the RCA.
(b) The hard lesion was pre-dilated with a 3.0mm Elipse™ balloon catheter.
(c) It was then stented with a 3.5mm, 18mm long Microstent II™. There was complete relief of symptoms.
(d) The stent is radio-opaque enough to be easily visible.

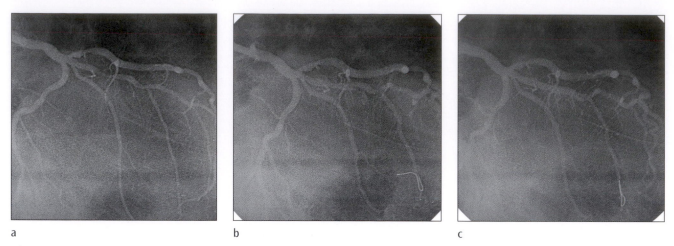

a   b   c

Figure 10.10

(a) A severe stenosis in the intermediate coronary artery of a 61-year-old man with unstable angina.
   The lesion was dilated with a 3.0mm Cheetah™ balloon.
(b) This resulted in a local dissection and a suboptimal result.
(c) A 3.0mm, 15mm long Multilink™ stent was deployed with an excellent angiographic result.

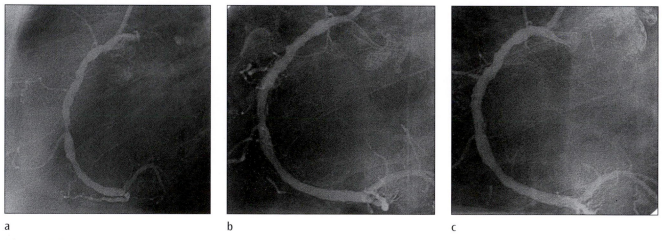

a   b   c

Figure 10.11

(a) A severe, calcified, balloon-resistant lesion in the middle third of the RCA of a 68-year-old man with a 10-year history of
angina.
   The lesion had failed to dilate significantly with a 3.5mm Goldie™ balloon at 18 atmospheres when the balloon ruptured.
(b) A 4.0mm Express NC™ balloon at 19 atmospheres dilated the stenosis and then ruptured.
Local dissection was evident and was treated by implantation of a 4.0mm, 18mm long Microstent II™.
(c) Final result.

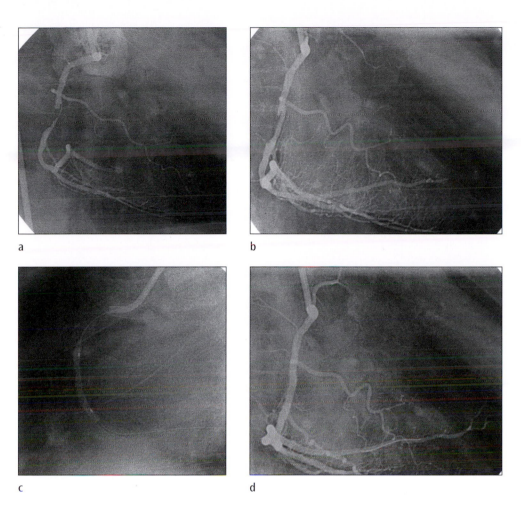

a

b

c

d

Figure 10.12
A 64-year-old retired joiner had undergone multivessel PTCA 8 years earlier including PTCA to his RCA. He then presented with severe unstable angina due to (a) a severe, eccentric restenosis in the RCA. The lesion was dilated with a 3.0mm Cheetah™ balloon leaving (b) a significant residual stenosis. (c) It was therefore stented with a 3.0mm, 25mm long Multilink™ stent. (d) This gave a good result and immediate relief of symptoms.

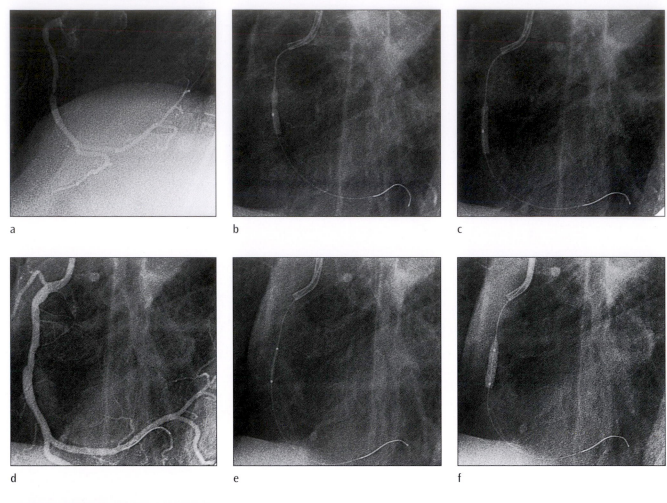

a

b

c

d

e

f

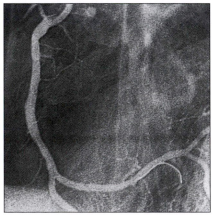

g

Figure 10.13

A 46-year-old man with unstable angina. (a) He had a severe, short, discrete stenosis in a dominant RCA.

(b, c) The hard stenosis was dilated at 10 atmospheres with a 3.0mm Cheetah™ balloon.

(d) However, this left a residual stenosis.

(e, f) A 3.5mm, 15mm long Palmaz-Schatz™ stent was implanted, with (g) an excellent result.

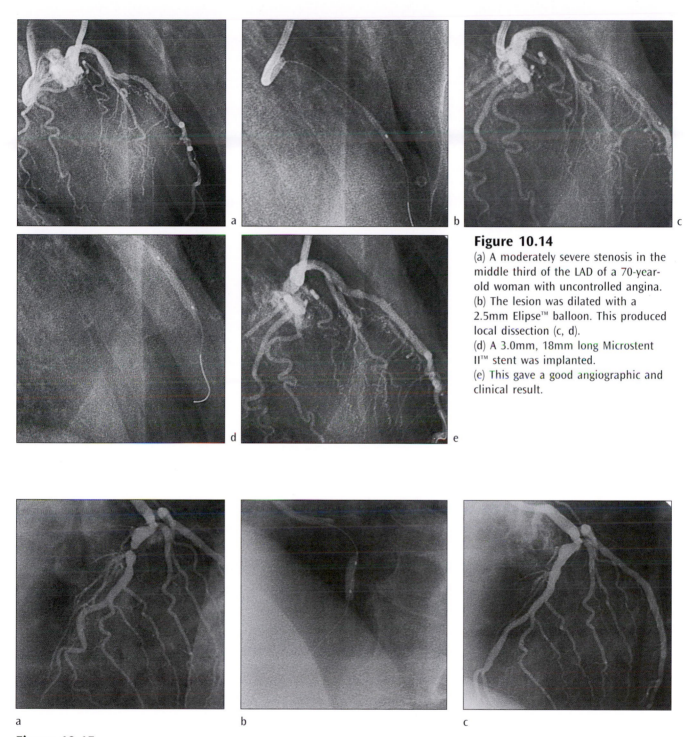

Figure 10.14
(a) A moderately severe stenosis in the middle third of the LAD of a 70-year-old woman with uncontrolled angina.
(b) The lesion was dilated with a 2.5mm Elipse™ balloon. This produced local dissection (c, d).
(d) A 3.0mm, 18mm long Microstent II™ stent was implanted.
(e) This gave a good angiographic and clinical result.

Figure 10.15
A 54-year-old executive with moderate angina had (a) a severe stenosis in the proximal LAD 2 years after PTCA (LAO projection). After PTCA with a 3.0mm Samba® balloon, a 3.0mm, 15mm Multilink™ stent was implanted (b), with (c) a good result.

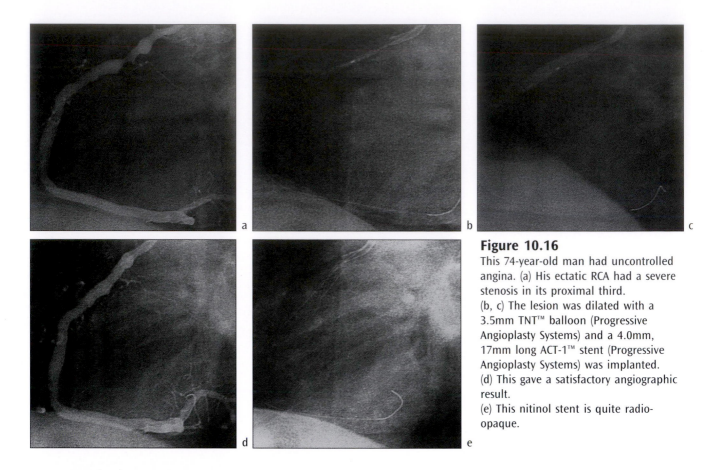

a

b

c

d

e

Figure 10.16
This 74-year-old man had uncontrolled angina. (a) His ectatic RCA had a severe stenosis in its proximal third.
(b, c) The lesion was dilated with a 3.5mm TNT™ balloon (Progressive Angioplasty Systems) and a 4.0mm, 17mm long ACT-1™ stent (Progressive Angioplasty Systems) was implanted.
(d) This gave a satisfactory angiographic result.
(e) This nitinol stent is quite radio-opaque.

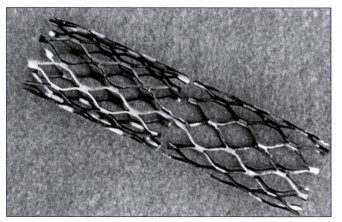

Figure 10.17
The ACT-1™ stent, which originally had to be finger-crimped on to a balloon catheter and was relatively inflexible. It was replaced by the Paragon™ stent.

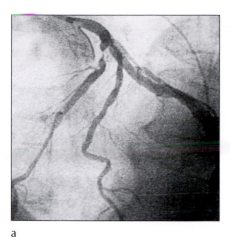

a

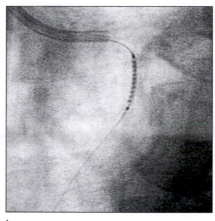

b

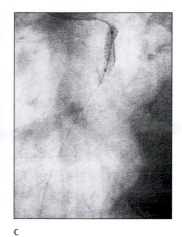

c

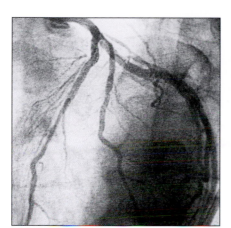

d

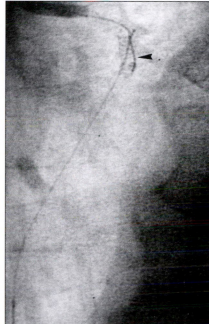

e

Figure 10.18
A 68-year-old man with unstable angina and ST-T-wave ECG abnormalities in leads V1-V6 was found to have (a) a severe stenosis in the proximal LAD.
(b, c) The lesion was pre-dilated with a 3.0mm Worldpass™ balloon and stented with a 3.0 mm, 24mm long Bard XT™ stent (CR Bard).
(d) The final result was good.
(e) The stent is characterized by its radio-opaque spine (arrow).

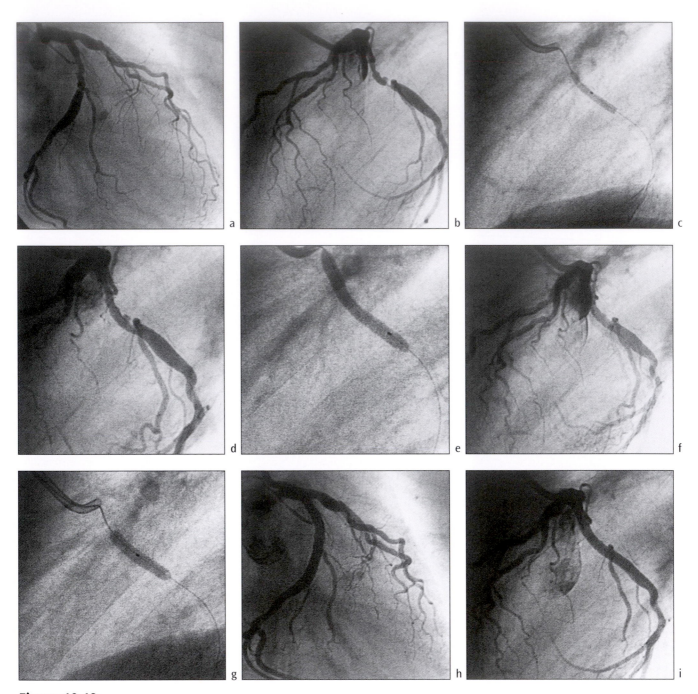

Figure 10.19

(a, b) A severe eccentric ulcerated lesion in the proximal LCx of a 55-year-old woman with moderately severe angina.

(c, d) The lesion was dilated with a 3.0mm Worldpass™ balloon with some improvement.

(e) It was then stented with a 3.5mm, 25mm long Multilink™ stent at 10 atmospheres.

(f) However, the result was unsatisfactory.

(g) Therefore, the stent was further dilated with a 4.0mm/4.5mm CAT™ balloon up to a pressure of 12 atmospheres.

(h, i) Final result.

The CAT™ balloon (Cardiovascular Dynamics) (now discontinued) was a hybrid balloon that was composed of an outer non-compliant portion embracing a central compliant portion. At 6 atmospheres, the whole balloon was at nominal size, but at 12 atmospheres the central portion was 0.5mm larger than the outer portion. This design was a help in trying to prevent 'edge dissection' during high-pressure balloon inflation in order to appose the stent struts completely against the wall of the artery.

Bail-out stenting

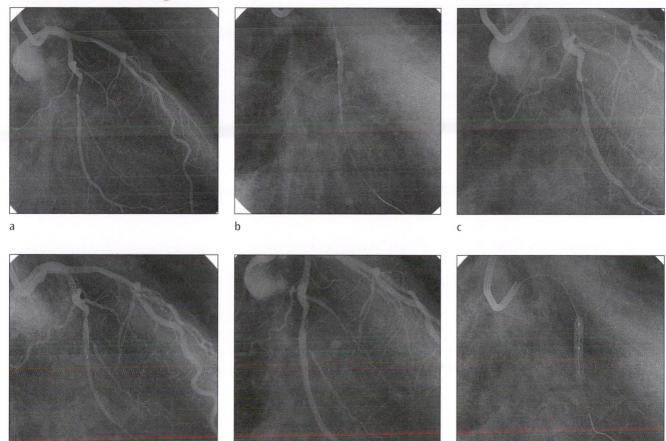

a

b

c

d

e

f

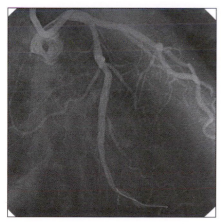

g

Figure 10.20

A 58-year-old building contractor presented with chest pain and collapse as a result of ventricular fibrillation. (a) Angiography after resuscitation revealed a severe stenosis in the OMCx.

(b) PTCA with a 2.5mm Elipse™ balloon left a significant residual stenosis.

(c) However, after inflation at a pressure of 10 atmospheres, a significant local dissection almost occluded the artery.

The dissection became an occlusion and the vessel was reopened with a 3.0mm Express™ balloon and stented first with a 3.0mm, 18mm long Microstent II™ to its distal half (d, e) and then a 12mm long Microstent II™ stent proximally (f).

The balloon was then advanced inside the 12mm stent to avoid dissection proximal to the 12mm stent and fully inflated to 14 atmospheres.

(g) Final result.

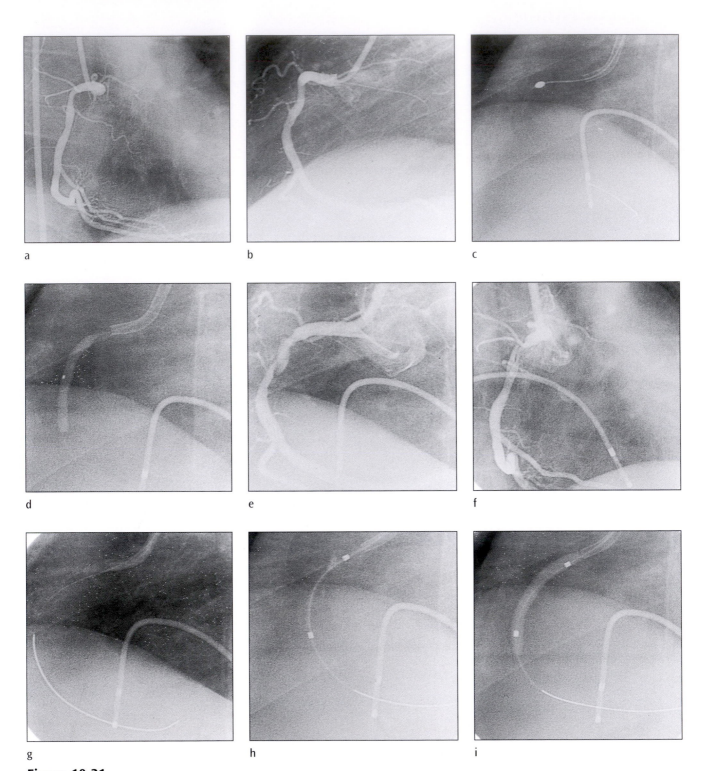

Figure 10.21
(a, b) A relatively innocuous looking eccentric stenosis in the proximal RCA of a 53-year-old man with severe angina.
   However, the artery was shown to be severely stenosed by IVUS.
(c) Rotablator® atherectomy produced an improved IVUS result.
(d) However, adjunctive PTCA caused a subtotal occlusive dissection (e, f).
(g) A Cook® guidewire was placed down the RCA.
   A 4.0mm Gianturco-Roubin® (Cook) stent was (h) positioned and (i) deployed.

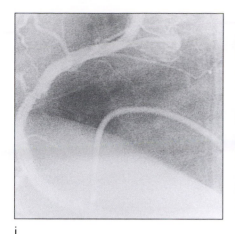

j

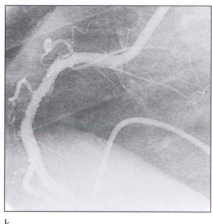

k

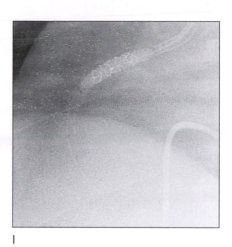

l

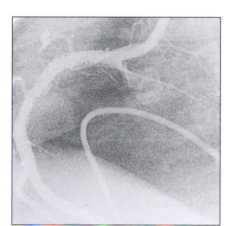

m

Figure 10.21 *continued*

(j) The angiographic result was improved.

(k) However, a small dissection was evident on the proximal bend of the RCA.

(l) A 4.0mm Wiktor® stent was therefore deployed.

(m) This gave a good angiographic result and abolition of symptoms.

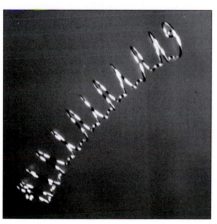

a

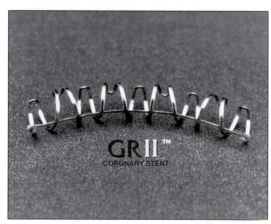

b

Figure 10.22

(a) The original Gianturco-Roubin (GR) Flexstent® (implanted in Fig. 10.21).

(b) The subsequent GR II™ (Cook), with its flexible spine.

Both of these stents were flexible coil stents, but they have now been withdrawn.

'Spot stenting'

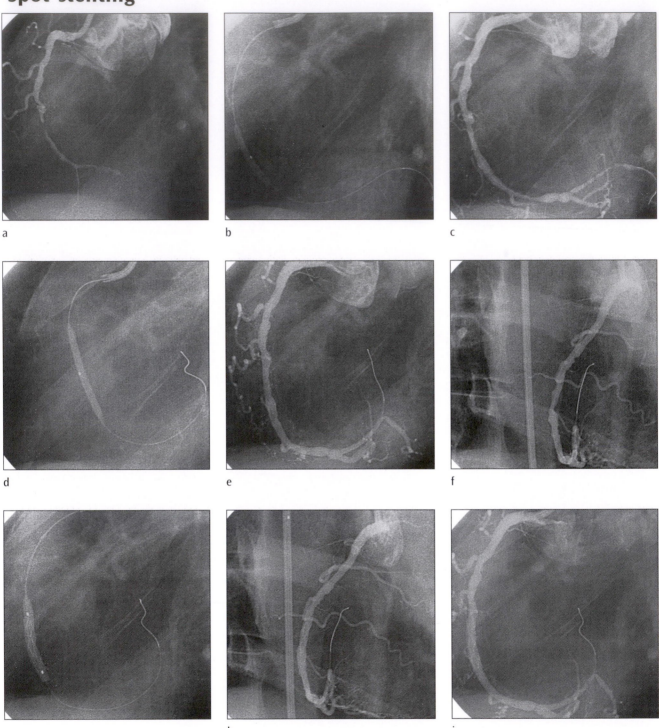

Figure 10.23

A 47-year-old maintenance technician presented with severe unstable angina and (a) a subtotally occluded dominant RCA with diffuse disease.

(b) The RCA was reopened by PTCA with a 3.0mm, 20mm long Elipse™ balloon catheter.

(c) This revealed several areas of significant stenosis.

(d) A 3.5mm, 30mm long Elipse™ balloon was used to dilate these areas in the mid- and distal thirds of the vessel.

Although (e) the LAO view shows a reasonable result, (f) the RAO view still shows significant residual stenosis.

(g) A 3.5mm, 18mm long Microstent II™ was implanted on the most severe 'spot'.

This produced a satisfactory result – (h) RAO view; (i) LAO view .

Whether 'spot stenting' to the most severe and threatening segment is as safe acutely as stenting the whole length of the diseased segment with a long stent or with multiple stents, and whether it is less likely to be associated with late restenosis, remains to be determined by a controlled clinical trial.

Short stents

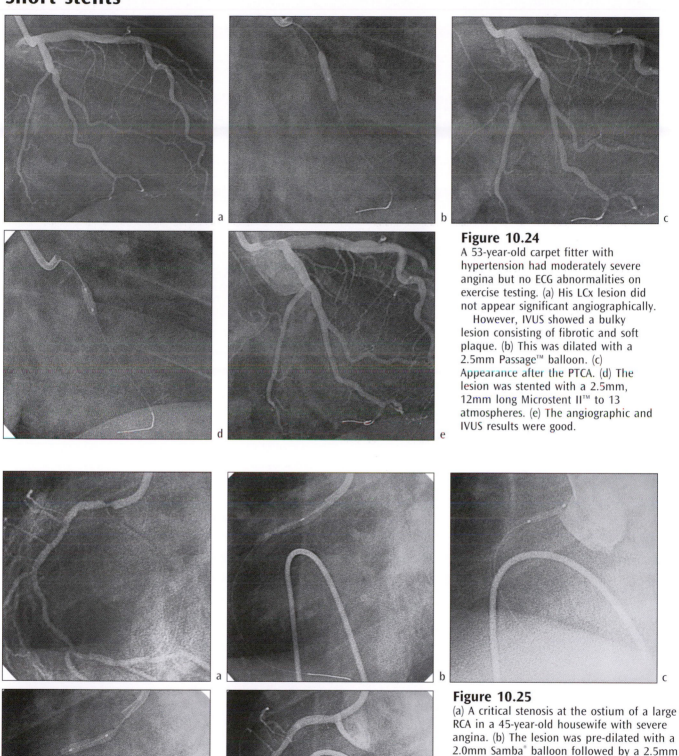

Figure 10.24
A 53-year-old carpet fitter with hypertension had moderately severe angina but no ECG abnormalities on exercise testing. (a) His LCx lesion did not appear significant angiographically.

However, IVUS showed a bulky lesion consisting of fibrotic and soft plaque. (b) This was dilated with a 2.5mm Passage™ balloon. (c) Appearance after the PTCA. (d) The lesion was stented with a 2.5mm, 12mm long Microstent II™ to 13 atmospheres. (e) The angiographic and IVUS results were good.

Figure 10.25
(a) A critical stenosis at the ostium of a large RCA in a 45-year-old housewife with severe angina. (b) The lesion was pre-dilated with a 2.0mm Samba® balloon followed by a 2.5mm Samba® balloon up to 10 atmospheres. As is often the case with such tough aorta-ostial lesions, significant recoil occurs, leaving an unacceptable residual stenosis. (c, d) Therefore, a 3.0mm, 12mm long Multilink™ stent was placed. (e) This gave an excellent angiographic result. Note how the tip of the guiding catheter must be carefully disengaged from the ostium during placement and deployment of the stent, and that re-engagement must be avoided during final check angiography in order to prevent damage to the stent.

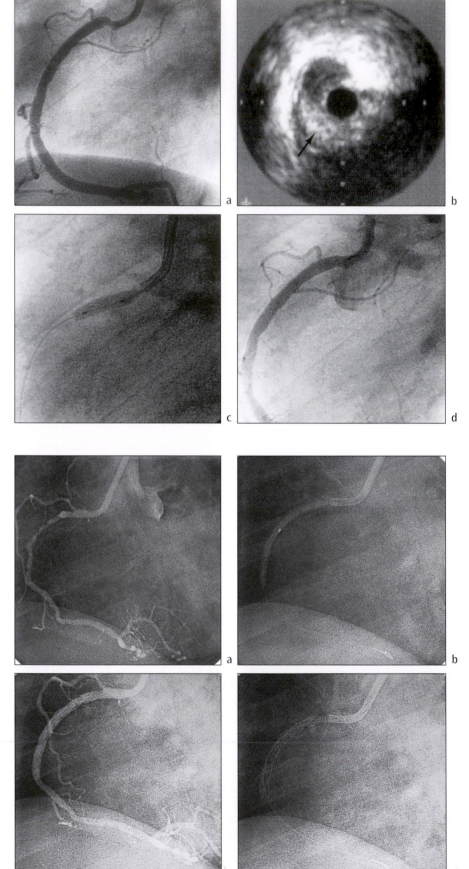

Figure 10.26

A 53-year-old lady with frequent angina and a positive exercise stress test was found to have (a) only an ostial RCA lesion of less than 50% of the vessel diameter on angiography.

It was decided to study the lesion further by IVUS. A 2.5–3.5F Visions® FX (Endosonics) IVUS catheter was used over a 0.014-inch guidewire via a 3.5JR guide catheter with side holes. (b) IVUS confirmed that bulky, dense plaque (arrow) was eccentrically obstructing the ostium of the RCA. The lesion was pre-dilated with a 3.5mm Cruiser II balloon. (c) It was stented with a 9mm long NIR™ stent that had been premounted on a 4.0mm Viva Primo™ balloon. This balloon was inflated up to 15 atmospheres, giving an estimated balloon diameter of 4.2mm. Note how the tip of the guide catheter has to be withdrawn into the aorta during stent deployment. This is a critical manoeuvre that is made particularly difficult because it is then difficult to check the stent-lesion relationship by contrast injections through a displaced guide catheter with side holes. (d) The final result shows a significant angiographic improvement. Repeat IVUS examination was not performed for fear of damaging the back of the stent.

Long stents

Figure 10.27

A 43-year-old woman with frequent atypical angina was found to have (a) a long segment of severe disease in the proximal and middle thirds of the RCA. (b) The lesion was dilated with a 2.5mm, 40mm long Elipse™ balloon. (c) Local dissection necessitated implantation of a 3.0mm, 39mm long Microstent II™, with a good final result. (d) The stent is radio-opaque.

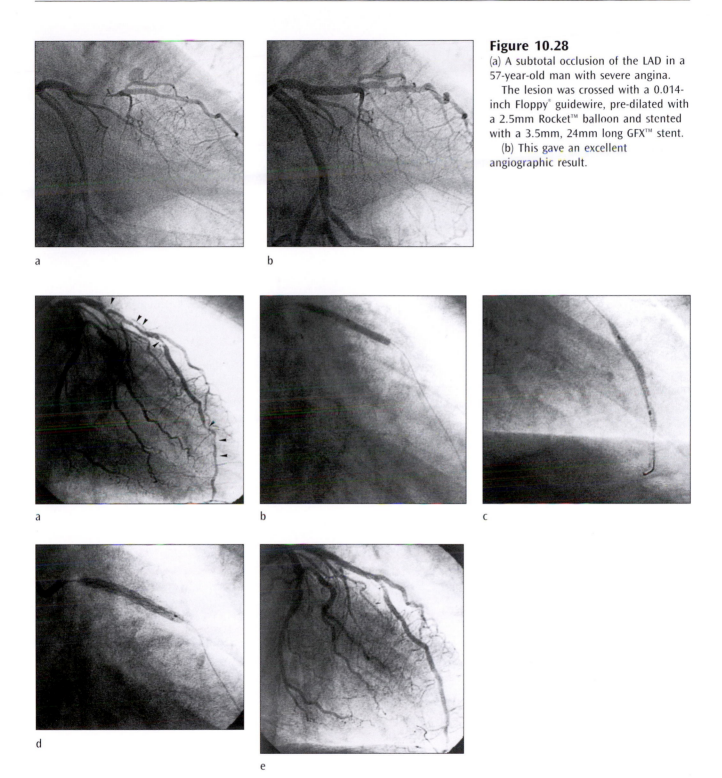

Figure 10.28
(a) A subtotal occlusion of the LAD in a 57-year-old man with severe angina.

The lesion was crossed with a 0.014-inch Floppy® guidewire, pre-dilated with a 2.5mm Rocket™ balloon and stented with a 3.5mm, 24mm long GFX™ stent.

(b) This gave an excellent angiographic result.

Figure 10.29
A 60-year-old man presented with persisting unstable angina 3 weeks after receiving thrombolytic therapy for acute anteroseptal myocardial infarction. Left ventriculography showed normal contractility. (a) Coronary arteriography showed a severe, bulky, complex stenosis in the proximal LAD with a long segment of significant narrowing immediately beyond and a long segment of significant disease in its distal third (arrows).
(b, c) Both segments were dilated with a 3.0mm, 30mm long Elipse™ balloon.
This produced some improvement but there was a residual stenosis proximally and local dissection distally.
The distal segment was treated with a 3.0mm, 25mm long Multilink™ stent and (d) the proximal segment was treated with a 3.0mm, 30mm long Microstent GFX™.
(e) The final result was good.

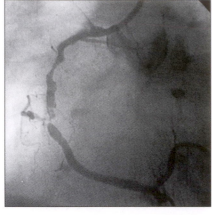

a

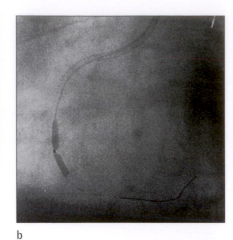

b

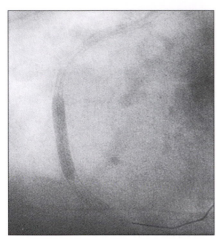

c

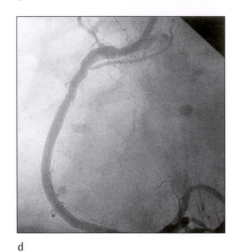

d

Figure 10.30
(a) A long segment of severe disease in the mid-RCA in a 62-year-old man with a 1-year history of stable angina.
(b) The segments were pre-dilated with a 2.5mm Europass™ balloon (Cordis). A 3.5 48mm self-expanding Magic Wallstent™ was deployed in order to cover the entire length of disease. (c) The stent, which is visible, was then finally expanded with a 3.5mm Bonnie™ balloon inflated up to 14 atmospheres.
(d) The final angiographic result indicated occlusion of only a small right ventricular branch. The patient was asymptomatic 7 months later.
Courtesy of Dr MS Norell, Hull Royal Infirmary, Hull, UK.

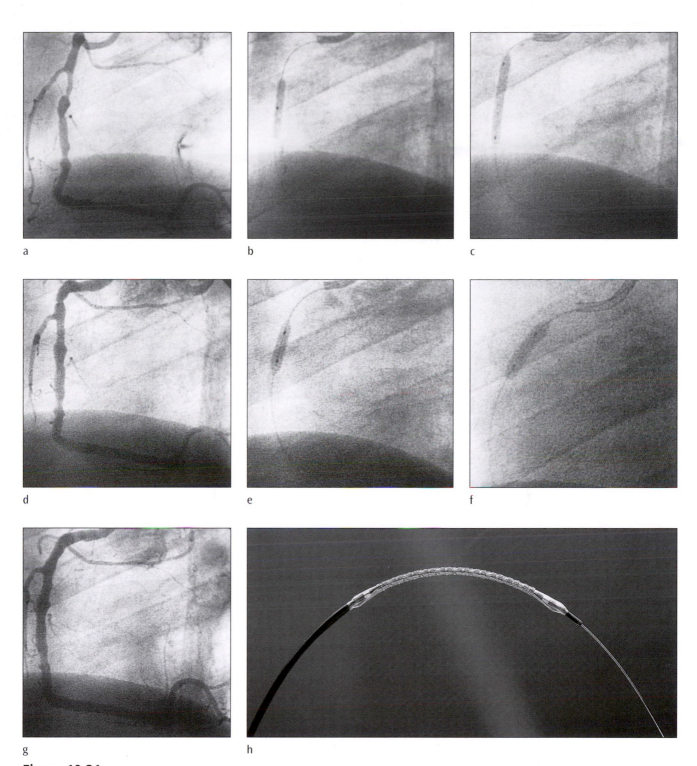

Figure 10.31

(a) A long segment of disease in the RCA of a 57-year-old man with exertional angina.

(b) A 3.0mm, 20mm long LTX™ balloon (AVE) was used to dilate the most severe proximal lesion.

(c) A 3.5mm, 24mm long V-flex Plus™ stent (Cook) was deployed over the diseased segment.

Because of residual stenosis (d), a 3.5mm, 12mm long Cruiser® balloon was used to post-dilate the stent by serial inflations along its length (e).

(f) A 3.5mm, 9mm long NIR™ stent was then implanted over the most proximal lesion.

(g) The final angiographic result was very satisfactory.

(h) The V-flex Plus™ stent is a tubular stent that is based on crown units linked by alternating V-bridge and tie bars to improve the compromise between radial force and flexibility/conformability.

Use of single long stent to cover lesions in series

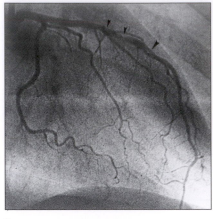

a

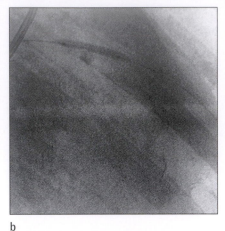

b

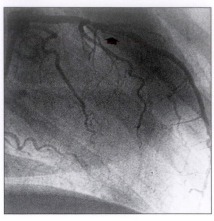

c

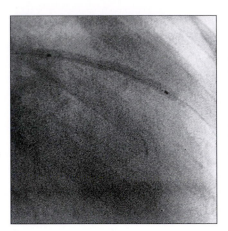

d

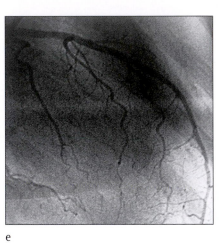

e

Figure 10.32

(a) A series of three lesions in the mid-third of the LAD (arrows) in a 54-year-old lady with moderately severe angina.

(b) The lesions were dilated with a 3.0mm Rocket™ balloon.

(c) However, local dissection was evident (arrow).

(d) A single 3.0mm, 35mm long Multilink™ stent was therefore deployed over the three lesions.

The stent was then post-dilated with a 3.0mm Rocket™ balloon up to 14 atmospheres followed by a 3.5mm Cruiser® balloon up to 10 atmospheres.

(e) The final angiographic result was excellent.

Spot-stenting, when only the segments of a long lesion that appear significant (cross-sectional area less than 5.5mm² or less than 50% of reference diameter at the site of the lesion on IVUS) are stented with short stents, may have a better long-term outcome with lower restenosis rates than the use of long stents with full lesion coverage. A randomized clinical trial is necessary, however, to answer this question.

Long stents in series for long segments of disease

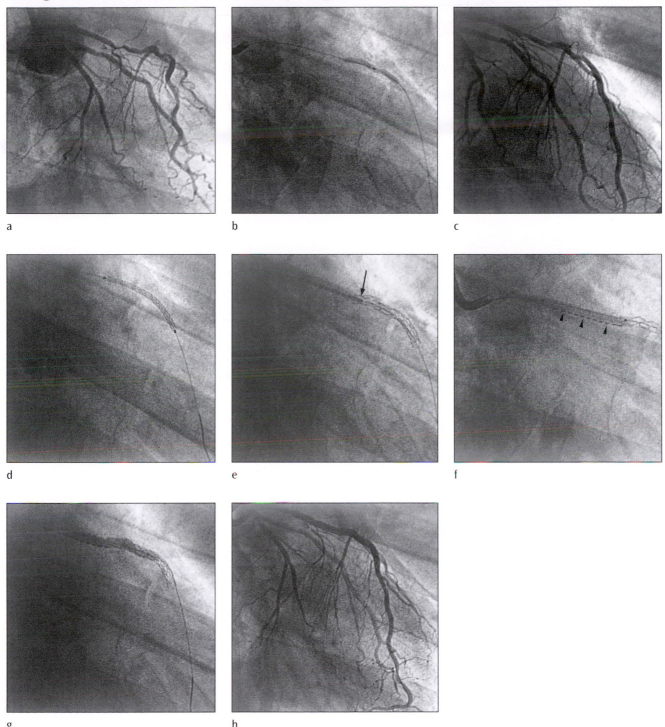

Figure 10.33

A 56-year-old man. (a) A long segment (55mm) of disease in the middle third of the LAD, which was also tortuous.

(b) A 2.5mm, 30mm long Elipse™ balloon was used to dilate the lesions with two separate inflations.

(c) Only a modest improvement was achieved.

(d) A 3.0mm, 39mm long Microstent™ was implanted over the distal half of the lesion.

(e, f) A 3.0mm, 24mm long Bard XT™ stent was implanted over the proximal half of the lesion. Care was taken to ensure overlapping of the two stents (arrow). The characteristic radio-opaque spine of the Bard XT™ stent is clearly visible (arrowheads).

(g) The long balloon was then advanced within the Microstent™ to dilate the two stents and the overlap.

After further dilatation at intervals along the stents with a 3.0mm, 20mm long Samba™ balloon up to 14 atmospheres, the final angiographic appearance (h) is excellent.

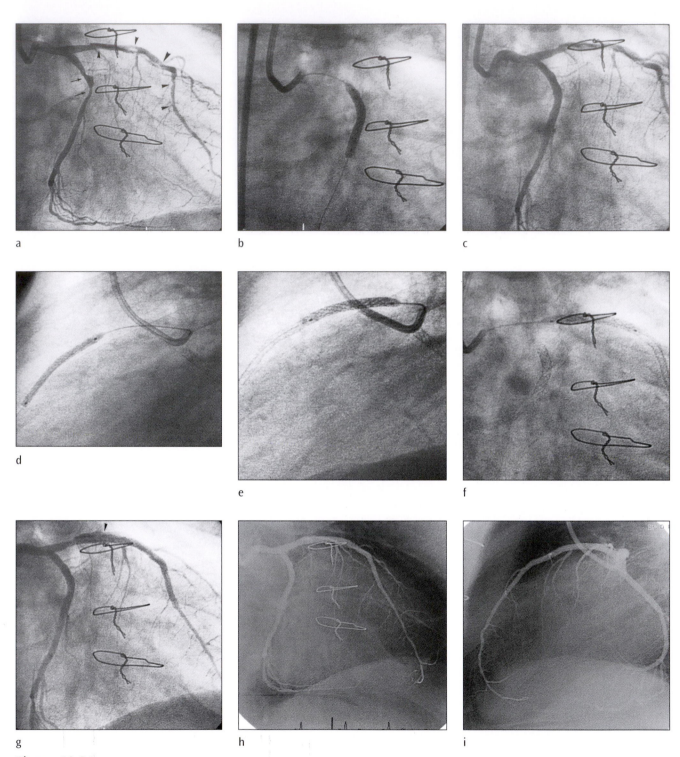

a

b

c

d

e

f

g

h

i

Figure 10.34

A 49-year-old man with unstable angina 5 years after CABG surgery was found to have (a) an occluded OMCx SVG, a severe stenosis of the RCA SVG as well as severe disease in the proximal LCx (arrows) and a series of significant lesions in the LAD (arrowheads).

Since the first OMCx and the distal RCA appeared diffusely diseased, the cardiac surgeons considered that he was suitable only for grafting the left internal mammary artery to the LAD. It was decided to attempt PTCA and stenting to the LAD, the LCx and the SVG to the RCA.

The LCx was crossed with an 0.014-inch Floppy® guidewire and (b) 'primarily stented' without pre-dilatation with a 3.5mm, 32mm long NIRoyal™ stent.

(c) This gave a good result.

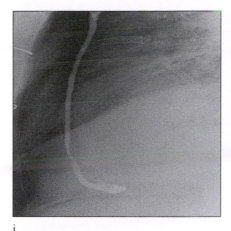

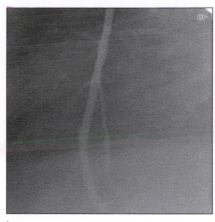

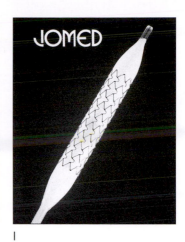

j

k

l

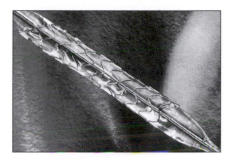

m

Figure 10.34 *continued*

The LAD lesions were crossed with a 0.014-inch Floppy® guidewire and pre-dilated with a 2.5mm, 20mm long Rocket™ balloon.

(d) A 3.0mm, 35mm long Crossflex™ stent was deployed over the distal lesions.

(e, f) This stent was overlapped with a 3.0mm, 32mm long NIRoyal™ stent over the proximal lesions.

A 3.5mm, 16mm long JoStent® flex stent was placed most proximally and the 'overlaps' were post-dilated up to 15 atmospheres with a 3.0mm, 20mm long Worldpass™ balloon.

(g) The final result was excellent. A small diagonal vessel (arrowhead) exits the most proximal stent, giving the appearance of a dissection. However, other views confirm that this is not the case (h, i).

(j) The stenosis in the RCA SVG underwent 'primary stenting' with a 3.0mm, 19mm long Jostent® flex stent.

(k) This gave an excellent result. The Jostent® flex stent (l) and the Crossflex™ stent (m) are shown.

Stents in small vessels

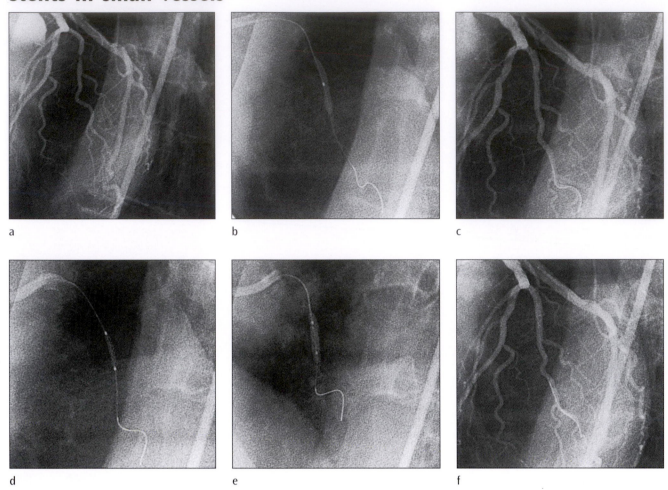

a   b   c

d   e   f

Figure 10.35

A 65-year-old lady with moderate angina. (a) There was a severe discrete stenosis in the middle third of the diagonal branch of LAD.

(b) The lesion was pre-dilated with a 2.5mm Elipse™ balloon.

   Because of significant recoil (c), the lesion was stented with a 2.5mm, 12mm long Microstent II™ (d, e).

(f) Final result.

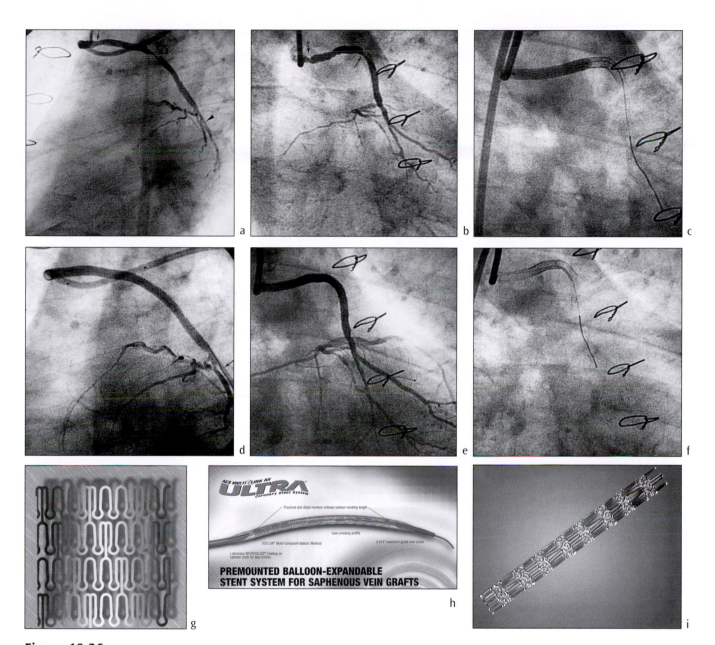

Figure 10.36

A 61-year-old retired bus driver presented with unstable angina 7 years after CABG surgery.

The OMCx SVG was found to have a significant proximal and a severe mid-third stenosis (arrows), but severe disease in the native OMCx just beyond the insertion point of the graft (arrowhead) – (a) LLAT projection; (b) RAO projection.

The lesions were crossed with a 0.014-inch Floppy® guidewire. The mid-third SVG lesion and the stenosis in the native vessel were pre-dilated with a 2.0mm Adante™ balloon and a 2.0mm, 10mm long divYsio™ SV PC-coated stent (Biocompatibles) was placed over the distal stenosis in the native vessel. The mid-third SVG lesion was then dilated with a 3.0mm Freeway® (JoMed) balloon and a 3.5mm, 18mm long Ultra™ stent (Guidant) was deployed to this site.

(c) A 3.5mm, 28mm long Ultra™ stent was then deployed more proximally (overlapping) and a third 4.0mm, 28mm long Ultra™ stent placed proximal to this and covering the ostium of the SVG.

The final result was excellent and shows improved distal run-off with much improvement in the segment of stented native vessel (arrow) – (d) LLAT projection; (e) RAO projection.

(f) The Ultra™ stent is very radio-opaque by virtue of its high metal-artery ratio (19% for a 3.5mm stent).

(g, h) The high wall coverage is ideal for implantation in SVGs and the Ultra™-smooth surface transitions and crimping process and the flexible delivery system enhance its passage through tight lesions.

The divYsio™ PC stent (i) is coated with phosphorylcholine to help reduce thrombosis.

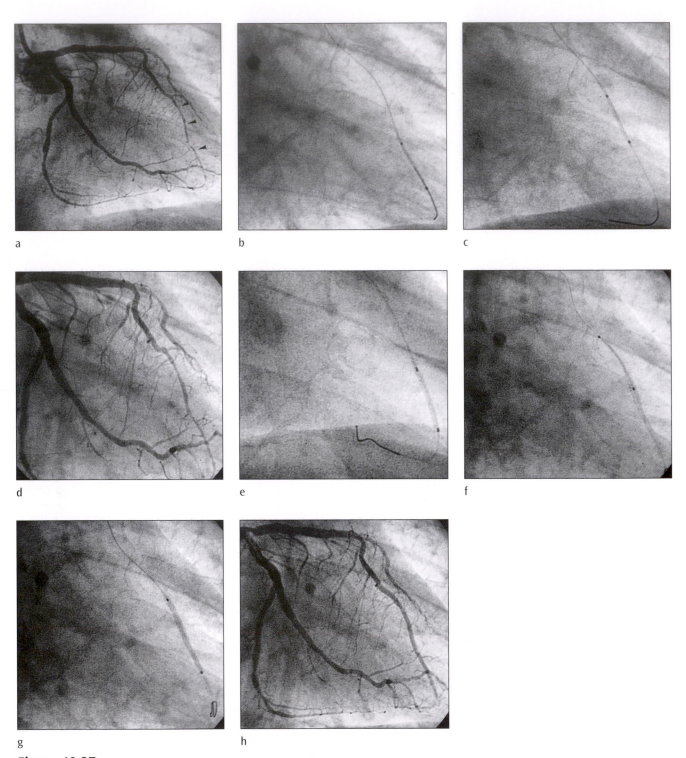

Figure 10.37

A 52-year-old man with moderately severe angina had previously undergone Rotablator® atherectomy to the OMCx 4 years earlier with a good angiographic and clinical result. (a) However, he had now developed diffuse disease in the distal half of the LAD, which measured approximately 1.6mm in diameter (arrowheads).

(b, c) The whole segment was pre-dilated with a 1.5mm Rocket™ balloon.

(d) This produced a marginal improvement.

(e) A 2.0mm, 18mm long divYsio™ Penchant SV™ stent was placed distally.

(f, g) A 2.5mm, 23mm long Duet™ stent was then placed more proximally to overlap the two stents and a further 2.5mm, 28mm long Duet® stent was placed more proximally again.

(h) The angiographic result was good.

Restenosis is more of a problem in stented small vessels than in stented vessels of 3mm in diameter or more. Randomized clinical trials such as the BESMART study are evaluating the benefits of stenting in small vessels (less than 3.0mm in diameter) compared with PTCA alone.

Stents after acute myocardial infarction

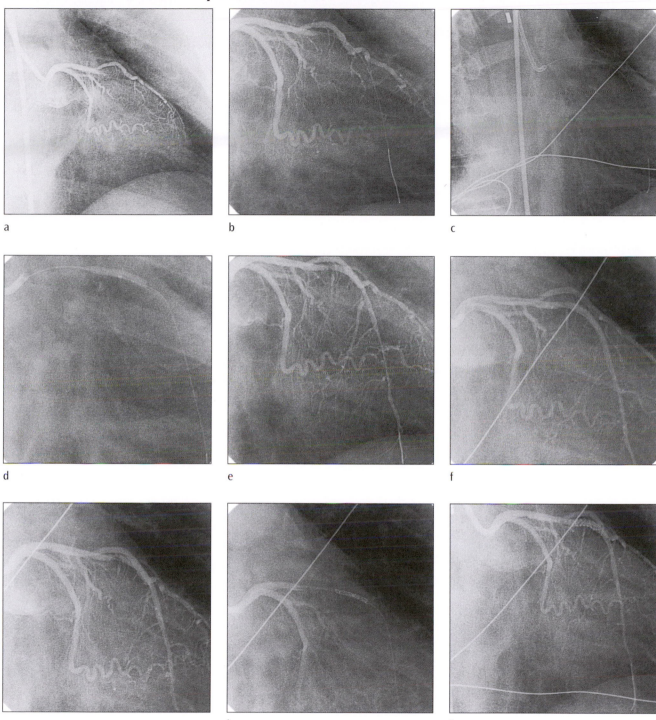

Figure 10.38

(a) An acute occlusion of the proximal and mid-LAD was associated with cardiogenic shock in this 64-year-old woman within 2 hours of an acute anterior myocardial infarction.

(b) Occlusion was easily crossed by a guidewire but with little antegrade flow.

(c) The intra-aortic balloon can be seen to be inflated and was essential in providing some haemodynamic stability once the vessel had been reopened and some blood pressure had been restored.

(d) PTCA was performed with a 3.0mm Samba™ balloon.

(e) Antegrade flow with distal spasm was now evident.

(f) After intracoronary glyceryl trinitrate, the spasm resolves and the flow improves.

(g) A residual stenosis was evident and the result became suboptimal (owing to recoil) within 5 minutes of the last inflation.

(h) A 3.0mm Wiktor® stent was carefully placed at the lesion site and deployed successfully.

This produced an excellent angiographic (i) and clinical result.

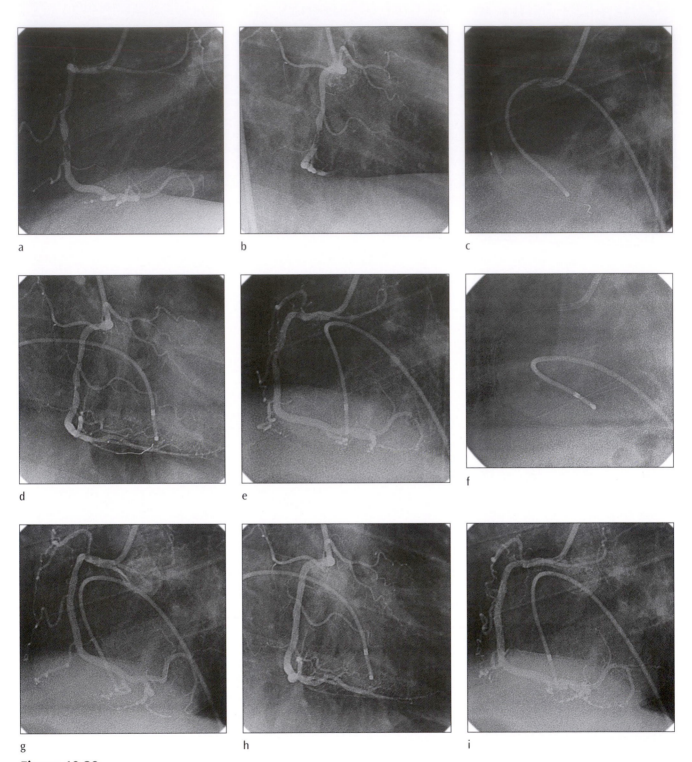

Figure 10.39

A 41-year-old social worker developed an acute inferior myocardial infarction while pushing his car. An ECG showed ST-segment elevation in the inferior leads and angiography showed acute subtotal occlusion of a dominant RCA. (a, b) There was a large thrombus that was producing severe flow limitation.

(c) The lesion was crossed with a 0.014-inch Floppy® guidewire and dilated with a 3.0mm Cheetah™ balloon.

(d) A significant residual stenosis was evident.

(e) Thrombus was also seen to have embolized into the distal posterolateral branch of the RCA.

(f) A 3.5mm, 30mm long Microstent II™ was implanted at the lesion site.

(g, h) This gave a good angiographic result.

(i) The distal thrombus resolved with the aid of 20mg of intracoronary rtPA.

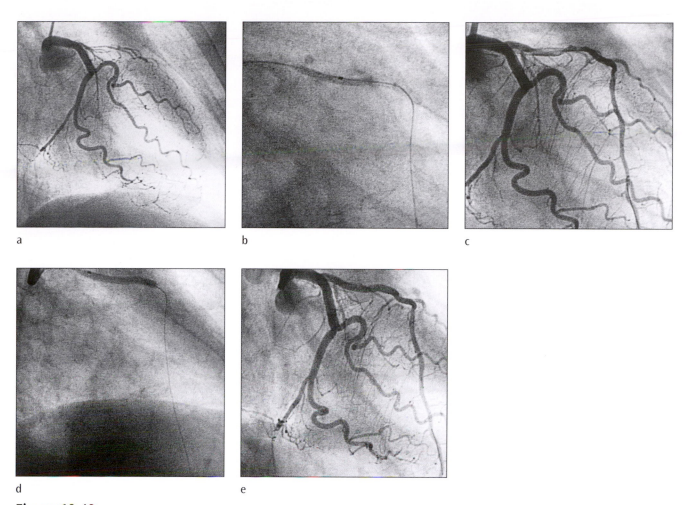

a b c

d e

Figure 10.40
This 82-year-old woman presented 3 weeks after the onset of severe chest pain and dyspnoea. The ECG and left ventricular angiogram suggested recent anteroseptal myocardial infarction. (a) Coronary arteriography showed a proximally occluded LAD. (b) The vessel was reopened with a 2.5mm Passage® balloon over a 0.014-inch Floppy® guidewire. (c) There appeared to be dissection at the lesion site. (d) A 3.0mm, 25mm long Multilink™ stent was implanted. (e) This gave an excellent angiographic and clinical result.

Use of stents in saphenous vein grafts

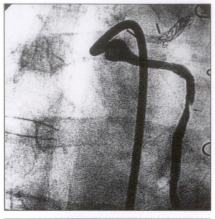 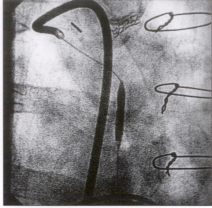 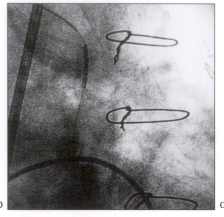

a   b   c

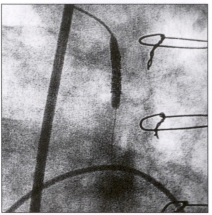 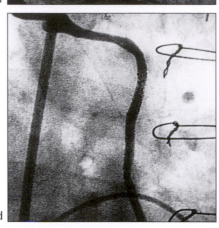

Figure 10.41
(a) This 9-year-old RCA SVG had an eccentric stenosis in the body of the graft.
(b) The stenosis was pre-dilated with a 3.5mm balloon.
(c) A Wiktor® stent was positioned and deployed (d).
(e) The final result is acceptable but would have been improved by a larger stent.

Note the presence of another Wiktor® stent in the aorta-ostial position of an OMCx SVG (a).

d   e

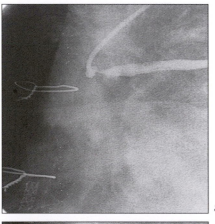 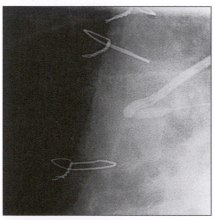 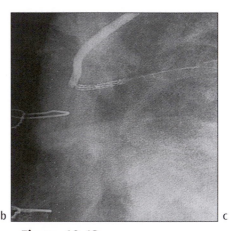

a   b   c

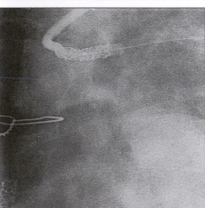 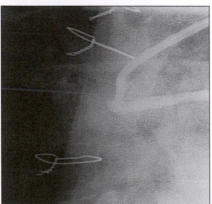

Figure 10.42
A 63-year-old male restaurateur had (a) a severe ostial stenosis in an 8-year-old LAD SVG, which was causing limiting angina.
(b) The stenosis was pre-dilated with a 3.5mm Elipse™ balloon.
(c, d) A 3.5mm Wiktor® stent was implanted with a good final result (e).

d   e

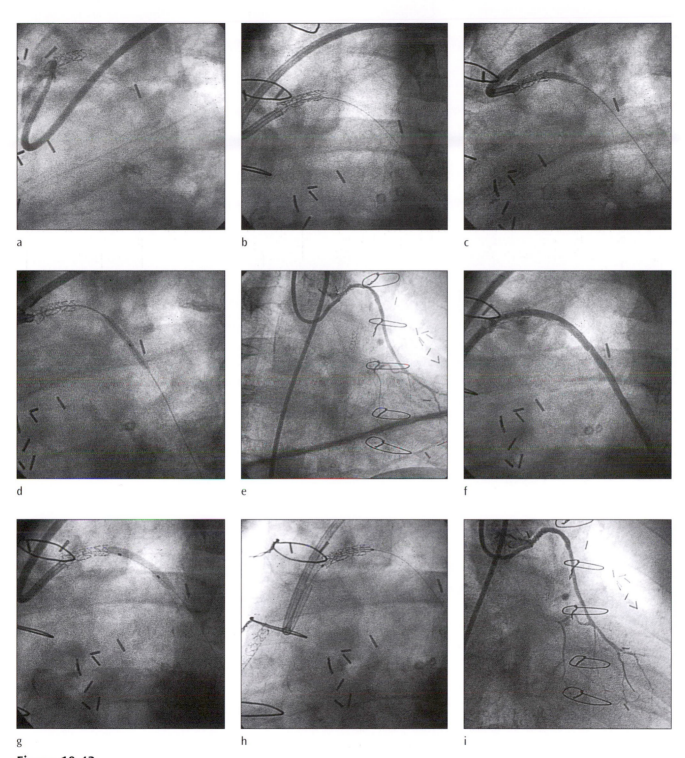

a

b

c

d

e

f

g

h

i

Figure 10.43

This 3.0mm Wiktor® stent in the aorta-ostial position of a 9-year-old OMCx SVG developed a restenosis within the stent 5 months after implant and was initially successfully dilated. (a) However within 2 months it had become totally occluded.

The graft was reopened by PTCA with a 2.0mm Goldie™ balloon within the stent (b, c) and along the length of the SVG (d).

(e) This produced a reasonable angiographic result after similar inflations with a 3.0mm Express NC™ balloon up to 18 atmospheres.

(f) However, there was local dissection within the proximal third of the graft.

This necessitated a 3.5mm Multilink™ stent implant (g), which was followed by the use of a 3.5mm, 18mm long Microstent™ within the Wiktor® stent (h).

(i) The final angiographic result.

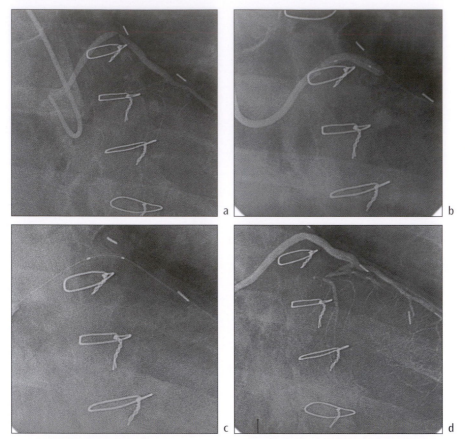

a   b

c   d

Figure 10.44
A 63-year-old ophthalmic surgeon had only mild angina but he had (a) a subtotal occlusion of an 11-year-old SVG to a diagonal branch of the LAD.
(b) The lesion was pre-dilated with a 3.0mm Cheetah™ balloon.
(c) A 4.0mm Multilink™ stent was implanted.
(d) Final result.

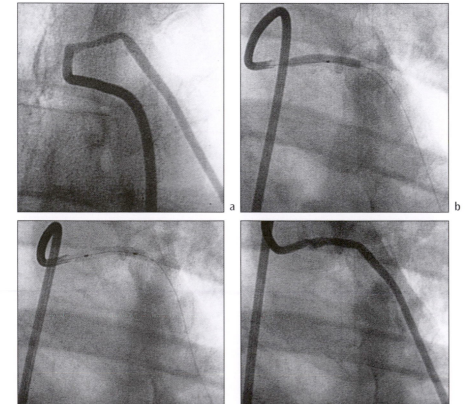

a   b

c   d

Figure 10.45
(a) A stenosis in the proximal third of an OMCx SVG in a 48-year-old man.
(b) The lesion was dilated with a 3.0mm Worldpass™ balloon.
(c) It was stented with a 3.5mm, 15mm long Multilink™ stent.
(d) This gave a good angiographic result.

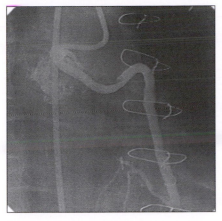

a

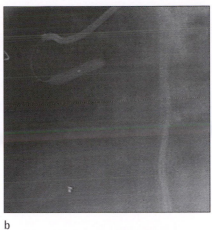

b

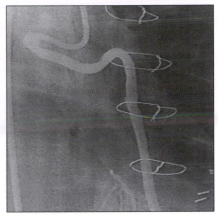

c

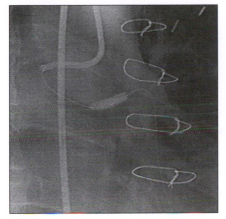

d

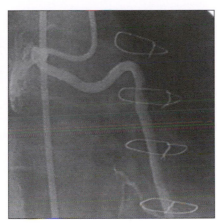

e

Figure 10.46
A 63-year-old man presented with sudden onset of severe chest pain 9 years after CABG surgery. (a) Angiography showed an eccentric lesion of the OMCx SVG with the appearance of a ruptured atherosclerotic plaque.
(b) The lesion was pre-dilated with a 3.0mm balloon.
(c) This produced some improvement.
(d) Two 7mm Palmaz-Schatz™ stents were then implanted.

This gave an excellent final result (e) and complete relief of symptoms.

Use of Wallstents for large SVGs

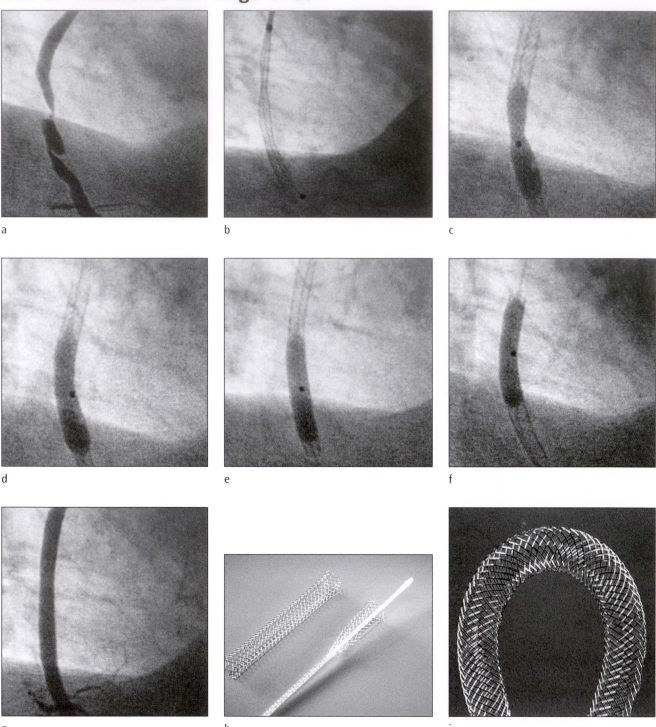

a

b

c

d

e

f

g

h

i

Figure 10.47

A 69-year-old man had had CABG surgery 9 years earlier. Recurrent angina was associated with (a) severe lesions in the body of an RCA SVG.

(b) The disease was stented with a 5.0mm, 47mm long Magic Wallstent™ without pre-dilatation.

The distal lesion was well dilated by the self-expanding action of the stent, whereas the proximal lesion was only moderately dilated.

(c, d) The proximal lesion was then dilated with a 4.5mm Bypass Speedy™ balloon at 12 atmospheres.

(e, f) The stent was dilated again distally and proximally.

(g) A good final result was achieved.

(h) The Wallstent™ self-expands as its restraining membrane is retracted.

(i) It is a mesh stent with a high metal-space ratio.

Courtesy of Dr U Sigwart, Royal Brompton Hospital, London, UK.

The WINS randomized trial established the equivalency of the Wallstent with the Palmaz-Schatz™ stent for the prevention of restenosis in patients with a de-novo or restenotic lesion in an SVG.

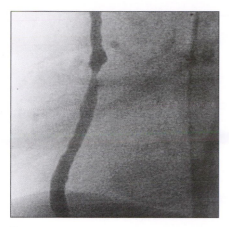

a

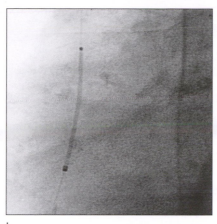

b

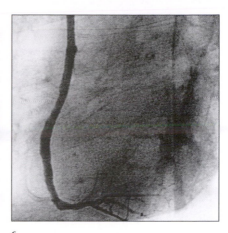

c

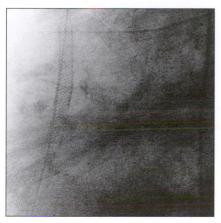

d

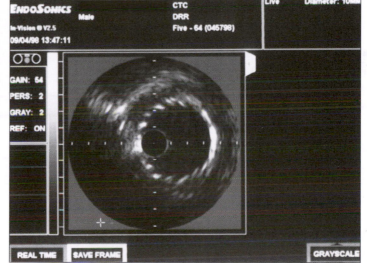

e

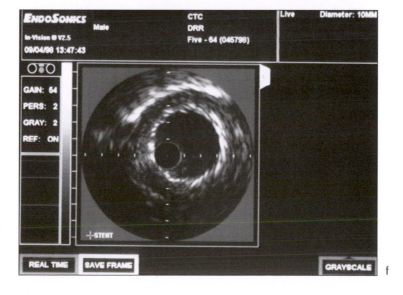

f

Figure 10.48

A 65-year-old man developed angina 8 years after CABG surgery.

(a) Angiography showed an eccentric stenosis in the middle third of the RCA SVG.

(b) The lesion was stented with a 4.5mm Magic Wallstent™ (3.5mm, 33mm long) without pre-dilatation.

Unfortunately, this self-expanding mesh stent shortens significantly on deployment and the distal edge of the stent appeared to be placed in the distal end of the stenosis.

It was decided to deploy a second shorter 4.5mm Magic Wallstent™ (3.5mm, 24mm long) distally and overlap the two stents.

(c) The stents were then post-dilated with a 4.5mm Speedy™ balloon at 12 atmospheres to produce an excellent final angiographic result.

(d) The stent is very radio-opaque.

(e) IVUS showed excellent concentric deployment of the stent with the typical appearance of the Wallstent™ with its obliquely positioned struts.

(f) IVUS over the overlap shows twice the number of struts.

Use of biliary stents for large SVGs

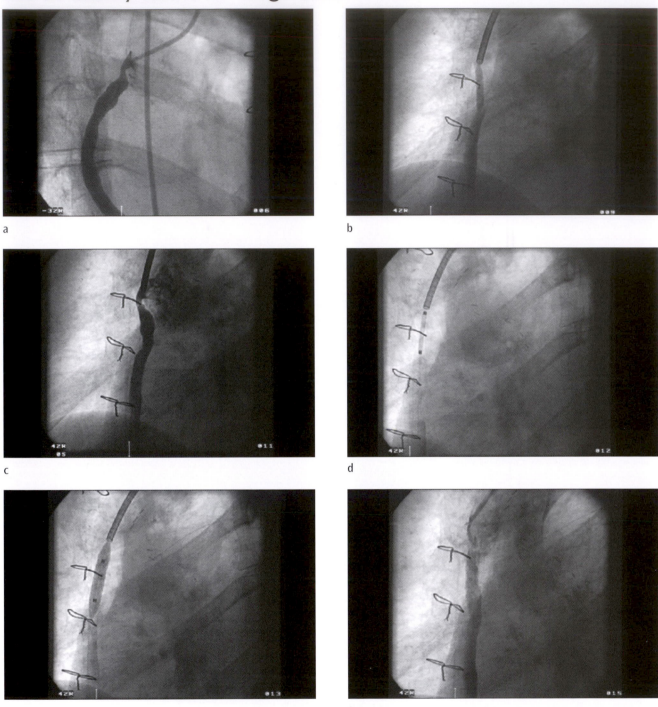

a

b

c

d

e

f

Figure 10.49

A 60-year-old male driving instructor presented with unstable angina 9 years after CABG surgery. (a) Angiography demonstrated a severe eccentric stenosis in the proximal third of a very large SVG to the RCA.

(b) With the use of a 10F guiding catheter, a 300cm, 0.014-inch extra-support guidewire was passed into the distal vessel and the lesion was pre-dilated with a 4.0mm Express™ balloon.

(c) A significant residual stenosis persisted.

(d) A Biliary stent (Johnson and Johnson) was therefore deployed on a 6mm Blue Max™ balloon (Boston Scientific) inflated to 14 atmospheres (e).

(f) Final angiographic result.

Courtesy of Drs P Schofield and P Ludman, Papworth Hospital, Cambridge, UK.

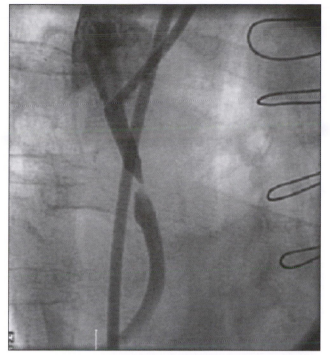

a

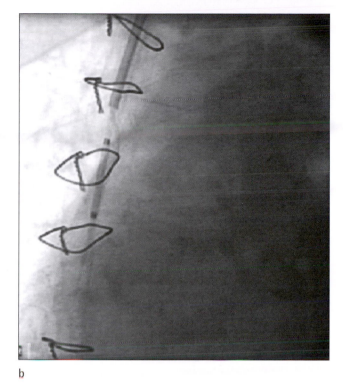

b

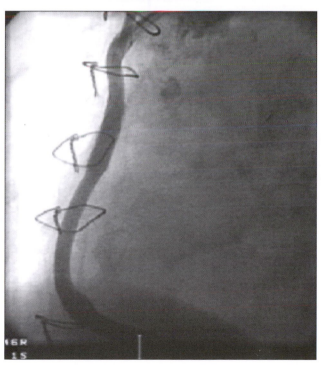

c

Figure 10.50

A 65-year-old retired prison officer presented with unstable angina 5 years after CABG surgery. (a) Angiography showed a severe stenosis in the proximal third of an RCA SVG.

(b) The lesion was pre-dilated with a 3.5mm Passage™ balloon and a Biliary stent (Johnson and Johnson) was deployed on a 5mm Blue Max™ balloon inflated to 14 atmospheres.

The stent was then dilated further with a 5mm Chubby™ balloon (Schneider) inflated to 16 atmospheres.

(c) Final result.

Courtesy of Drs P Schofield and P Ludman, Papworth Hospital, Cambridge, UK.

The SAVED trial showed that stenting of focal SVG lesions results in an improved event-free survival compared with PTCA despite similar angiographic restenosis rates.

Use of multiple stents in series in a single vessel

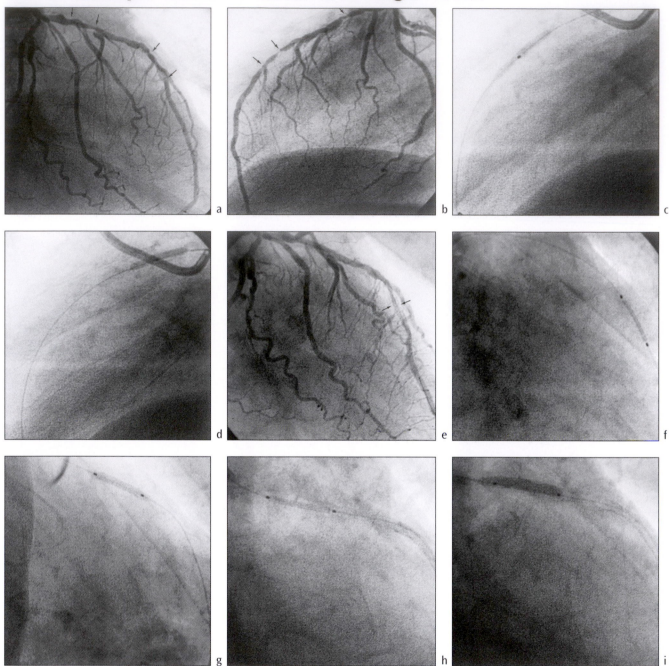

Figure 10.51

A 46-year-old banker with moderate angina. There was a diffusely irregular LAD with multiple stenoses in its proximal and middle third (arrows) – (a) RAO projection; (b) LLAT projection.

(c, d) The lesions were dilated with a 2.5mm, 20mm long balloon.

(e) Significant dissection occurred (arrows).

(f) A 2.75mm, 16mm long Paragon™ stent (Vascular Therapies) was deployed distally. This stent covered a diagonal branch that had ostial disease. A 3.0mm, 16mm long Paragon™ stent was deployed proximal to the first stent.

(g) A 3.0mm, 25mm long Multilink™ stent was then deployed proximal to the Paragon™ stent.

(h, i) A 3.0mm, 18mm long Microstent II™ was deployed most proximally in the LAD.

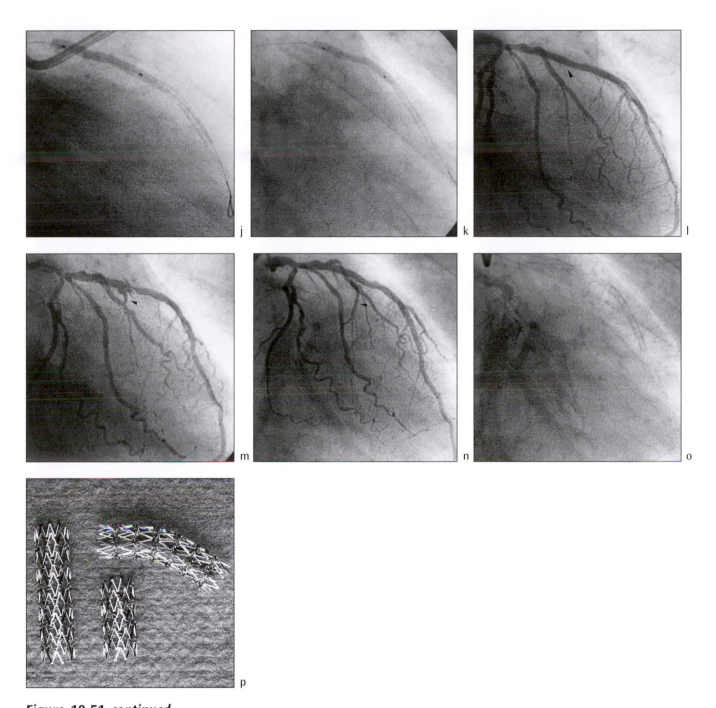

Figure 10.51 *continued*

(j, k) A 3.0mm, 40mm long Elipse™ balloon was then serially dilated along and within the stents.

(l) A septal branch with an ostial stenosis closed after deployment of the Multilink™ stent across it (arrowheads).

(m, n) However, this septal branch reopened (arrowheads) without any noticeable event or enzyme rise.

Care was taken to ensure that no 'gaps' existed between the stents by overlapping the individual stents end-to-end.

(o) The varied radio-opacity of the four stents is evident.

(p) The extremely flexible Paragon™ stent was made of nitinol and was the successor to the ACT-1™ stent. It was radio-opaque and strong and came well crimped on its delivery balloon. It has now been discontinued.

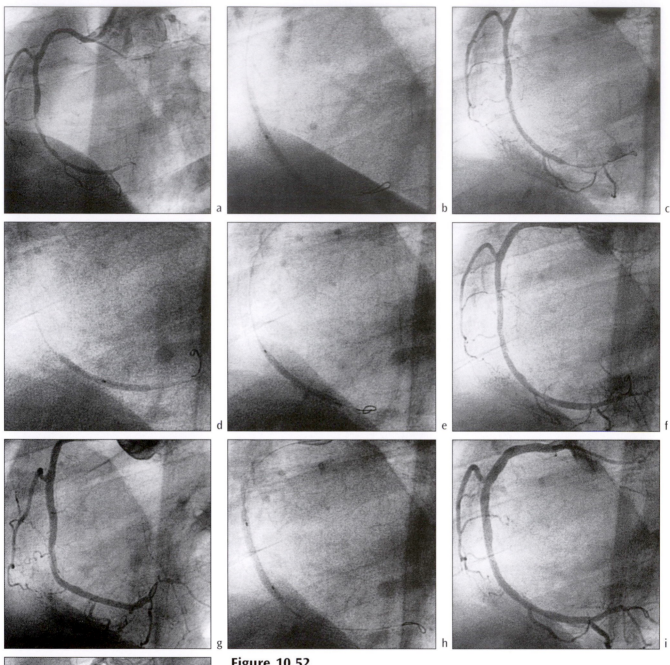

Figure 10.52

(a) A subtotally occluded RCA in a 53-year-old man with severe angina.

(b, c) The occlusion was crossed with an 0.014-inch Floppy® guidewire with the backup support of a 2.5mm, 30mm long Elipse™ balloon.

After PTCA with the long balloon more distally (d), the vessel was stented with a 2.5mm, 32mm long NIR™ stent placed at the crux (e–g) and a 3.0mm, 25mm long Multilink™ stent placed more proximally (h, i).

(j) The stents are overlapped slightly to ensure that no 'gaps' exist between them and a good final result is produced.

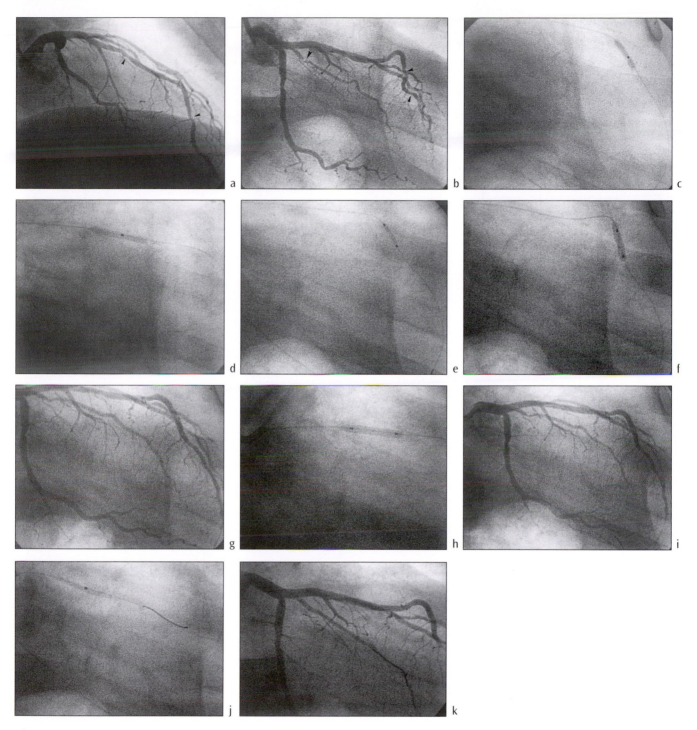

Figure 10.53

A 47-year-old architect with severe unstable angina after myocardial infarction. (a) There is a 70% stenosis in the proximal LAD (arrow) and a 75% lesion beyond an acute bend (arrow).

(b) The intermediate artery had a significant proximal lesion (arrow). There are two lesions in the LAD that are located distally (arrows).

(c) The distal LAD lesions were dilated with a 2.5mm Worldpass™ balloon.

(d) The proximal lesion was dilated with a 3.0mm Worldpass™ balloon.

(e, f) A 2.5mm, 12mm long Microstent II™ was placed in one of the more distal lesions.

(g) This produced a good result.

(h) A 3.0mm, 16mm long NIR™ stent was placed in the proximal lesion.

(i) This produced a similarly good result.

(j) The stenosis in the intermediate artery was dilated with a 2.0mm Worldpass™ balloon.

(k) This too produced a good result. Stenting was not necessary.

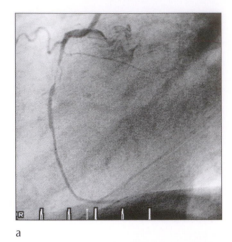

a

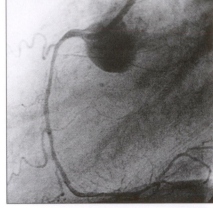

b

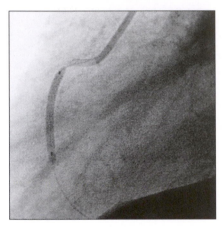

c

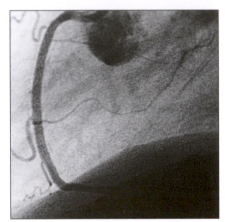

d

Figure 10.54

A 48-year-old man with limiting stable angina was found to have (a) a subtotal occlusion of the proximal RCA.

A 0.014-inch Floppy® guidewire crossed the stenosis with the support of a 2.0mm Adante® balloon.

(b) There was improvement after dilatation with the 2.0mm balloon.

(c) The artery was then stented with a 2.5mm, 32mm long NIRoyal™ stent proximally.

A 2.5mm, 18mm long Duet™ stent was delivered through the first stent and placed at its distal end, overlapping the two stents.

(d) The final result was excellent.

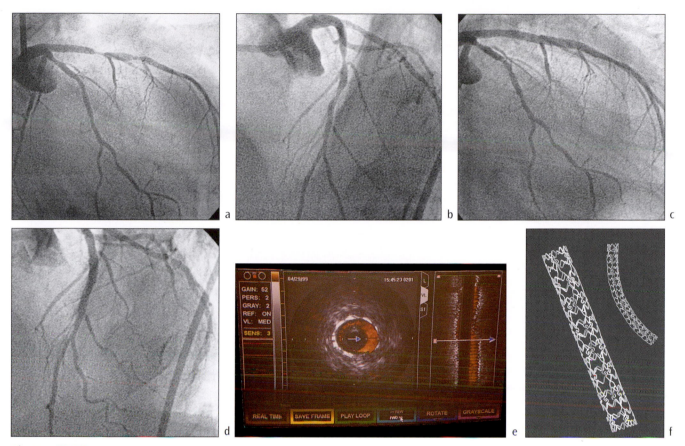

Figure 10.55

A 72-year-old man with uncontrolled angina. (a, b) There is a severe proximal LAD stenosis and a less severe stenosis in the middle third of the LAD.

IVUS showed quite marked, deep calcification in the proximal stenosis; however, this was not superficial enough to warrant rotational atherectomy. The lesions were both dilated with a 3.0mm Worldpass™ balloon. The distal lesion was then stented with a 3.5mm, 26mm long JoStent® flex stent and a 3.5mm, 16mm long JoStent® flex stent was placed over the proximal lesion overlapping the stents.

(c, d) Both stents were post-dilated with a 3.5mm, 9mm long Maxxum™ balloon up to 18 atmospheres with an excellent angiographic result.

(e) IVUS using the In-Vision Chromaflo™ facility (EndoSonics) clearly showed full stent deployment with good strut apposition and excellent blood flow between the stent struts and the central catheter artefact.

(f) The geometric design of the JoStent® flex stent is shown. The cells are connected with unique spiral bridges and the stent is designed to combine flexibility with high radial strength.

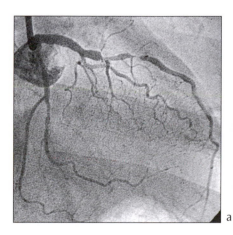
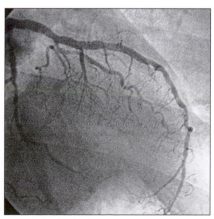

Figure 10.56

A 60-year-old man with rest pain and ST-segment depression in leads V1–V6 had (a) a long segment of severe disease in the proximal and middle thirds of the LAD.

The lesions were dilated with a 2.5mm and then a 3.0mm Vital™ balloon (Blue Medical) and stented with a 4.0mm, 25mm long Phytis™ stent (Phytis).

The stent was post-dilated with a 4.0mm, 9mm long Maxxum™ balloon at 12 atmospheres.

(b) This gave a good angiographic result.

Variations in the radio-opacity of stents

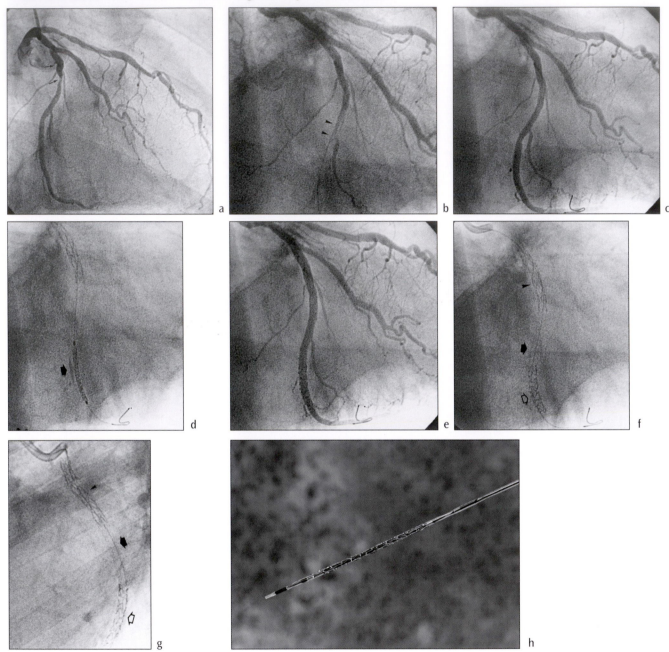

Figure 10.57
A 50-year-old man with moderately severe angina had undergone Rotablator® atherectomy to the LAD and OMCx 2 years earlier. (a) He was found to have two significant stenoses in the LCx itself (arrows) but there was no significant restenosis in the vessels previously addressed.

(b) The lesion in the mid-third was dilated first with a 3.0mm Seajet® (Nycomed) balloon, which resulted in distal occlusive coronary dissection (arrowheads).

After dilatation of the proximal lesion, a 3.0mm, 25mm long Multilink™ stent was placed in the middle third with marked angiographic improvement and restoration of distal flow.

(c) The proximal segment was stented with a 3.5mm, 30mm long Microstent II™ with a similar excellent result.

(d) However, there appeared to be a small dissection beyond the distal end of the Multilink stent (arrow).

A 3.0mm, 16mm long Wiktor-i™ stent was therefore passed through the first two stents and placed distally.

This gave an excellent angiographic (e) and clinical result.

(f, g) The varied radio-opacity of the three stents can be appreciated. The centrally placed Multilink stent is barely visible (broad arrow), whereas the Microstent™ (arrowhead) is more obvious and the tantalum Wiktor-i™ stent (open arrow) is very radio-opaque.

(h) The Wiktor-i™ stent is shown crimped on to its rapid-exchange balloon catheter. However, it has been superseded by more modern stents that are just as flexible and provide better wall coverage.

Radio-opaque stents to aid accurate overlapping of two stents

The use of radio-opaque stents to aid accurate overlapping of
two stents is shown in Fig. 4.28.

11

Intracoronary stenting II: complex stenting techniques

Over the past few years, as technology has developed and low-profile, modern machine-crimped stents have become available to interventional cardiologists, difficult anatomy and complex lesion morphology are no longer absolute contraindications to stenting. Thus, patients who have multilesion or multivessel disease, including bifurcation lesions, ostial lesions, total occlusions, SVG disease or any combination of these unfavourable characteristics can now be treated by PTCA and coronary stenting with the use of complex techniques that often involve other technologies.

Such cases are frequently challenging and they demand patience and special expertise and an understanding from the outset on the part of the patient that staged procedures may be required for safety and that further procedures may be required for long-term success. Procedures are usually associated with prolonged radiation exposure to the operator, and this may become an important issue for high-volume interventionists.

CABG surgery will often be a real alternative for these patients. However, if PTCA and stenting are successful, they should have a lower operative morbidity, require a shorter hospital stay and be associated with a more rapid return to normal activity. Moreover, the waiting time to receive catheter-based intervention will be shorter than the waiting time for surgery.

Multivessel stenting

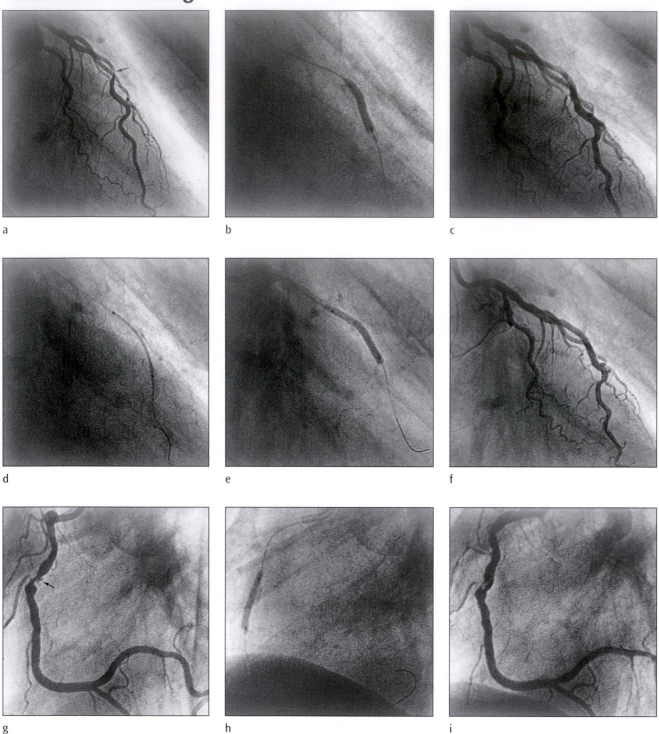

a

b

c

d

e

f

g

h

i

Figure 11.1

A 62-year-old artist had a severe, discrete lesion on a bend in the mid-LAD and an ulcerated complex stenosis in the proximal RCA. (a) The LAD stenosis (arrow) was addressed first.

(b) The lesion was crossed with a 0.014-inch Floppy® guidewire and dilated with a 2.5mm Activa™ balloon (Scimed).

(c) Although there was improvement there was local dissection.

(d, e) A 3.0mm, 32mm long NIR™ stent was implanted, since the disease appeared to extend above the lesion site.

(f) The final angiographic result was excellent.

(g) A floppy guidewire would not cross the lesion in the RCA but continued to enter the ulcerated plaque (arrow). A 0.014-inch Intermediate® guidewire crossed the lesion and then the RCA became occluded.

(h) However, it was possible to reopen the vessel with a 2.5mm Activa™ balloon followed by a 3.0mm Worldpass™ balloon.

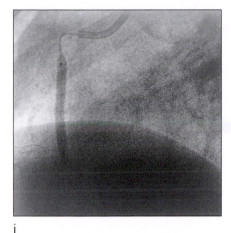

j

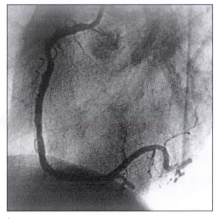

k

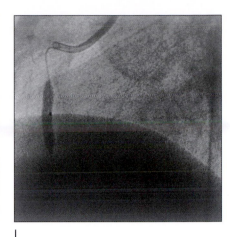

l

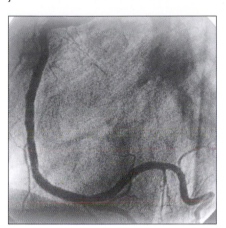

m

Figure 11.1 *continued*

(i) The stenosis had been abolished but there was clearly material occluding the lumen of the RCA.

(j) A 3.5mm, 32mm long NIR™ stent was therefore implanted.

(k) This gave a good angiographic result.

(l) A 4.0mm Viva™ balloon was then dilated within the stent up to 6 atmospheres.

(m) This yielded an excellent final result.

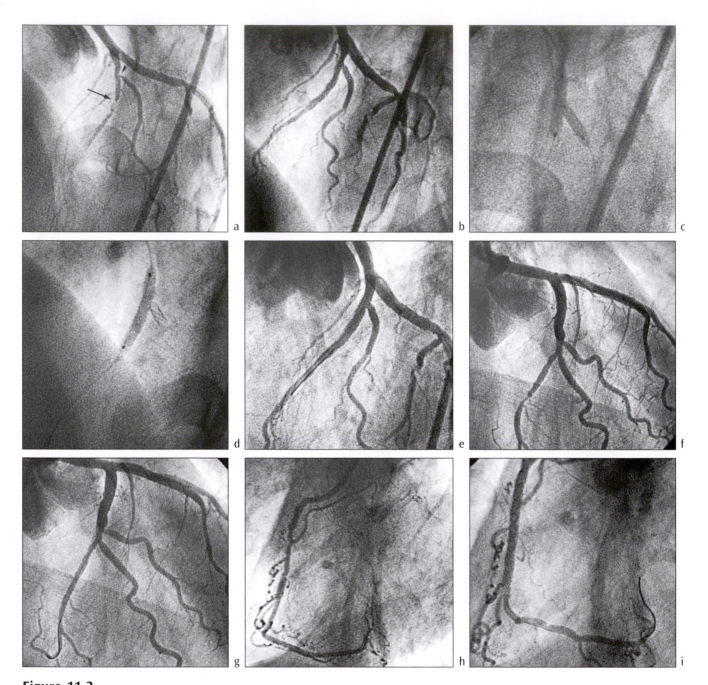

Figure 11.2
A 59-year-old minister had a 3-month history of unstable angina and a 1-week history of rest pain without ECG changes. (a) Coronary angiography showed an occluded LAD (arrow) and a severe first DG ostial stenosis (arrowhead).

The angiograms also showed a severe LCx stenosis and a long segment of moderately severe disease in the RCA.

(a) The LAD occlusion was crossed with a 0.014-inch Intermediate® guidewire and the vessel was reopened with a 2.5mm Adante™ balloon. The ostium of the first DG was similarly dilated with a 2.5mm Adante™ balloon over a 0.014-inch Floppy® guidewire. (b) This produced a good result. The mid-LAD was stented with a 3.0mm, 16mm long JoStent® flex stent. (c) The ostium of the first DG was then stented with a 2.5mm, 9mm long NIRoyal™ stent with a 3.0mm Freeway™ balloon positioned in the LAD across the ostium of the first DG in an attempt to prevent struts being deposited in the lumen of LAD.

After removal of the guidewire from the first DG, the LAD was stented across the ostium of the first DG using a 3.0mm, 23mm long Duet Multilink™ stent.

(d) It can be seen that the ostium of the first DG is not totally covered by the NIRoyal™ stent because of the acute angle of take-off of the first DG from the LAD. After further dilatation of the ostium of the first DG via the side wall of the Duet Multilink™ stent in the LAD and further dilatation of the Multilink™ stent with a 3.0mm balloon at high pressure, the final result was considered acceptable (e). (f) The LCx stenosis was dilated with a 2.0mm Adante™ balloon over a 0.014-inch Floppy® guidewire and stented with a 2.0mm, 10mm long PC-coated divYsio™ SV stent. (g) This produed a good result. (h) Finally, the long segment of disease in the RCA was crossed with a 0.014-inch Floppy® guidewire and dilated with a 2.5mm Adante™ balloon and stented with a 2.5mm, 18mm long GFX™ stent in its middle third, and a 2.5mm, 12mm long GFX™ stent was placed more proximally with stent overlap. (i) After post-dilatation of the stents up to 13 atmospheres, the angiographic result was excellent.

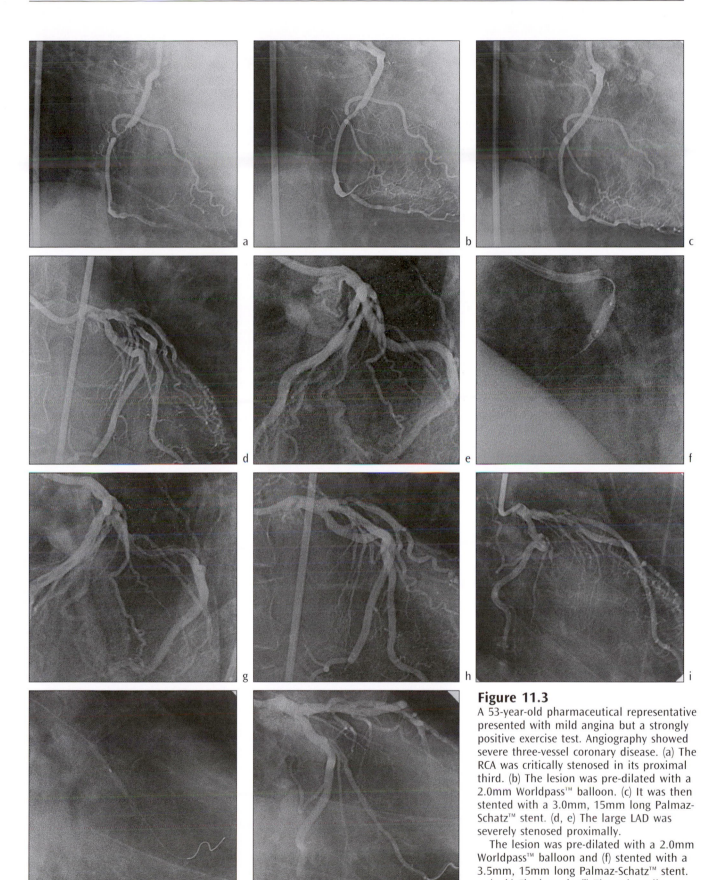

Figure 11.3

A 53-year-old pharmaceutical representative presented with mild angina but a strongly positive exercise test. Angiography showed severe three-vessel coronary disease. (a) The RCA was critically stenosed in its proximal third. (b) The lesion was pre-dilated with a 2.0mm Worldpass™ balloon. (c) It was then stented with a 3.0mm, 15mm long Palmaz-Schatz™ stent. (d, e) The large LAD was severely stenosed proximally.

The lesion was pre-dilated with a 2.0mm Worldpass™ balloon and (f) stented with a 3.5mm, 15mm long Palmaz-Schatz™ stent.

(g, h) Final result. (i) The subtotally occluded OMCx was reopened by PTCA with serial inflations with a 2.5mm, 30mm long Elipse™ balloon (j). (k) Final result shows dissection proximally but good anterograde flow and an improved angiographic result.

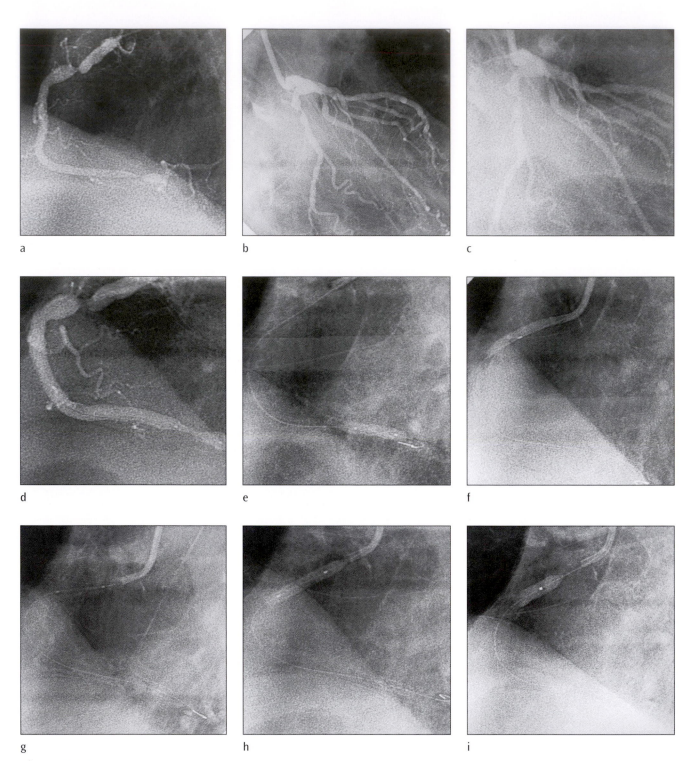

a

b

c

d

e

f

g

h

i

Figure 11.4

A 64-year-old retired police officer had a 4-week history of severe limiting angina. His exercise stress test showed ST-segment elevation in leads II, III and aVF and ST-segment depression in leads V1-V5. (a) Coronary arteriography showed a severe stenosis in the proximal third of a large, dominant RCA and a critical stenosis just above the crux.

(b, c) A large intermediate artery and the LCx also had severe eccentric stenoses proximally.

(d, e) The distal RCA stenosis was dilated with a 3.5mm Samba™ balloon and a 3.5mm, 12mm long GFX™ stent was implanted (because of recoil), with a good result.

(f–h) The proximal lesion was dilated with a 3.5mm Samba™ balloon and because of significant recoil a 4.0mm NIR™ stent on a Primo Viva™ balloon was deployed.

(i) This was post-dilated with a 5.0mm Chubby™ balloon.

j

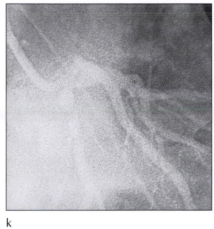

k

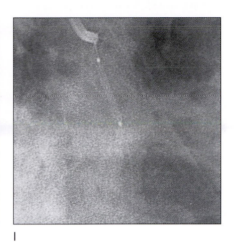

l

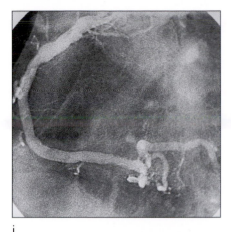

m

Figure 11.4 *continued*

(j) Final result.

The intermediate artery stenosis was then dilated with a 3.0mm Samba™ balloon and a 3.0mm, 12mm long GFX™ stent was implanted.

(k) Good final result.

Finally, the LCx stenosis was dilated with a 3.0mm Passage™ balloon over an intermediate guidewire and a 3.0mm, 18mm long GFX™ stent was then passed around a sharp bend in the proximal LCx (l) and deployed with a good angiographic result (m).

Flexible stents such as the GFX™ stent are essential for tracking around sharp angulated segments.

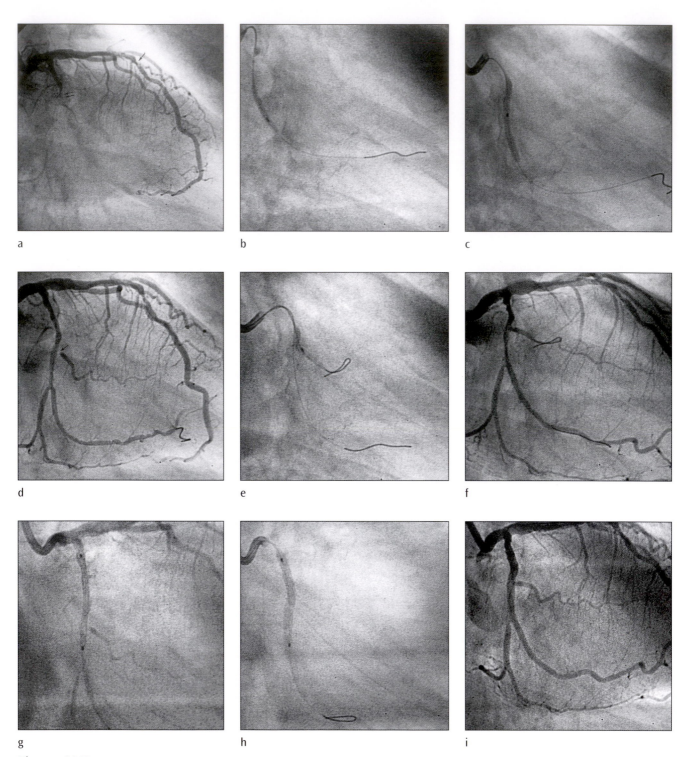

a
b
c
d
e
f
g
h
i

Figure 11.5

This 56-year-old female general practitioner with limiting angina had (a) an occluded LCx (arrows) and a severe stenosis in the mid-LAD (arrow).

There was also significant proximal disease in the RCA.

The strategy was to attempt to reopen the LCx by PTCA and to stent the vessel electively, then to perform PTCA and stent implantation to the LAD lesion at one session, and finally to perform PTCA and possible stent implantation to the RCA at a second session 2 weeks later.

The LCx occlusion proved difficult to cross.

(b) Once the distal vessel was entered with a floppy guidewire, the artery was opened with a 2.0mm Samba® balloon serially inflated along its length.

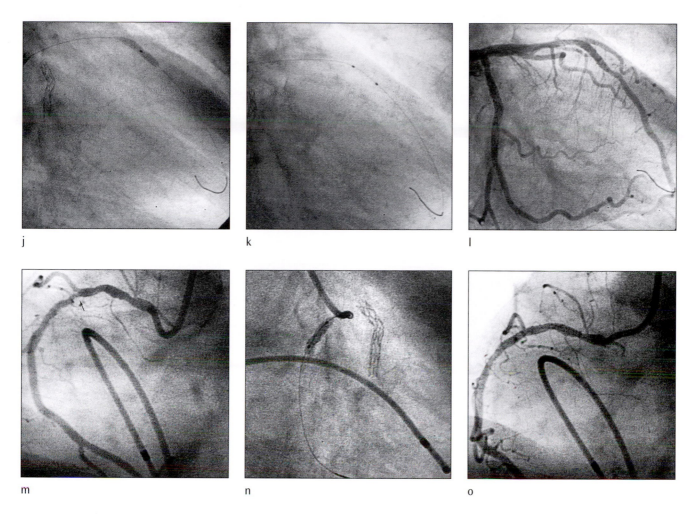

j   k   l

m   n   o

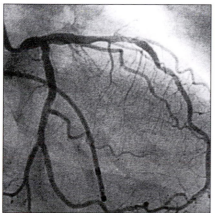

p

Figure 11.5 *continued*

(c) This was followed by a 2.5mm, 30mm long Elipse balloon.
This gave a very good result with local dissection.
(d) An OMCx was revealed that had a tight ostial stenosis.
(e) The OMCx was dilated with a 2.0mm Samba™ balloon with a good result (f).
(g, h) The LCx was stented with a 3.0mm, 39mm long Microstent™.
(i) Result.
(j) The LAD stenosis was dilated with a 3.0mm Elipse™ balloon and (k, l) a 3.0mm, 15mm long Multilink™ stent was then implanted with an excellent result.
(m) Two weeks later, the most severe lesion in the proximal RCA (arrow) was dilated with a 2.5mm Passage® balloon via a 6F guiding catheter.
(n) Because of recoil, a 2.5mm, 12mm long Microstent™ was implanted.
(o) Final result.
(p) The LAD and LCx were unchanged.

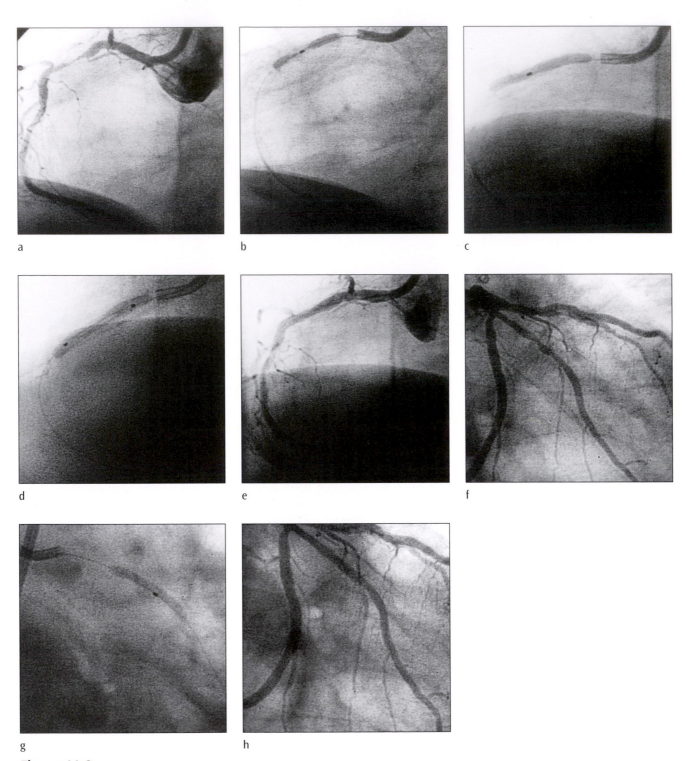

Figure 11.6
A 50-year-old butcher with cold-induced angina had significant disease in the RCA and intermediate artery.

The severe stenosis in the proximal RCA (a) did not dilate at 10 atmospheres (b) but yielded at 11 atmospheres with a 2.5mm Express™ balloon (c).

Ventricular fibrillation followed balloon deflation.

(d) A 3.0mm, 18mm long Microstent™ was then implanted with significant improvement (e).

The intermediate artery stenosis (f) was crossed with a 0.014-inch TEC° guidewire and dilated with the same 2.5mm Express™ balloon.

(g) Because of residual stenosis a 3.0mm, 15mm long Palmaz-Schatz™ stent was implanted with an excellent angiographic result (h).

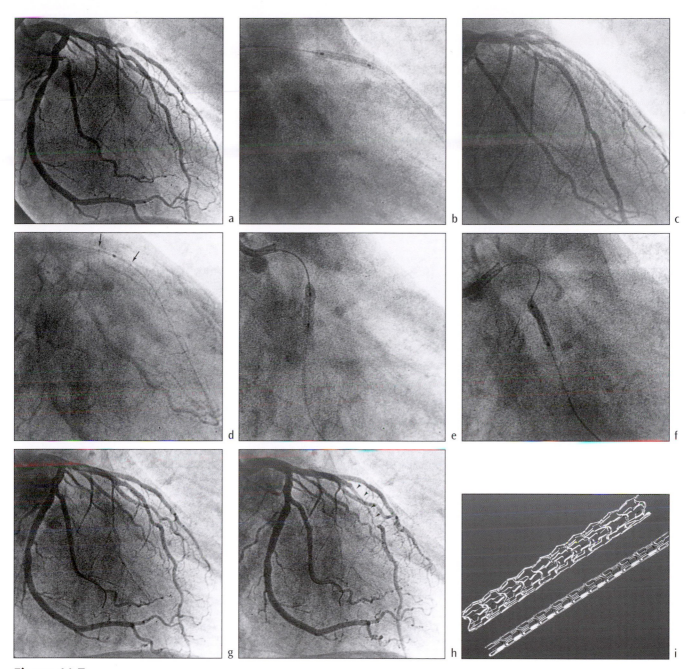

Figure 11.7

A 59-year-old man with mild stable angina. (a) He had a severe stenosis in the proximal LAD at the origin of the second septal branch and in the large first diagonal artery. There was also a significant eccentric lesion in the LCx and a severe lesion in the proximal third of the OMCx. The OMCx lesion was situated on a sharp bend.

(b) The diagonal stenosis was pre-dilated with a 2.5mm Worldpass™ balloon over a 0.014-inch Floppy® guidewire and stented with a 2.5mm, 16mm long NIR™ stent.

(c) The LAD stenosis is best seen in the caudal RAO projection.

(d) This stenosis was pre-dilated with a 3.0mm Worldpass™ balloon and stented with a 3.0mm, 15mm long beStent™ (Medtronic). Note the radio-opaque markers (arrows) on either end of the stent and the balloon's central marker.

(e) The LCx was then stented with a 12mm long 3.5mm GFX™ stent without pre-dilatation.

(f) The OMCx stenosis was crossed with a 0.014-inch Intermediate® guidewire, pre-dilated with a 2.0mm and then a 2.5mm Worldpass™ balloon and stented with a 18mm long 2.5mm GFX™ stent.

(g) There was a good final result.

(h) The LAD had a long segment of myocardial bridging beyond its proximal lesion, and it is clearly visible in systole (arrows). The LAD stent stops short of this segment.

(i) The beStent™ has two radio-opaque terminal gold markers to make the ends of the stent visible for precise positioning.

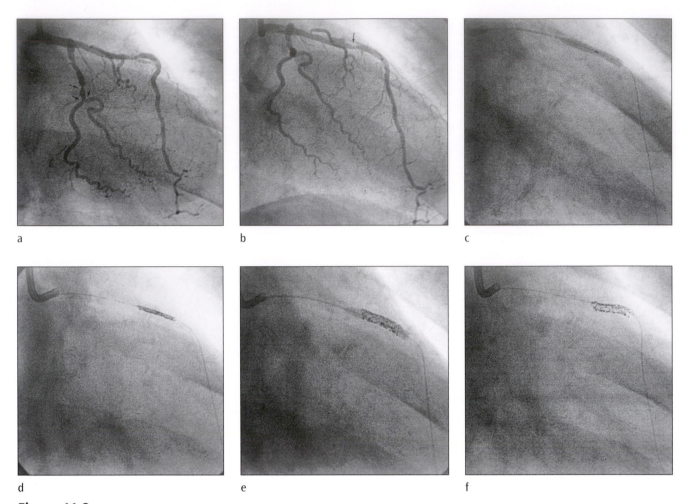

a

b

c

d

e

f

Figure 11.8

A 59-year-old woman with severe angina. (a, b) There are significant stenoses in the LAD, in the proximal LCx and at the AVCx and OMCx bifurcation point (arrows).

(c) The LAD stenosis was dilated with a 3.0mm Cruiser II® balloon and (d, e) stented with a 3.0mm Angiostent® (Nycomed).

(f) The stent is very radio-opaque.

(g) The LCx and the OMCx were dilated with a 2.5mm Cruiser II® balloon.

(h) A second floppy guidewire was then placed down the AVCx and its bifurcation point dilated with the same balloon.

(i) Interestingly, the bend in the OMCx is straightened out by the guidewire and the 'concertina effect' suggests that lesions have been created.

(j) When the floppy part of the guidewire is pulled back into the bend, the artery takes up its normal shape and the appearance returns to normal.

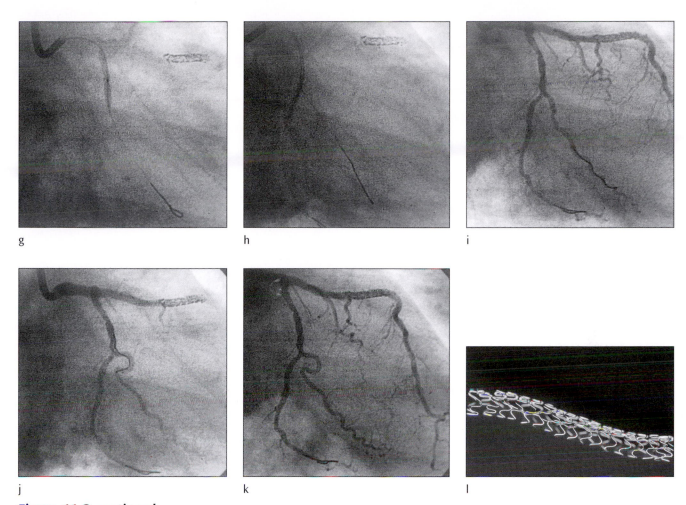

g

h

i

j

k

l

Figure 11.8 *continued*

(k) The final result is satisfactory in both vessels.

(l) The Angiostent™ was made of a single platinum-iridium alloy wire, which was sinusoidal in form and was wrapped helically and connected end to end by a second longitudinal wire.

Although, like other coil stents, the Angiostent™ had the advantage of flexibility and side-branch accessibility, it had the disadvantage of uneven expansion in lesions with uneven profiles.

The SOS trial in Europe and the ARTS trial in the USA have evaluated the cost and efficacy of stenting versus CABG surgery for the treatment of multivessel disease.

The SOS trial is still recruiting but 1-year follow-up results from the ARTS trial showed that major adverse events occurred with similar frequency in patients undergoing stenting to those undergoing CABG surgery. Although stented patients required further intervention more often (14%) (as a result of restenosis), stented patients received treatment more quickly, had less morbidity and shorter hospital stays and had a more rapid return to full activity. Moreover, stenting was cheaper.

Complex multivessel stenting

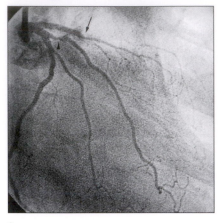

a

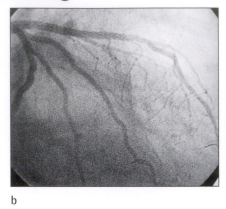

b

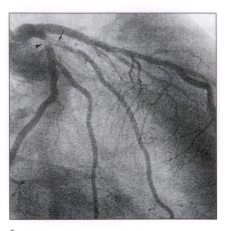

c

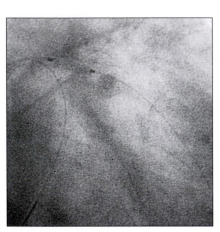

d

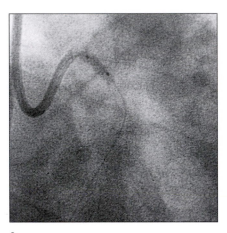

e

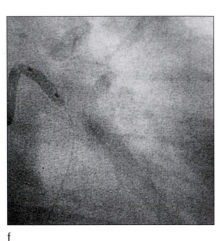

f

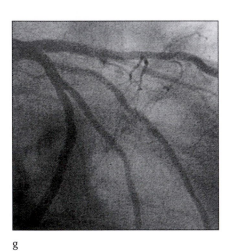

g

Figure 11.9

A 52-year-old man with a 4-month history of angina and a history of myocardial infarction 11 years earlier had a positive exercise test. (a) He was found to have an occluded LAD (arrow) and a severe stenosis in the first OMCx (arrowhead).

The stenosis in the first OMCx was crossed with a 0.014-inch Floppy® guidewire and dilated with a 2.0mm Vital™ balloon and stented with a 2.5mm, 13mm long Multilink Duet™ stent with an excellent result.

The LAD occlusion could not be crossed with a floppy guidewire, but a 0.014-inch Intermediate® guidewire crossed into the distal vessel. A 2.0mm Adante™ balloon was forced across the occlusion, and dilatation opened the LAD to reveal a long stenosed segment. The site was further dilated with a 3.0mm, 30mm long Rocket™ balloon and stented with a 3.0mm, 32mm NIR Primo™ stent.

(b) An overlapping 3.5mm, 12mm long GFX™ stent was then deployed in the most proximal segment of the LAD with an excellent final result.

(c) The LAD result persisted at 6 months but the first OMCx stent developed in-stent restenosis. The severe in-stent restenosis (arrow) can be seen to have extended backwards to involve the main LCx itself (arrowhead) – a very worrying situation.

Both lesions were crossed with 0.014-inch Floppy® guidewires.

(d) The first OMCx in-stent restenosis was treated with a 2.5mm, 10mm long Barath™ cutting balloon, with a good result.

(e) The main LCx lesion was then dilated with a 2.5mm, 10mm long Worldpass™ balloon.

(f) It was stented with a 3.0mm, 9mm long NIRoyal™ stent with an excellent angiographic (g) and clinical result.

Complex multivessel stenting, including primary stenting

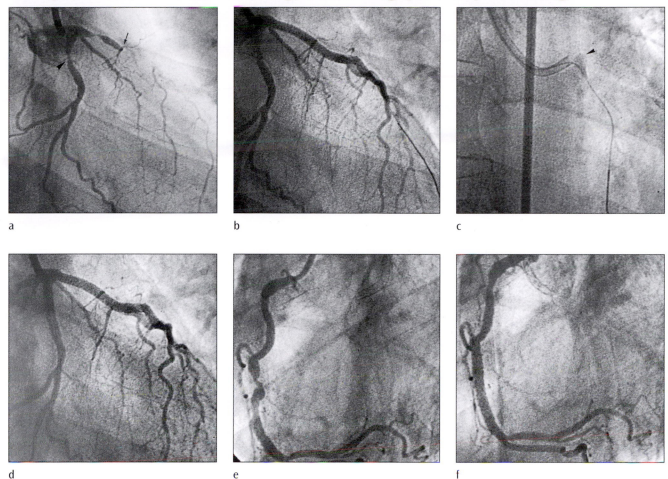

a   b   c

d   e   f

Figure 11.10

A 50-year-old man was transferred with unstable angina and non-Q-wave myocardial infarction (his troponin-T level was 0.11U per litre) while awaiting multivessel coronary intervention. (a) Coronary arteriography showed that the LAD had occluded (arrow) beyond the severe proximal stenosis. There was a severe proximal LCx stenosis (arrowhead) and the RCA had a severe stenosis in its middle third.

The LAD occlusion was crossed with a 0.014-inch Intermediate® guidewire and reopened with a 2.5mm Adante™ balloon and stented with a 3.0mm, 25mm long Duet® stent. A further 3.0mm, 18mm long GFX™ stent was passed through this stent and placed more distally to a significant stenosis in the mid-third of the LAD beyond the DG1.

(b) The result was excellent.

(c) Contrast staining was evident (arrowhead) in the very proximal portion of the LCx; this was possibly caused by entry of the intermediate guidewire into the LCx plaque during the attempt to cross the LAD lesion.

A 0.014-inch Floppy® guidewire crossed the LCx stenosis and the lesion was 'primary stented' without pre-dilatation using a 3.0mm, 18mm long Multilink Duet™ stent placed from the ostium of the LCx to beyond the lesion.

(d) The result was excellent and the contrast staining disappeared.

Because the procedure was uncomplicated, it was decided to proceed to the RCA during the same session.

The lesion in the RCA (e) was crossed with a 0.014-inch Floppy® guidewire, pre-dilated with a 2.5mm Adante™ balloon and stented with a 3.5mm, 25mm long NIRoyal™ stent. The stent was post-dilated with a 3.5mm, 12mm long Seajet® balloon up to 16 atmospheres with an excellent final result (f).

Primary (or direct) stenting without balloon pre-dilatation has been shown to be safe and effective in well-defined subgroups. Highly calcified lesions, lesions in tortuous vessels and chronic total occlusions should be contraindications. If successful, the procedure is cheaper and quicker and associated with less radiation exposure than conventional stenting after pre-dilatation by PTCA. Randomized studies such as SWAP and SLIDE have carefully assessed this technique. The results are awaited.

Complex multivessel stenting involving total occlusion and bifurcation lesion in high-risk patient with unstable angina

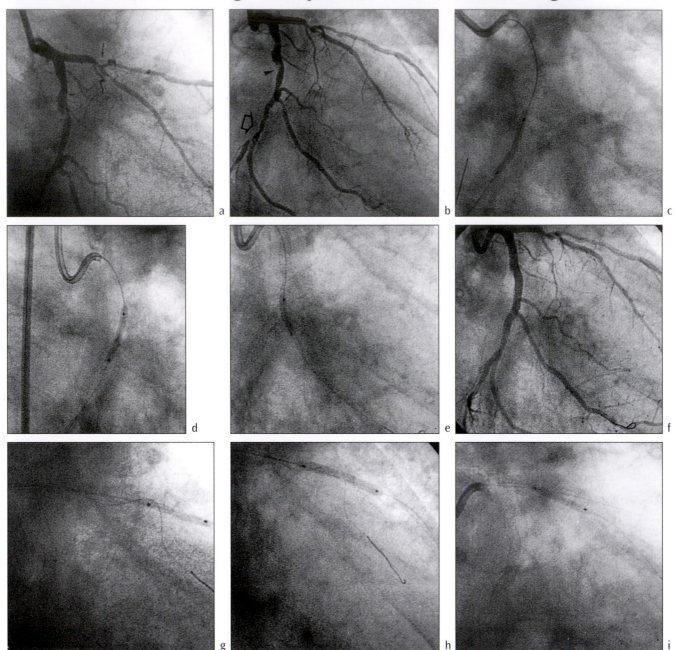

Figure 11.11

A 58-year-old man was transferred with severe unstable angina and pulmonary oedema 4 days after an inferior myocardial infarction, which had been treated with rtPA. He was unable to take aspirin and was therefore given clopidogrel 75mg daily. After treatment with diuretics and intravenous nitrates and heparin, coronary arteriography was performed.

Left ventricular angiography showed a markedly impaired left ventricle, owing to anteroapical infarction. Coronary arteriography showed (a) severe proximal and mid-LAD disease, including a bifurcation lesion involving the first DG (arrow), (b) a severely stenosed, ulcerated lesion in the proximal LCx (arrowhead) and more severe disease in the mid- and distal AVCx (open arrow).

There was an ostial stenosis in the OMCx (arrow). The RCA was occluded proximally.

The cardiac surgeon rejected the patient for emergency CABG surgery because of an unacceptable mortality risk; however, because of ongoing ischaemia (pain and extensive anterior ST-segment depression), the patient was offered emergency multivessel PTCA and stenting.

The LCx lesions were addressed first. (c, d) The lesions were crossed with a 0.014-inch Floppy® guidewire and dilated with a 2.5mm Worldpass™ balloon and then a 3.0mm Worldpass™ balloon.

A 2.5mm, 23mm long Multilink Duet™ stent was first placed in the distal segment, a 3.0mm, 18mm long Multilink Duet™ was placed in the middle segment and a 3.5mm, 23mm long Multilink Duet™ was placed more proximally over the severe complex proximal stenosis. All the stents overlapped each other.

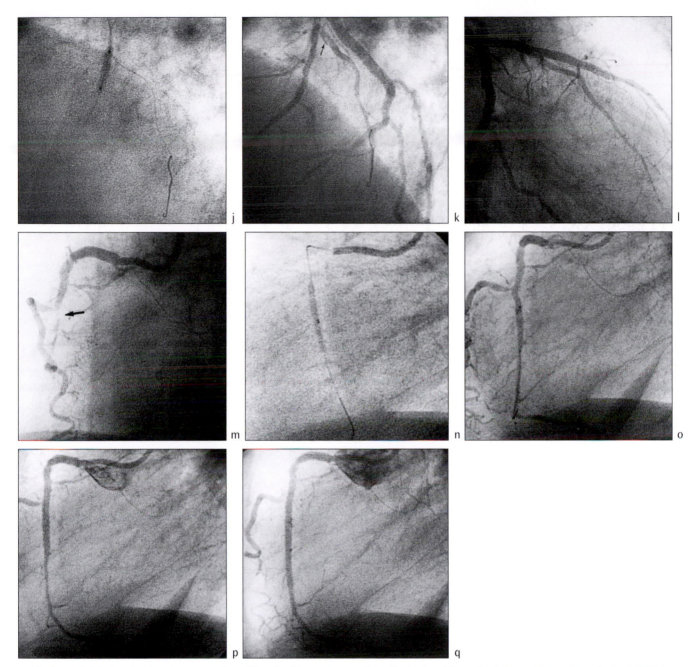

(e) The ostial lesion in the OMCx was then dilated with a 2.5mm Adante™ via the side wall of the 3.0mm, 18mm long Multilink Duet™ stent using the same 0.014-inch Floppy® guidewire.

(f) The result was excellent.

The LAD and first DG lesions were crossed with a 0.014-inch Floppy® and 0.014-inch Intermediate® guidewire respectively.

(g) The LAD lesions were dilated first with a 2.5mm and then a 3.0mm Worldpass™ balloon.

(h) The mid- and distal lesions were then stented with a 3.0mm, 20mm long Multilink Duet™ stent.

The more proximal lesion at the bifurcation point of the LAD and the first DG was stented with a 3.0mm, 18mm long Multilink Duet™ stent.

(i) The first DG was then dilated with a 2.5mm Worldpass™ balloon via the side-wall of the stent. With a 3.0 mm balloon inflated within the LAD stent, the 2.5 mm Worldpass balloon is pulled back into the ostium of the DG, (j) before kissing balloon PTCA is performed (cranial LAO projection).

(k, l) This gave a very good result. There was local dissection (arrow) but this was not flow-limiting and was not stented.

(m) The RCA occlusion (arrow) was crossed with a 0.014-inch Intermediate® guidewire and opened with a 2.0mm Adante™ balloon (n).

The stenosis was then dilated with a 3.0mm Worldpass™ balloon, with significant improvement (o).

(p) The occlusion site was then stented with a 3.0mm, 22mm long Crossflex LC™ stent (Cordis/Johnson and Johnson).

A 2.5mm, 13mm long Multilink Duet™ stent was then passed through the Crossflex LC™ stent and deployed at its distal end.

(q) The final angiographic result was excellent.

This patient had no further angina and was discharged home 5 days later. Eighteen months later he remains asymptomatic with normal exercise tolerance.

Complex multivessel stenting combined with Rotastenting

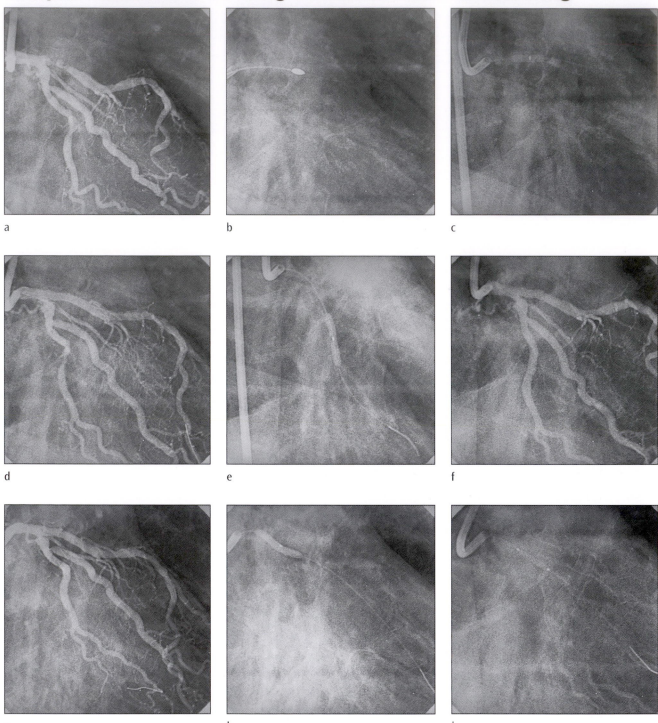

Figure 11.12

A 62-year-old insurance agent with severe angina was found to have severe three-vessel disease. (a) There was a bulky, calcified lesion in the proximal and ostial LAD.

(b) This was first ablated with a 1.75mm Rotablator® burr followed by a 2.25mm Rotablator® burr.

(c) It was then dilated with a 3.0mm, 10mm long Finale™ balloon.

(d) A 3.5mm, 15mm long Multilink™ stent was deployed with an excellent result.

The severe stenosis in the LCx (d) was then dilated with a 3.0mm Cheetah™ balloon (e).

(f) It was stented with a 3.5mm, 15mm long Multilink™ stent with a good result.

(g) The severe ostial OMCx lesion is best seen in the caudal RAO view.

(h) It was dilated with a 3.0mm Passage® balloon.

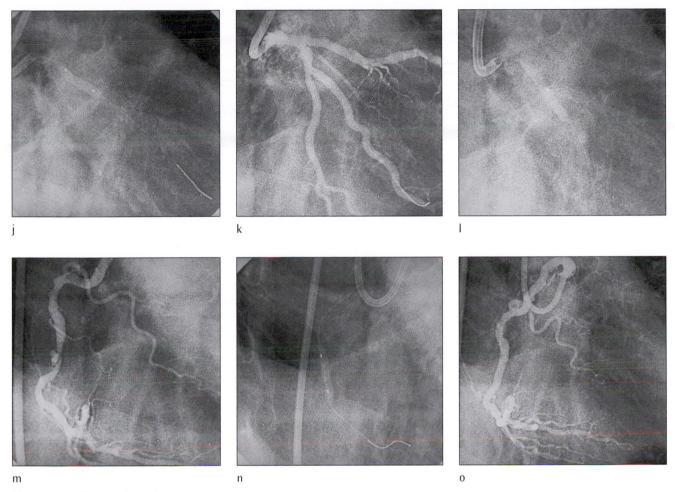

j

k

l

m

n

o

Figure 11.12 *continued*

(i, j) Because there was a lot of recoil (which is not unusual with ostial lesions) a 3.5mm, 12mm long Microstent II™ was implanted.

(k) This gave an excellent final result.

(l) A final inflation in the main LCx across the ostium of the OMCx was made with the 3.0mm balloon to ensure that no struts were left protruding into the lumen of the LCx.

Two weeks later, the patient returned for intervention to the tortuous RCA.

(m) The RCA had an ulcerated, severe and eccentric lesion in its mid-third. A small coronary artery aneurysm was associated with the stenosis. (n) An 8F Amplatz Left 2 guiding catheter was necessary to enable guidewire crossing and the lesion was dilated with a 3.0mm Passage® balloon.

The guiding catheter had to be deeply engaged to enable deployment of a 3.5mm, 15mm long Multilink™ stent.

(o) An excellent angiographic result was obtained.

The patient remains asymptomatic 12 months later.

It is often wise to stage multivessel procedures such as this, although this adds further to what is already an expensive procedure.

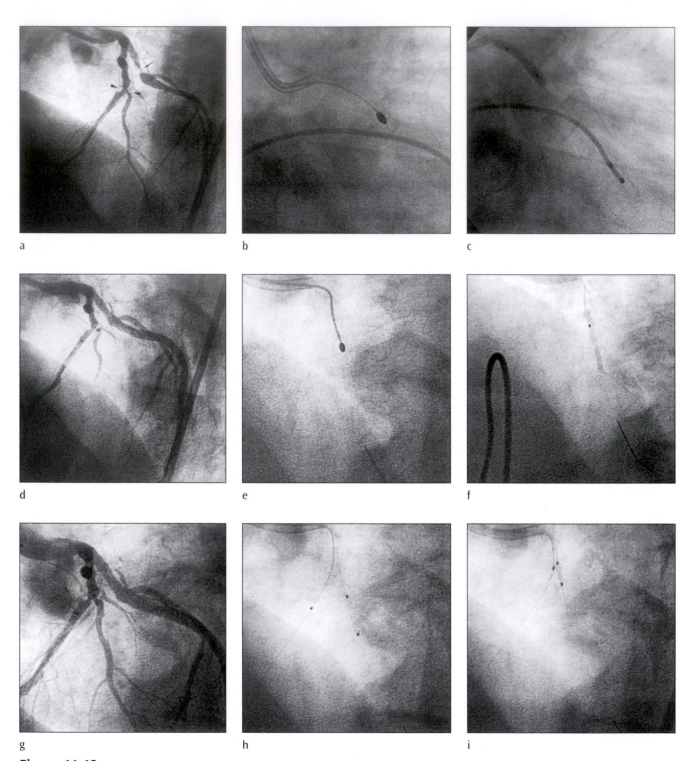

a

b

c

d

e

f

g

h

i

Figure 11.13

A 52-year-old man with angina. (a) There is a severe, bulky, eccentric lesion in the proximal LCx (arrow) as well as a severe bifurcation lesion involving LAD and its diagonal branch (arrowheads) (cranial LAO projection).

(b) The calcified LCx lesion was first ablated with a 1.75mm and then a 2.25mm Rotablator® burr over a 0.009-inch Rotawire™

(c) A 3.5mm, 15mm long Multilink™ stent was then implanted.

(d) This achieved a satisfactory result (cranial LAO projection).

(e) The ostial lesion in the diagonal artery was then ablated with a 1.75mm burr.

(f, g) It was post-dilated with a 2.5mm Worldpass™ balloon and then (h–j) stented with a 2.5mm, 12mm long Microstent II™. (h) A balloon catheter was placed in the LAD, as was a stent mounted on a balloon in the DG.

(i) The stent is then positioned and deployed (j) in the ostium of the DG and then a kissing balloon manoeuvre performed (not shown).

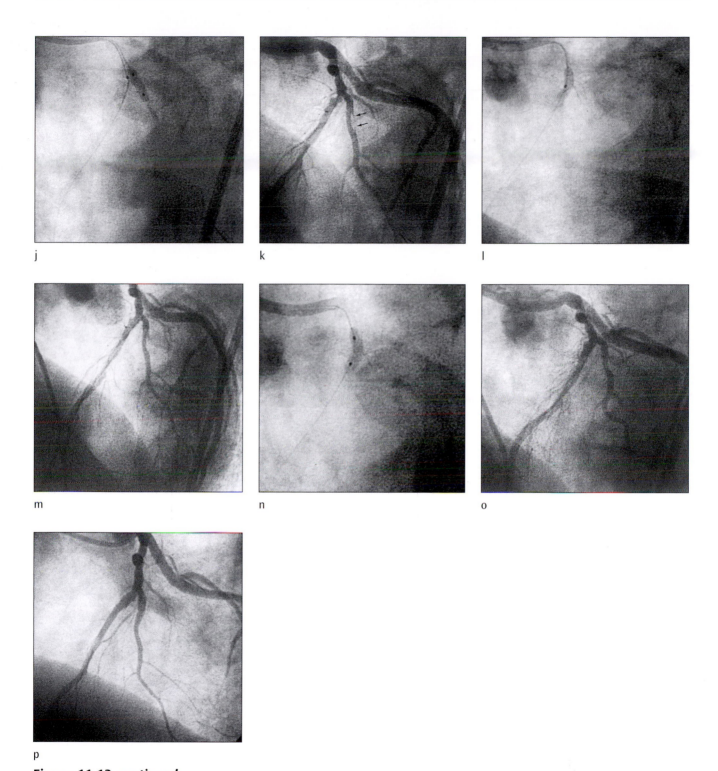

j

k

l

m

n

o

p

Figure 11.13 *continued*

(k) There appeared to be local dissection beyond the stent which did not improve with low-pressure balloon inflation. However, flow was not compromised and it was left alone.

(l, m) The LAD was then dilated with a 3.0mm Worldpass™ balloon over a 0.014-inch Floppy® guidewire and

(n) a 3.0mm, 15mm long Multilink™ stent was deployed.

(o) This gave a good final result.

(p) Two weeks later, repeat angiography showed that the dissection in the diagonal artery had healed satisfactorily.

Complex multivessel stenting involving kissing balloons via the side wall of a mesh stent for a bifurcation lesion

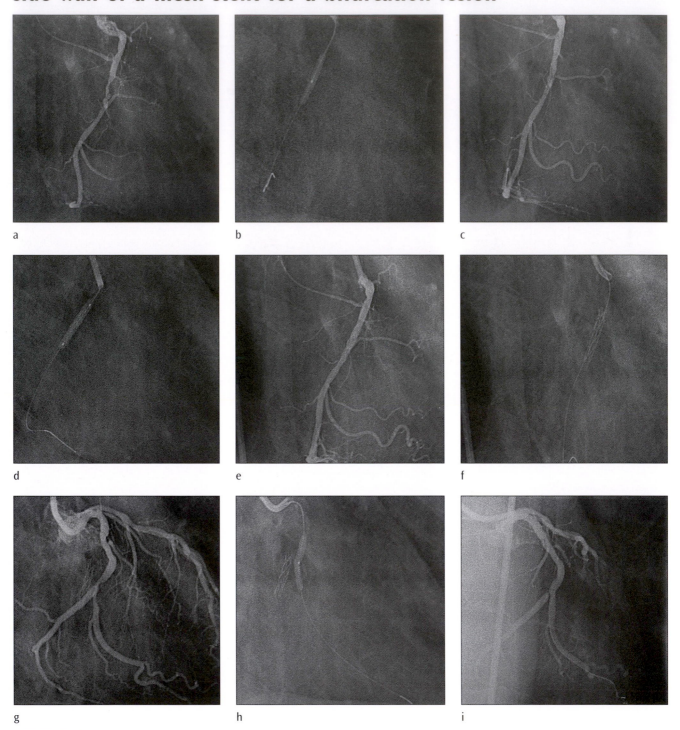

Figure 11.14

A 58-year-old retired car worker and keen long-distance cyclist presented with mild angina and a strongly positive exercise test (indicating inferolateral ischaemia) 3 years after PTCA to disease in the mid-third of the RCA. (a) Angiography showed a long severe stenosis in the mid-third of the RCA. There was also a significant lesion in the proximal portion of the OMCx.

(b) The RCA stenosis was pre-dilated with a 2.5mm Worldpass™ balloon.

(c, d) It was stented with a 3.0mm, 24mm long Microstent II™.

(e) Final result.

(f) The stent is easily visualized.

(g) The lesion in the OMCx-LCx bifurcation was more troublesome.

(h) After pre-dilatation with a 3.0mm Worldpass™ balloon, there was much recoil.

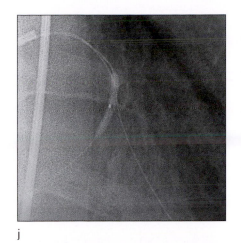

j

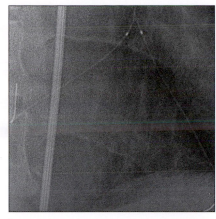

k

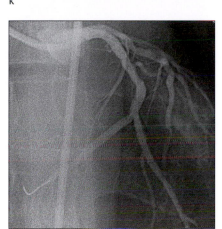

l

m

(i) A 3.5mm, 15mm long Multilink™ stent was therefore implanted across the bifurcation and down the proximal portion of the OMCx.

However, after stent deployment, angiography showed that atheromatous material had been displaced into the LCx.

(j) The vessel was entered with a 0.014-inch Floppy® guidewire via the side wall of the stent and the stent and stenosis were dilated with a 2.5mm Passage® balloon (j). A 3.0mm Passage® balloon was then inflated across the stenosis but this caused displacement of the stent.

A 3.0mm Tacker™ balloon (Cordis) was inflated within the stent, followed by kissing balloons.

(k, l) A 2.5mm Worldpass™ balloon was placed in the LCx (via the stent's side wall) and a 3.0mm Passage® balloon placed in the stent proper and down the OMCx.

(m) This produced a satisfactory final result.

Bifurcation stenting

Bifurcation PTCA using kissing balloon technique and stenting of single limb using an open coil Wiktor stent

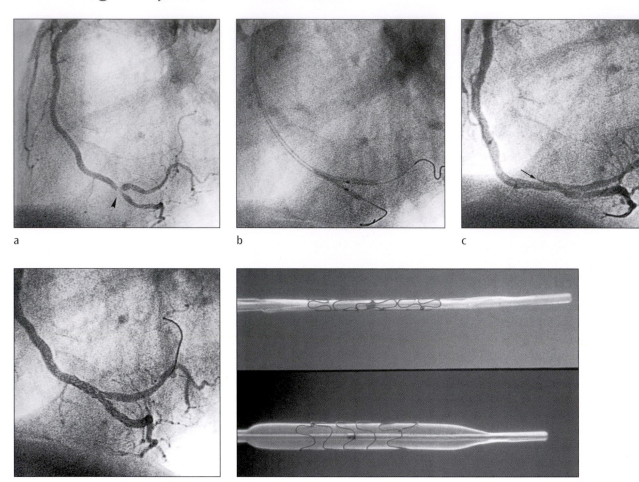

a

b

c

d

e

Figure 11.15

A 60-year-old man with moderate angina. (a) There is a severe stenosis at the crux of an RCA that involves the origins of both the PDA and the posterolateral branches (arrowhead).

Two 0.014-inch Floppy® guidewires were placed down each branch and the stenosis was dilated with a 2.5mm Worldpass™ balloon placed along each wire in turn.

(b) Local dissection was evident and so the stenosis was then further dilated using two 2.0mm Adante™ balloons in 'kissing' fashion.

(c) Although an acceptable result was obtained, local dissection was still visible (arrow).

(d) Therefore it was decided to place a 2.5mm, 20mm long Wiktor-i™ stent with the distal end of the stent in the PDA.

The ostium of the posterolateral branch was then further dilated through the side wall of the Wiktor-i™ stent using a 2.5mm Worldpass™ balloon without any complication.

(e) The open coil-design of the expanded Wiktor-i™ stent makes it easy to cross the side wall with a balloon in order to gain access to side branches and of course this stent is less likely to occlude them.

Bifurcation stenting using the 'kissing' stenting technique

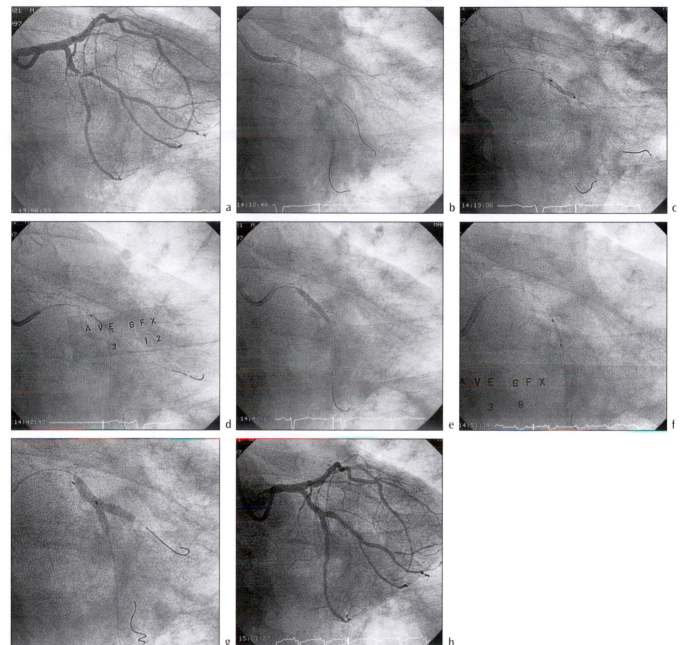

Figure 11.16
A 76-year-old man had unstable and rest angina. (a) Coronary arteriography showed a complex and severe stenosis at the bifurcation of the LCx and first OMCx. (b) Via a transradial approach and a 7F guiding catheter, 0.014-inch floppy ExtraSupport™ guidewires were placed into each vessel. (c) A 3.0mm, 15mm long Bonnie® balloon was used to first dilate the lesion in the LCx and then in the OMCx. (d) The guidewire in the LCx was removed so that a 3.0mm, 12mm long GFX™ stent could be implanted in the OMCx artery. (e) After replacing the wire down the LCx via the side wall of the stent, the LCx lesion was dilated with the same balloon through the stent struts. (f) A 3.0mm, 8mm long GFX™ stent was then placed in the LCx lesion through the side wall of the first stent. (g) Simultaneous inflation of the first balloon in the LCx and of a 3.0mm Pivot™ balloon (Scimed) in the OMCx was performed using the 'kissing' technique. (h) The final angiographic result showed a diameter of 3.25mm in the LCx and 3.29mm in the OMCx.

Treatment of bifurcation lesions with the 'kissing coronary stenting technique' requires stents with specific characteristics, which include:

- *a strut design that allows easy access to the side branch;*
- *a low profile to permit crossing through the first stent; and*
- *good radio-opacity to facilitate a precise implantation so as to avoid both the occurrence of gaps between the two stents and in-stent stenting.*

The procedure should be completed using the 'kissing' balloon technique to optimize the final result.

Courtesy of Dr T Joseph, Assistance Publique, Hôpitaux de Paris, Hôpital Ambroise Pare, Paris, and Drs R Cortina and J Marco, Clinique Pasteur, Toulouse, France.

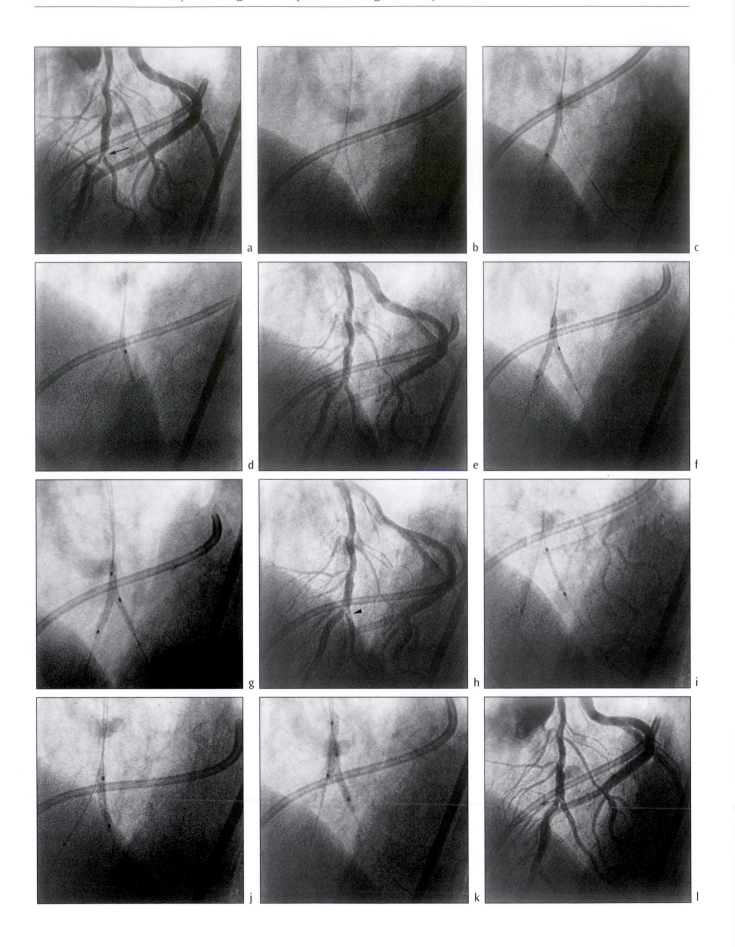

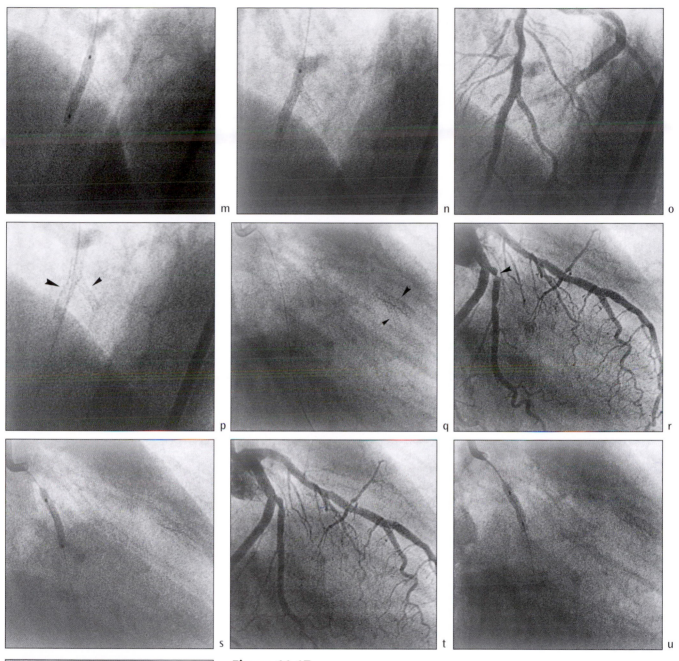

Figure 11.17

A 67-year-old woman with moderately severe angina. (a) There was a diffusely diseased LAD with a severe bifurcation stenosis affecting the LAD and the DG (arrow). There was also a severe stenosis in the proximal third of the OMCx. (b) High-torque Floppy® guidewires (0.014 inch) were placed down both LAD and diagonal branches. (c) The LAD limb was first dilated with a 2.5mm Worldpass™ balloon. (d) The DG limb was then dilated with a 2.0mm LTX™ balloon (AVE). (e) The improvement was marginal. (f, g) The 'kissing' balloon technique, using the same balloons, was applied to the bifurcation. (h) This resulted in local dissection in the DG limb (arrowhead). (i) With the deflated 2.5mm Worldpass™ balloon placed distally in the LAD, a 2.5mm, 12mm long GFX™ stent was placed in the DG limb. (j) It was then pulled back into the ostium of DG and deployed. (k) The 2.5mm Worldpass™ was then withdrawn to the exit point of the DG and again a 'kissing' balloon technique performed in order to ensure that the stented DG ostium was not distorted by the LAD balloon. (l) The result appears good in the DG limb but it is suboptimal in the LAD. (m, n) A 3.0mm, 18mm long Microstent™ was then deployed in the LAD opposite the ostium of the DG. (o) 'Kissing' balloons were again employed at high pressure in both stents to produce a satisfactory final result. The radio-opaque Microstents™ can be seen in both (p) the LAO view and (q) the RAO view. (r) Finally, the OMCx stenosis (arrowhead) is dilated with a 2.5mm Worldpass™ balloon over a 0.014-inch Intermediate® guidewire (s). (t) The result is suboptimal. (u) This leads to the deployment of a 2.75mm, 9mm long Paragon™ stent. (v) This achieves a good final result. The patient was rendered asymptomatic and remained free of symptoms 12 months after the procedure.

Bifurcation stenting using 'reverse Y' technique

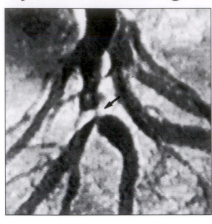
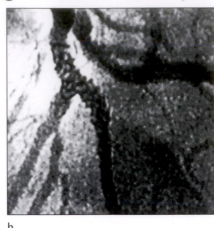
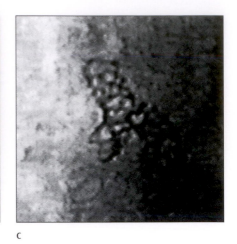

a   b   c

Figure 11.18

A 46-year-old man had unstable angina and T-wave inversion in leads V1-V4. (a) Coronary arteriography showed a severe, bulky bifurcation stenosis that involved the LAD and the first DG.

Floppy® guidewires (0.014 inch) were placed in both branches and a 3.0mm Europass® balloon was used to dilate the DG and then the LAD stenosis. Leaving the two guidewires in place, a 3.0mm, 15mm long Wiktor GX™ stent was deployed at the bifurcation, with the proximal half in the LAD and the distal half in the DG. Both guidewires were then removed and a guidewire was placed in the LAD passing through the mesh of the first stent. The mid-LAD was again pre-dilated at the bifurcation; this allowed a moderate expansion of the mesh of the Wiktor stent that was already in position and also allowed a second Wiktor GX™ stent to be placed in the mid-LAD through the side wall of the stent at the bifurcation with the DG.

(b) The final angiographic result was satisfactory.

(c) The radio-opaque stents can be seen in a 'reverse-Y' configuration that covers the bifurcation point without leaving any unstented gap.

Courtesy of Dr D Carrie, Purpan Hospital, Toulouse, France.

Bailout bifurcation stenting after DCA involving a stent delivered through the side wall of a stent

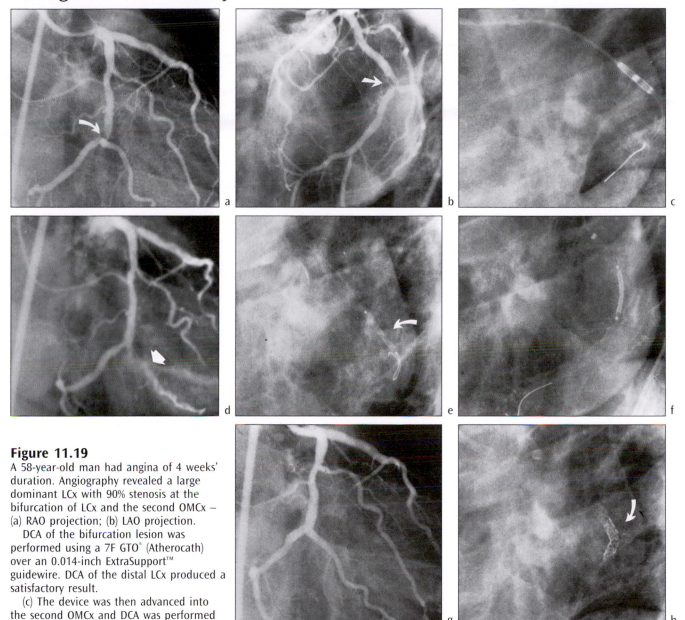

Figure 11.19

A 58-year-old man had angina of 4 weeks' duration. Angiography revealed a large dominant LCx with 90% stenosis at the bifurcation of LCx and the second OMCx – (a) RAO projection; (b) LAO projection.

DCA of the bifurcation lesion was performed using a 7F GTO® (Atherocath) over an 0.014-inch ExtraSupport™ guidewire. DCA of the distal LCx produced a satisfactory result.

(c) The device was then advanced into the second OMCx and DCA was performed to its ostium.

The patient experienced severe chest pain, and ST-segment elevation was evident on the ECG.

(d) Angiography showed TIMI I flow and contrast extravasation (type II perforation) (arrow).

(e) A 3.5mm, 18mm long Microstent™ (arrow) was deployed into the second OMCx, with the proximal half of the stent in the LCx and the distal half across the ostium of the second OMCx.

This resulted in restoration of flow into the second OMCx, with no evidence of contrast extravasation. However, recoil of the LCx stenosis occurred beyond the origin of the second OMCx. A 0.014-inch ExtraSupport™ guidewire was passed through the struts of the Microstent™ into the distal LCx, and the stent struts were then dilated using a 3.0mm balloon. An attempt to pass a second 3.5mm, 18mm long Microstent™ stent through these struts was unsuccessful.

(f) A 3.5mm, 15mm long Angiostent™ with stent delivery system was passed through the struts of the Microstent™.

This stent was deployed at 16 atmospheres; its proximal half overlapped the previously deployed Microstent™. The Angiostent™ is made of a single platinum wire that is wrapped helically and connected end to end by a longitudinal wire. It is very radio-opaque and flexible and has excellent radial strength.

(g) Angiography demonstrated no residual stenosis and normal flow in both vessels.

(h) The two stents can be seen to take-up a 'Y' configuration (arrow).

The advantages of the Angiostent™ in this case include its low-profile stent delivery system, which allowed delivery through the struts of the Microstent™ without snagging, its radio-opacity, which allowed precise positioning and the high-pressure-semicompliant nature of the balloon, which allowed high-pressure deployment without the need to recross.

Courtesy of Drs A Seth, R Salwan, P Chandra and ZM Hijazi, Escorts Heart Institute and Research Centre, New Delhi, India. (Seth A, Salwan R, Chandra P, Hijazi ZM. Bailout bifurcation stenting involving Angiostent through the struts of AVE Microstent™. J Invas Cardiol 1997;9:590-92.)

Bifurcation stenting assisted by atherectomy

Stenting of true bifurcation lesions can be technically very demanding. Debulking plaque before stent deployment can help avoid some of the potential complications such as uneven or incomplete stent deployment and movement of the stent during deployment.

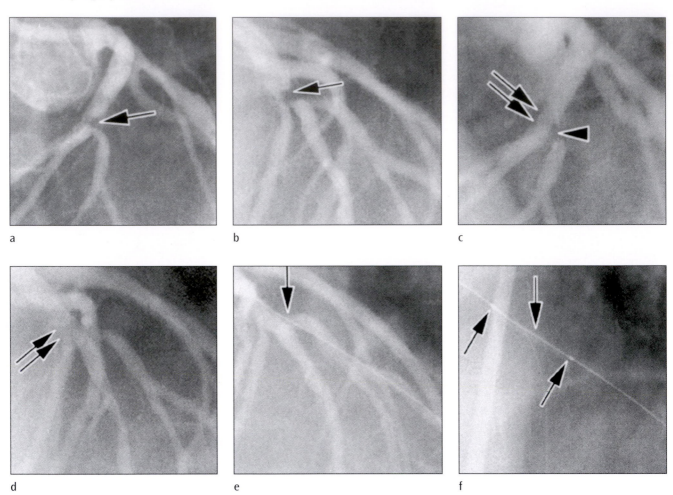

a   b   c

d   e   f

Figure 11.20

A 42-year-old man with severe angina had a bulky stenosis affecting the bifurcation of the LAD and first DG – (a) LSO projection; (b) cranial projection. It was decided to debulk the lesion by the Pullback Atherectomy Catheter™ (PAC) (Arrow International) and to follow this with 'culotte' stenting of the bifurcation to give proximal overlap of the two stents above the bifurcation point. The choice of a coil stent was aimed at minimizing the amount of metal in the overlap.

The PAC was placed over a 315cm Hannibal™ extra-support guidewire (Schneider) positioned in the LAD. The first DG cannot be protected by a guidewire because of the risk of cutting the wire with the atherectomy device.

(c, d) After two passes with a 2.4mm PAC device there was considerable improvement at the original lesion site (double arrow). However, there was a significant ostial stenosis of the large first diagonal (arrowhead).

(e) A 0.010-inch ACS TEN™ guidewire (Guidant) was then passed down the first DG.

The lesions in the LAD and the first DG were dilated in turn with a 3.0mm Viva™ balloon.

(f) A 3.0mm, 16mm long Freedom™ stent (Global Therapeutics) was then placed in the LAD/first DG. The radio-opaque markers on the balloon can be seen (arrows), demonstrating that the stent will be placed across the bifurcation.

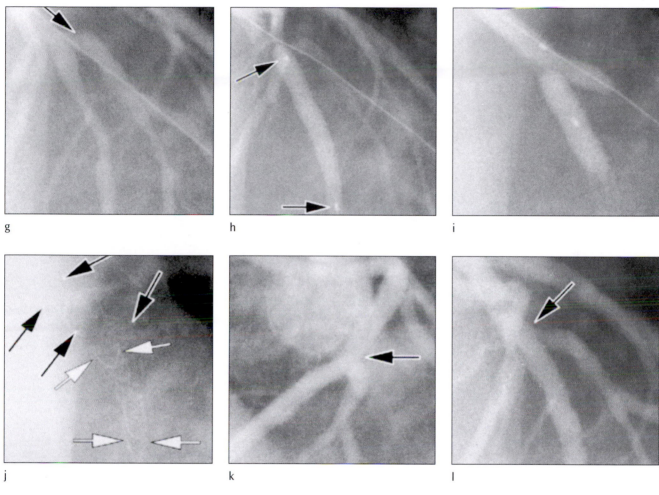

g

h

i

j

k

l

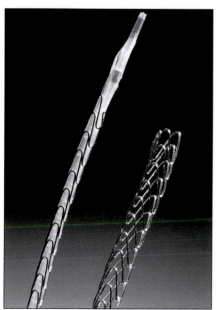

m

Figure 11.20 *continued*

(g) The immediate result was satisfactory.

The trapped guidewire in the LAD was then removed and placed back down the LAD through the side wall of the LAD/first DG Freedom™ stent. The struts were then dilated with a 3.5mm Viva™ balloon and a second 3.5mm, 30mm Freedom™ stent was advanced through the side wall into the LAD beyond the first DG ostium.

(h) The stent was deployed here because the diseased segment in the LAD could not be covered if it was extended back to cover the ostium of the first DG in true 'culotte' fashion.

The two stents were then simultaneously post-dilated using a 3.5mm, 15mm long Speedino™ balloon (Schneider) in the mid-LAD and a 3.0mm, 20mm long Viva™ balloon in the proximal LAD and first DG (i) – each to a pressure of 18 atmospheres. A 3.5mm balloon was again used to post-dilate the proximal LAD.

(j) The bifurcation stent can be seen faintly (arrows).

Final result – (k) LSO projection; (l) cranial projection.

(m) The Freedom™ stent had a unique 'fishscale' design (shown here) and it was premounted on a balloon. It has now been replaced by other, more modern stent designs.

Courtesy of Dr D Foley, Thoraxcenter, Rotterdam, The Netherlands.

Bifurcation Rotastenting using the 'T-stenting' technique

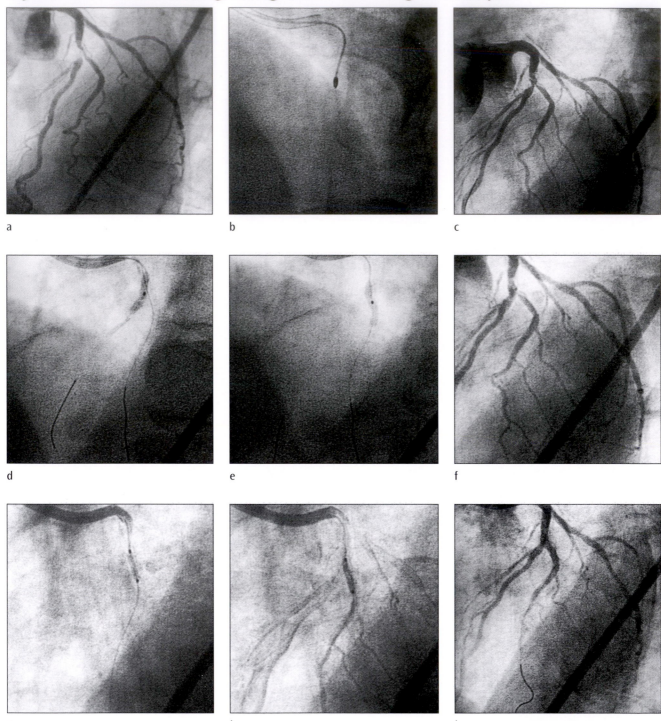

Figure 11.21

(a) A severe, bulky stenosis above, beyond and involving the origin of a large first DG in a 70-year-old lady with moderately severe angina.

(b) The LAD was most severely affected and was treated by Rotablator® atherectomy with a 1.5mm burr and a 2.0mm burr.

(c) This produced improvement but created a local dissection.

(d) After adjunctive PTCA with a 3.0mm Passage® balloon, the ostium of the first DG appeared more severely stenosed.

(e) The ostium was dilated with a 3.0mm Passage® balloon over a 0.014-inch Floppy® guidewire.

(f) This left a similar significant residual stenosis.

(g, h) A 2.5mm, 12mm long Microstent™ was therefore deployed at the ostium.

   This stent was chosen because its radio-opacity helps careful positioning of the proximal stent struts.

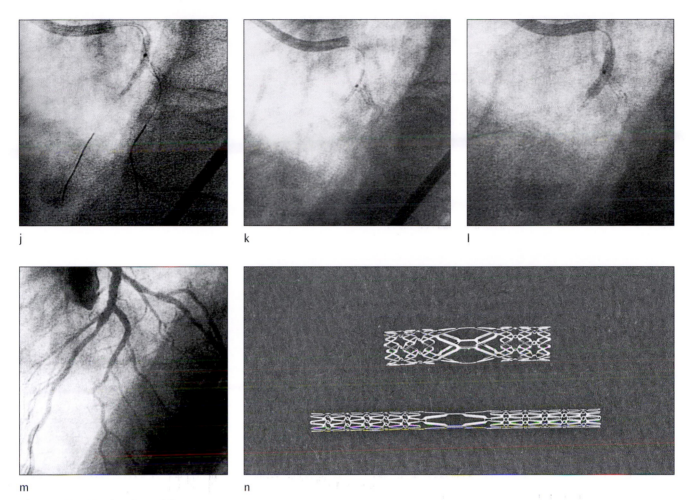

j

k

l

m

n

Figure 11.21 *continued*

(i, j) The residual LAD stenosis was then dilated with a 3.0mm Passage® balloon over the 0.009-inch Rotawire™ .

(k, l) A 17mm JoStent®-S (JoMed) side-branch stent mounted on the same balloon was placed with the open cells carefully positioned at the ostium of the first DG.

(m) The final result was excellent.

(n) The larger cells in the centre of the stent can be seen here.

Figure 11.22
A 48-year-old man was admitted with chest pain and ST-segment elevation in leads I, aVL, V5 and V6. The patient was given rtPA and became pain-free. His creatine phosphokinase level peaked at 600IU per litre and Q waves did not develop. Four days later an exercise stress test produced significant ST-segment depression in the same leads in which ST-segment elevation had previously been noted. (a) Coronary arteriography showed a severe stenosis in a large intermediate artery with two major marginal branches (open arrow) (RAO caudal projection).

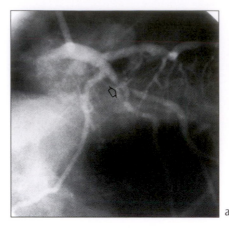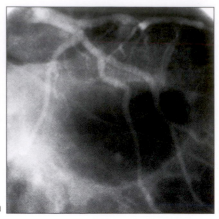

Two weeks later the patient was brought back for rotational atherectomy. A 9FL guiding catheter was used and Rotablator® atherectomy was performed with sequential 1.5mm and 2.0mm burrs placed over a C-wire™. Adjunctive PTCA of both limbs was performed using a non-compliant 3.0mm NC Bandit™ balloon (Scimed). After PTCA, a 3.0mm Palmaz-Schatz™ stent was placed in the inferior branch; care was taken to position it from the origin distally. The stent was subsequently dilated at high pressure. A 3.0mm Gianturco-Roubin™ stent was placed across the stent into the anterior branch in a 'T-stenting' fashion. The stent was post-dilated, and (b) this resulted in an excellent angiographic appearance.

Courtesy of Dr CS Rihal, Cardiovascular Diseases and Internal Medicine, Mayo Clinic, Rochester, Minnesota, USA.

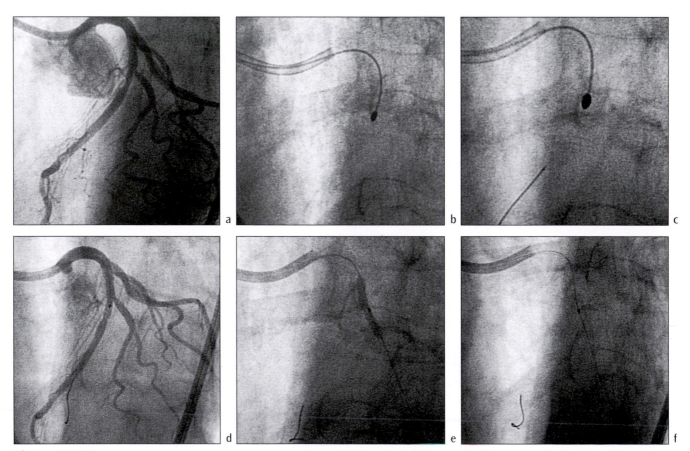

Figure 11.23
(a) A stenosis at the bifurcation of the LAD and first DG in a 67-year-old woman with frequent angina.
   The patient's symptoms far outweighed the angiographic severity of the stenosis, although the LAD was found to be calcified on fluoroscopy. IVUS showed a severe eccentric stenosis in the LAD just beyond the diagonal branch and less severe calcified plaque more proximally.
   (b, c) Rotablator® atherectomy was performed to the LAD using a 1.75mm burr and a 2.25mm burr.
   IVUS showed little change after this but (d) the angiogram showed improvement.
   (e) The ostium of the first DG was then dilated with a 2.5mm Worldpass™ balloon.
   (f, g) It was stented with a 2.5mm, 12mm long Microstent™ producing a good result (h).

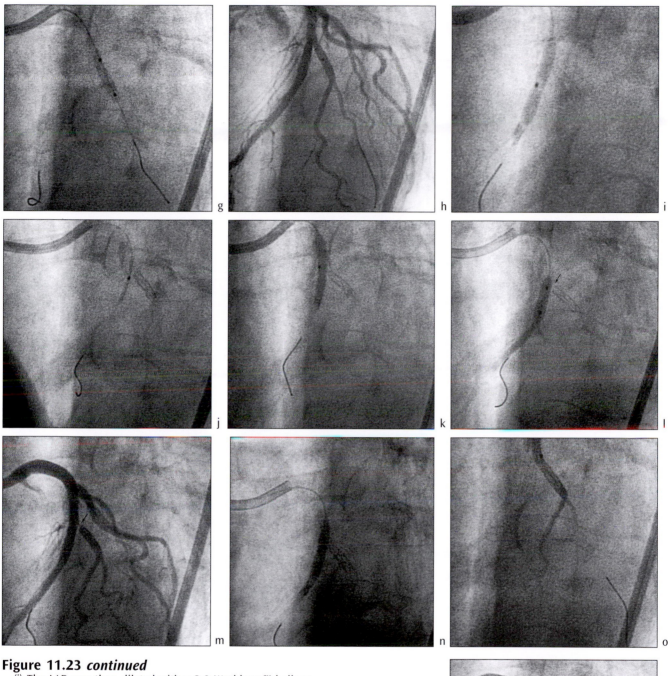

Figure 11.23 *continued*

(i) The LAD was then dilated with a 3.0 Worldpass™ balloon.

(j, k) It was stented with a 17mm long JoStent®-S side-branch stent mounted on the same balloon. Post dilation at high pressure clearly shows that the diagonal stent was not 'flush' with the LAD at the ostium of the first DG (arrow) (l).

(m) Although the LAD looked excellent, there was clearly prolapse of atheroma into the ostium of the diagonal branch (arrow).

(n) The LAD stent was then post-dilated with a 3.5mm, 13mm long Viva Primo™ balloon and (o) the first DG was dilated with the 3.0mm Worldpass™ balloon.

(p) This gave a good final result.

IVUS showed the eccentric plaque to be compressed laterally by the stent.

This problem of leaving an 'uncovered' segment at the very ostium of the side-branch during the technique of 'T-stenting' is not uncommon. It arises because one tries at all costs not to leave stent struts in the main vessel while simultaneously trying to cover all of the ostial segment. If the stent struts are left in the main vessel, it may prove impossible to then deliver a stent into the main vessel across the ostium of the side branch because of the protruding struts. The 'culotte' technique avoids this problem but leaves twice the density of struts in the proximal segment of the main vessel just above the bifurcation point and possibly increases the risk of restenosis. This, however, has not been shown to be an inevitable consequence.

'T-stenting' for bifurcation lesions

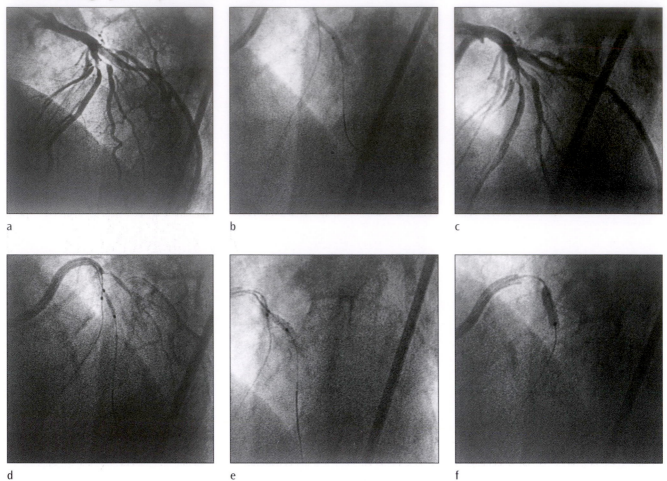

Figure 11.24

A 59-year-old man with severe angina had a severe stenosis in a dominant RCA and (a) a severe stenosis of the bifurcation of LAD and first DG (LAO cranial projection).

The RCA was addressed first and treated successfully by PTCA and stent implantation.

A 0.014-inch Floppy® guidewire was then placed down the LAD and a 0.014-inch Intermediate® guidewire was placed down the first DG.

(b) The first DG ostial lesion was first dilated with a 2.0mm Worldpass™ balloon.

(c) This produced local dissection and gave an inadequate result.

The first DG lesion was therefore stented with a 2.5mm, 12mm long GFX™ stent.

(d) The stent was positioned as close to the ostium as possible (with the proximal balloon marker just in the LAD). At the same time a 2.0mm, 20mm long Worldpass™ balloon was positioned in the LAD over the ostium of the first DG.

(e) The 2.0mm Worldpass™ balloon was first inflated and the GFX™ stent was then pulled up against the balloon and deployed in the DG ostium.

This manoeuvre is an attempt to bring the first DG stent exactly over the ostium without encroaching on the lumen of the LAD.

(f) The LAD lesion was then dilated with a 2.5mm and then a 3.0mm Worldpass™ balloon. This produced much improvement.

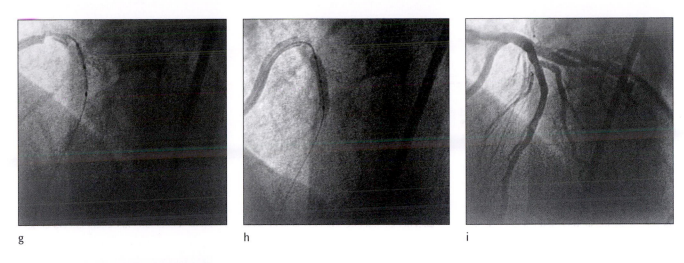

g   h   i

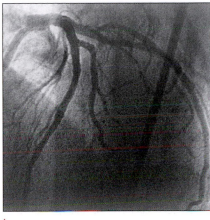

j

Figure 11.24 *continued*

(g) The LAD was then stented with a 3.0mm, 26mm long JoStent®, the balloon of which is characterized by three radio-opaque markers.

(h) In this case, care was taken to position the central marker distal to the first DG ostium.

The result was very good (i) but was improved further by post-dilatation to 20 atmospheres with a 3.0mm Calypso™ balloon (USCI) (j). This patient remains free of symptoms 2½ years later.

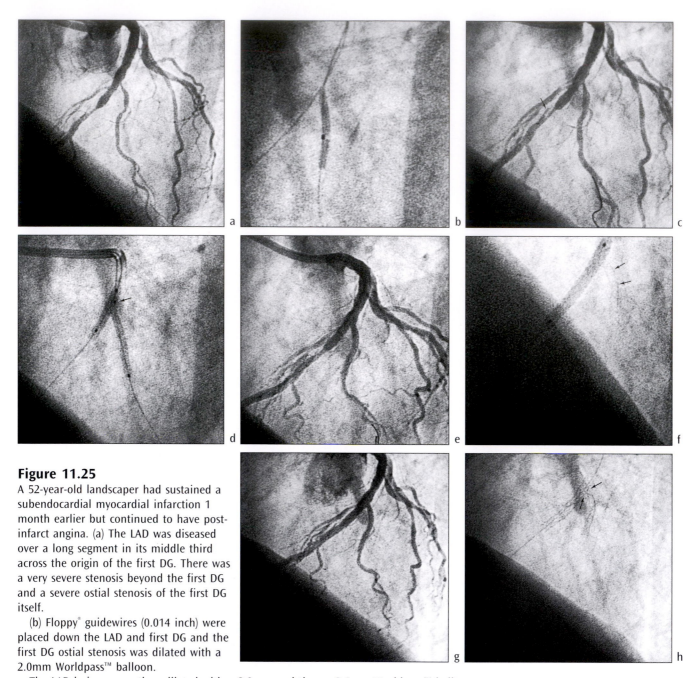

Figure 11.25

A 52-year-old landscaper had sustained a subendocardial myocardial infarction 1 month earlier but continued to have post-infarct angina. (a) The LAD was diseased over a long segment in its middle third across the origin of the first DG. There was a very severe stenosis beyond the first DG and a severe ostial stenosis of the first DG itself.

(b) Floppy® guidewires (0.014 inch) were placed down the LAD and first DG and the first DG ostial stenosis was dilated with a 2.0mm Worldpass™ balloon.

The LAD lesions were then dilated with a 2.0mm and then a 3.0mm Worldpass™ balloon.

(c) This gave an unsatisfactory result in both vessels. Dissection is clearly visible in the most distal lesion of the LAD (arrow). A 2.5mm, 23mm long Multilink Duet™ stent was then placed in the first DG and a 3.0mm balloon was placed in the LAD.

(d) With the 3.0mm balloon inflated in the LAD over the ostium of the first DG, the Duet™ stent was pulled up against the balloon until the proximal marker appeared in the shadow of the balloon in the LAD (arrow); the stent was then deployed in 'kissing fashion'.

(e) On removal of the balloon catheters, angiography showed an excellent result in the ostium of first DG but a suboptimal result in the LAD.

(f) A 3.5mm, 30mm long GFX™ stent was then deployed in the LAD to cover the bifurcation point and the most severe segment of disease more distally. The radio-opaque Duet™ in the first DG can be seen (arrows).

(g) The final result was very acceptable.

(h) The 'T-stent' shape could be seen on fluoroscopy. It would appear that the two stents abut closely on each other (arrows).

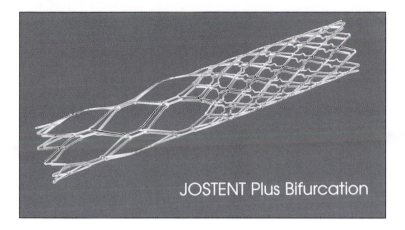

Figure 11.26
The JoStent®-B Bifurcation stent (JoMed) is shown here. It can be mounted and hand-crimped on to a balloon with the 'wide cells' proximal or distal, depending on the morphology of the bifurcation stenosis – the strategy would be to place the wide cells opposite the bifurcation point and the smaller cells in the most severe stenosis if it occurs distal or proximal to the bifurcation point.

'Culotte' stenting for bifurcation lesions

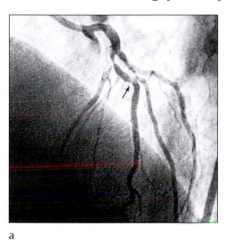
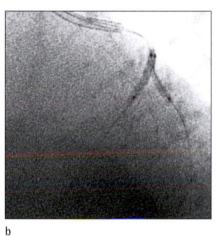
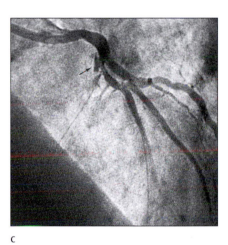

a   b   c

Figure 11.27
A 52-year-old company director presented with moderately severe angina and a positive exercise stress test at 4 minutes of Bruce protocol. (a) Coronary arteriography showed a critical stenosis at the bifurcation of the LAD and the first DG and a further more distal lesion in the first DG (arrow) (LAO cranial projection).
(b) An 0.014-inch Intermediate® guidewire was placed in the LAD and a 0.014-inch Floppy® guidewire was placed in the first DG. Negotiating the stenosis to gain entry into the distal LAD was difficult. The LAD site was dilated first with a 2.5mm Rocket™ balloon with only marginal improvement. A second 2.5mm Rocket™ balloon was placed in the first DG site and both simultaneously inflated to 6 atmospheres in 'kissing fashion'.
(c) Although there was improvement in the first DG, the LAD was dissected (arrow) and occluded.

continued

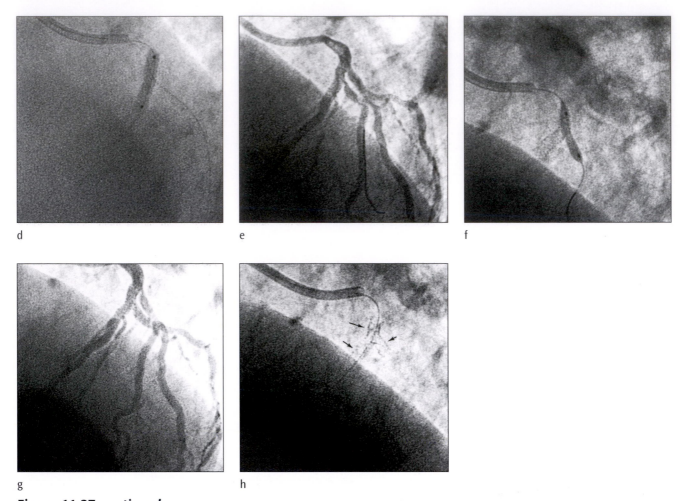

d

e

f

g

h

Figure 11.27 *continued*

(d) A 3.5mm, 18mm long Multilink Duet™ stent was then deployed in the proximal LAD across the ostium of first DG and post-dilated with a 3.0mm, 10mm long Worldpass™ balloon up to 18 atmospheres. The first DG then showed severe ostial and proximal lesions (e).

The 'jailed' floppy guidewire was then removed from the first DG and the intermediate guidewire in the LAD was withdrawn slightly and torqued into and down the first DG across the side wall of the LAD stent. (This manoeuvre prevented the operator from having to pass the proximal end of the LAD Duet™ stent and the risk of passing behind the struts between the struts and the wall of the artery.)

A 2.0mm Worldpass™ balloon was then used to dilate the struts of the side wall at the entry point into the first DG, which were then further dilated with a 3.0mm Rocket™ balloon. Unfortunately the result was poor, and so (f) a 3.0mm, 12mm long GFX™ stent was placed to cover the ostium of first DG and the proximal half of the Duet™ stent in a 'Y-shape' fashion.

This stent was post-dilated up to 13 atmospheres. The intermediate guidewire was then withdrawn out of the first DG and passed down the LAD through the side wall of the GFX™ stent and the stent was redilated with a 3.0mm Rocket™ balloon up to 14 atmospheres.

(g) The bifurcation result was very satisfactory.

(h) The 'Y-shape' of the stented bifurcation was evident fluoroscopically (arrows).

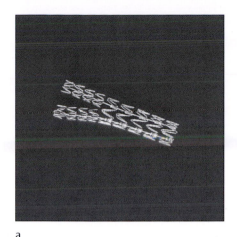

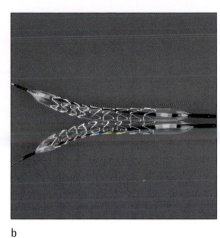

a   b

Figure 11.28
(a) The Bifurcate XT™ stent was a prototype, 'twin-limbed' stent that was developed by BARD for use in bifurcation lesions.
(b) It came mounted on two low-profile balloons.
Clearly this somewhat fixed geometrical design was only suitable for specific anatomy, although a range of customized, bifurcation stents similar to this stent might be made available in the future. The Bifurcate XT™ was not made commercially available.

Stenting of the main branch and PTCA of the side branch for bifurcation lesions

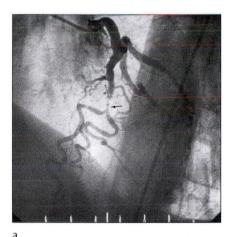

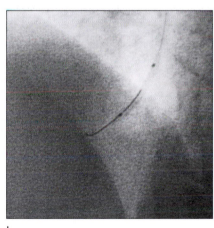

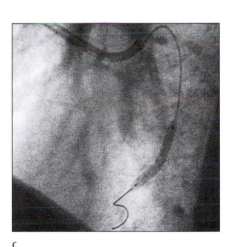

a   b   c

Figure 11.29
It is often sufficient simply to dilate the ostial lesion of the side branch and to stent the 'main' or 'most important' vessel, as in this case of a 60-year-old woman with severe unstable angina. (a) She had a severe bifurcation stenosis in the mid-LAD affecting the ostium of a large first DG (arrow).
(b) The LAD limb was first crossed with a 0.014-inch Floppy® guidewire and dilated with a 2.5mm Adante™ balloon.
(c) It was stented with a 3.0mm, 18mm long Tristar™ stent (Guidant).
   A further 2.75mm, 13mm long Tristar™ stent was placed at the distal end of the first stent with a good result in the LAD.

continued

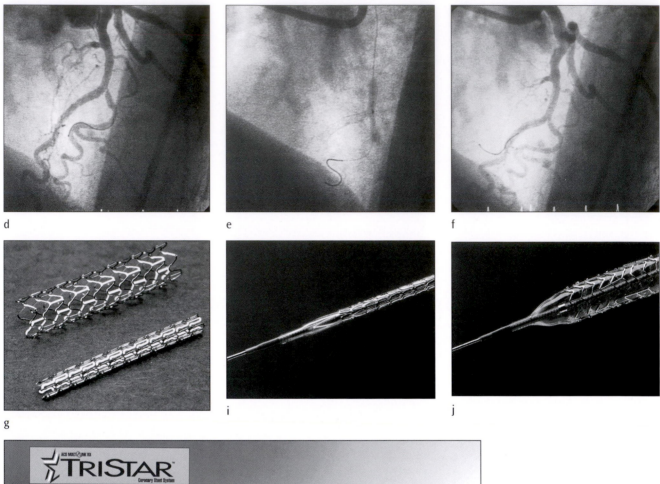

d

e

f

g

i

j

h

Figure 11.29 *continued*

(d) However, the ostium of first DG appeared to be severely stenosed.

(e) The first DG was entered with a 0.014-inch Floppy® guidewire via the side wall of the stent that was covering the ostium of first DG. The ostium was dilated with a 2.0mm Worldpass™ balloon and further dilated with a 2.5mm Adante™ balloon.

(f) The final result was excellent, and there was no need to stent the side branch.

Whenever possible, one should avoid stenting the side branch unless there is a very poor angiographic result or threatened closure. Restenosis that involves the origin of an unstented side branch is probably easier to deal with than dense in-stent restenosis that involves both limbs of a bifurcation stent.

(g) The Multilink Tristar™ stent has a very low profile and (h, i) comes mounted on a specially-shaped 'stepped' balloon.

(j) The 'steps' at the ends of the balloon may reduce the likelihood of proximal and distal edge tears after stent deployment and can be seen clearly as the stent-deployment balloon is inflated.

Data from the Mayo Clinic suggest that major adverse events (death, myocardial infarction, repeat revascularization) were more frequent after 'Y-stenting' than after 'T-stenting'.

Stenting of both branches appears to offer little advantage over stenting of one branch and performing PTCA to the other branch with or without atherectomy.

Stenting of protected left main coronary artery

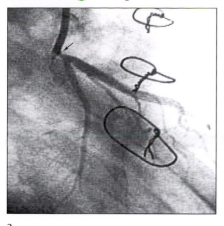

a

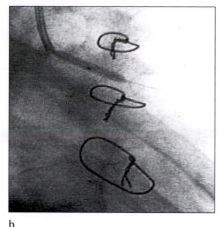

b

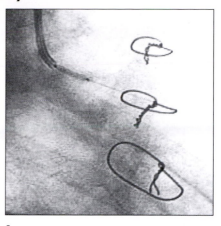

c

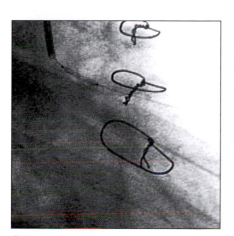

d

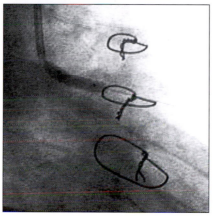

e

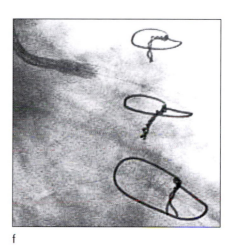

f

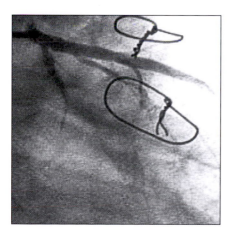

g

Figure 11.30

A 48-year-old woman with unstable angina had undergone CABG surgery one year earlier. The left internal mammary artery was patent but the SVG to the LCx was occluded. (a) Angiography showed a severe ostial stenosis of the left main coronary artery (arrow).

(b) The lesion was pre-dilated with a 2.0mm then a 3.0mm Worldpass™ balloon.

(c–e) It was stented with a 3.5mm, 12mm long stent. Note how the guiding catheter was disengaged before deployment (d, e).

(f) The stent was further dilated with a 4.0mm Finale™ balloon within the stent.

(g) Final result.

Courtesy of Dr L Morrison, Cardiothoracic Centre, Liverpool, UK.

Stenting of unprotected left main coronary artery

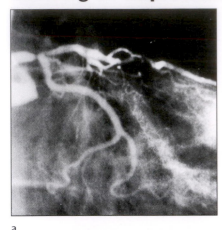

a

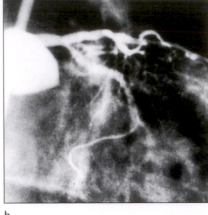

b

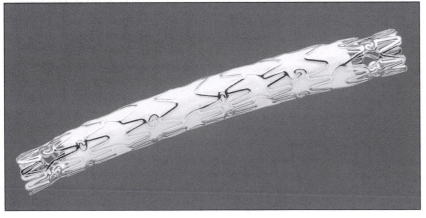

c

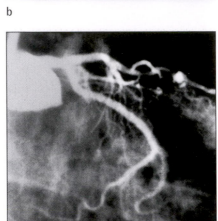

d

Figure 11.31
(a) A severe distal left main stem stenosis and an ostial LAD stenosis in an 86-year-old lady.
A 15mm long Palmaz-Schatz™ stent was placed with the articulation centred over the LCx 'take-off'.
(b) Spasm or plaque shift was noticed after high pressure inflation following stent implantation.
(c) A balloon was placed and dilated in the LCx via the side wall of the stent. (Note the two guidewires in the LAD and the LCx.)
(d) This gave an excellent angiographic result.
The next day a Wallstent™ was implanted into the right carotid artery for a high-grade stenosis. The patient recovered well and was rendered asymptomatic.
Courtesy of Dr PS Teirstein, Scripps Clinic and Research foundation, La Jolla, California, USA.

Covered stents

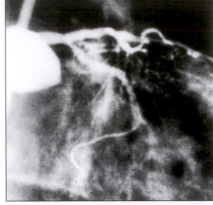

a

Figure 11.32
The JoStent® Coronary Stent Graft (JoMed) is constructed using a sandwich technique whereby an ultrathin layer of expandable PTFE is placed between two stents with reduced strut thickness. The stents can be dilated between 2.5 and 5.0mm and are available in lengths of 9, 12, 16, 19 and 26mm. The covered lengths are 2.0mm shorter than these lengths. This stent is now available premounted on a balloon catheter.

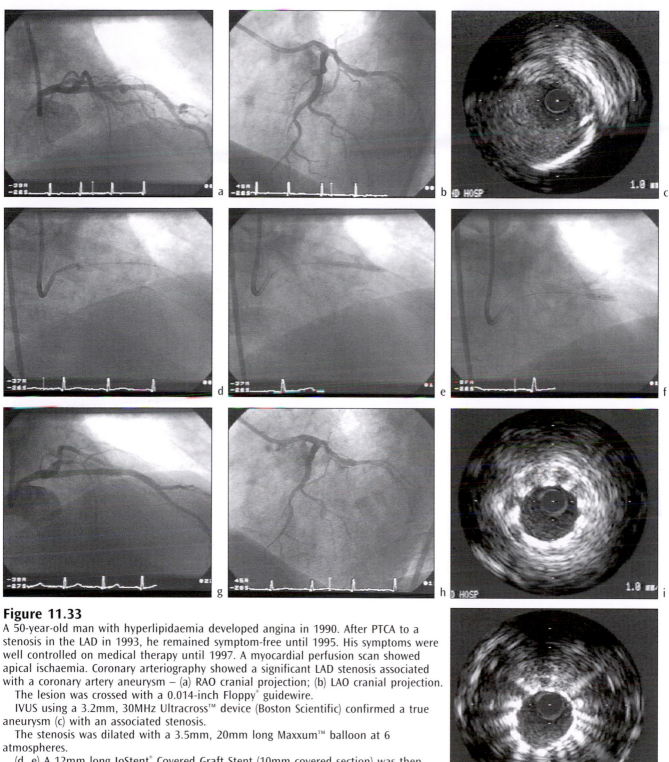

Figure 11.33

A 50-year-old man with hyperlipidaemia developed angina in 1990. After PTCA to a stenosis in the LAD in 1993, he remained symptom-free until 1995. His symptoms were well controlled on medical therapy until 1997. A myocardial perfusion scan showed apical ischaemia. Coronary arteriography showed a significant LAD stenosis associated with a coronary artery aneurysm – (a) RAO cranial projection; (b) LAO cranial projection.

The lesion was crossed with a 0.014-inch Floppy® guidewire.

IVUS using a 3.2mm, 30MHz Ultracross™ device (Boston Scientific) confirmed a true aneurysm (c) with an associated stenosis.

The stenosis was dilated with a 3.5mm, 20mm long Maxxum™ balloon at 6 atmospheres.

(d, e) A 12mm long JoStent® Covered Graft Stent (10mm covered section) was then hand-crimped on to the Maxxum® and placed across the aneurysm and the stenosis.

This stent was deployed at 12 atmospheres.

(f) A further stent dilatation was performed with a 3.5mm, 9mm long Chubby™ balloon at 18 atmospheres.

However, IVUS revealed suboptimal stent expansion. Further stent dilatation was then performed with a 4.0mm, 9mm long Chubby™ balloon at 18 atmospheres.

This resulted in a satisfactory angiographic (g, h) and IVUS appearance. The ultrasound images clearly show the uncovered stent segment (i) as well as the PTFE-covered section (j).

There were no complications and the patient was rendered asymptomatic.

Courtesy of Dr JA Hall, Cardiothoracic Unit, South Cleveland, UK.

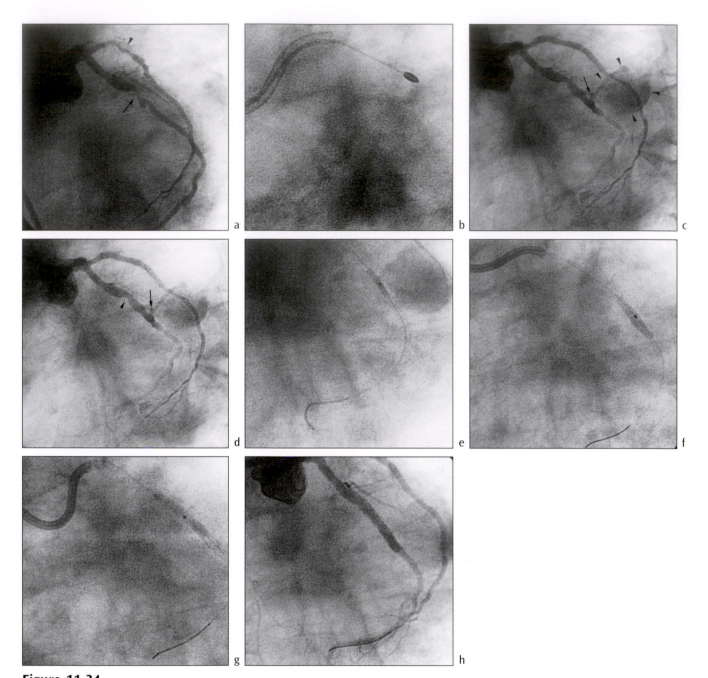

Figure 11.34

A 51-year-old man had uncontrolled angina 8 years after CABG surgery. (a) The LCx (arrow) and the intermediate artery (arrowhead) had undilatable calcified stenoses.

The intermediate artery was successfully treated by Rotablator® atherectomy and stent implantation (see (c)).

However, after Rotablator® atherectomy to the lesion in the LCx (b), a 3.5mm, 15mm long Multilink stent was implanted. On stent deployment, the vessel perforated at the distal end of the stent on a bend point in the artery.

(c) A false aneurysm was outlined by contrast (arrowheads) and the perforation point was easily visible (arrow).

(d) After high-pressure dilatation of the lesion within the stent (arrowhead), a 12mm JoStent® PTFE Covered Stent Graft was deployed initially at the perforation point (e, f).

A further 9mm JoStent® PTFE Covered Stent Graft was placed between the two stents (g) to obliterate flow into the false aneurysm (h).

Angiography at 6 weeks showed that the aneurysm was closed.

IVUS and stent deployment

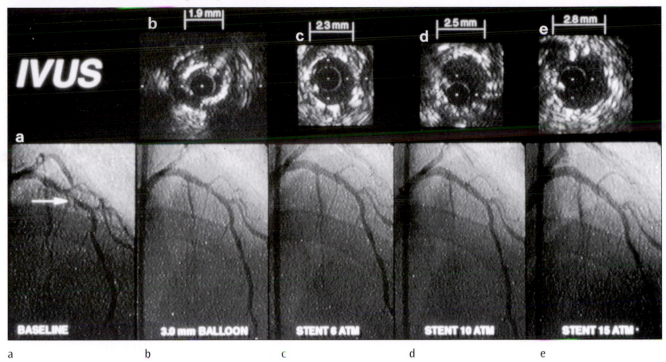

Figure 11.35

Figure 11.35
IVUS can more accurately assess the final result after PTCA and stent deployment than angiography. (a) In this illustration there is a 90% stenosis (arrow) in the LAD.

(b) There was a good angiographic result after PTCA with a 3.0mm balloon at 6 atmospheres. The IVUS showed an MLD of 1.9mm.

(c) The angiogram after deployment of a 3.0mm Wiktor GX™ stent at 6 atmospheres looked satisfactory. However, the IVUS showed an MLD of only 2.3mm.

(d) IVUS, after dilatation at 10 atmospheres, showed an MLD of 2.5mm; (e) after dilatation at 15 atmospheres, the MLD has increased to 2.8mm.

Courtesy of Dr C White, Ochsner Clinic, New Orleans, Louisiana, USA.

The OPTICUS study showed that IVUS-guided stent deployment was a safe procedure to optimize stent deployment.

The CRUISE study showed that IVUS-guided stent deployment results in a larger minimal stent diameter and area than angiography alone and that it reduces the 9-month target-vessel revascularization rate.

The MUSIC study showed that subacute stent thrombosis was rare when IVUS-guided stent deployment confirmed that the in-stent final minimal lumen area was more than 90% of the average proximal and distal reference cross-sectional area and that the minimum cross-sectional area was more than 9.0mm².

The SIPS trial showed that IVUS-guided PTCA or stenting results in reduced restenosis at 6 months.

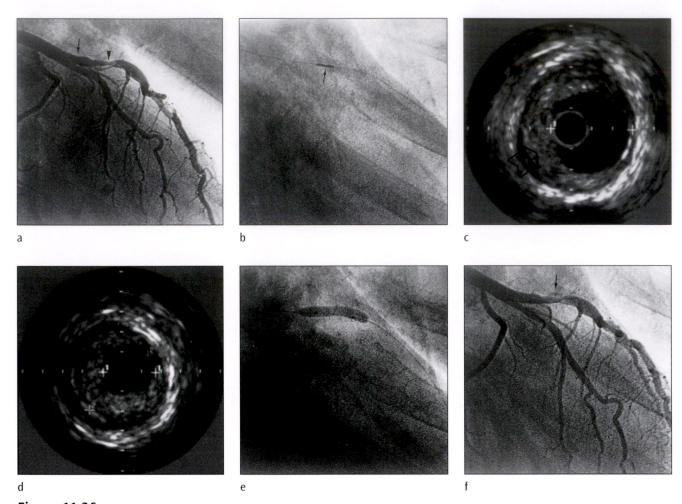

a

b

c

d

e

f

Figure 11.36

A 45-year-old asymptomatic soccer trainer with a positive exercise stress test had (a) a moderately severe stenosis in the LAD (arrowhead) and a minor stenosis more proximally (arrow) on coronary arteriography.

(b) IVUS was performed using the Visions® FX™ catheter (Endosonics). The transducer towards the distal end of the catheter can be seen (arrow).

(c) The most proximal 'minor' stenosis showed eccentric plaque over 300° of the circumference (open arrow). Although only the segment between 3 and 4 o'clock appears normal, the lumenal diameter measures 4.0mm.

(d) At the more severe stenosis (arrowhead), IVUS showed more dense stenosis occupying more than 330° of the circumference of the LAD. The lumenal diameter measured 2.6mm.

Moreover, IVUS demonstrated atheromatous plaque extending from the LAD's ostium to the more distal lesion.

(e) The second lesion was dilated with a 3.5mm Presario™ balloon (Medtronic).

(f) This resulted in local dissection (arrow).

continued

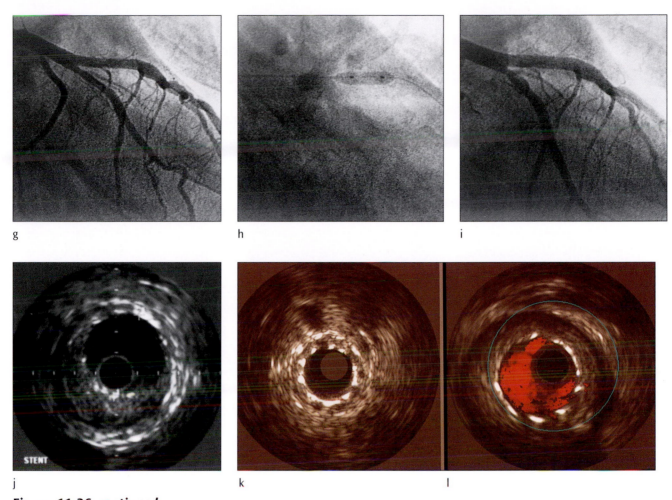

g   h   i

j   k   l

Figure 11.36 *continued*

(g) The lesion was therefore stented with a 4.0mm, 15mm long Multilink™ stent, with significant improvement.

(h) The stent was post-dilated with a 4.0mm, 12mm long Cruiser® balloon up to 18 atmospheres.

(i) The final angiographic result was excellent.

(j) IVUS showed a stent diameter of 4.1mm, with the eccentric plaque compressed by the stent. The proximal disease was left alone.

The In-Vision™ ChromaFlo™ visually depicts blood flow through the vessel. Colour maps blood flow velocity on the IVUS image and is helpful in detecting underexpanded stents and dissections. (k) Standard IVUS image of stent. (l) ChromaFlo™ image of stent showing area of blood flow.

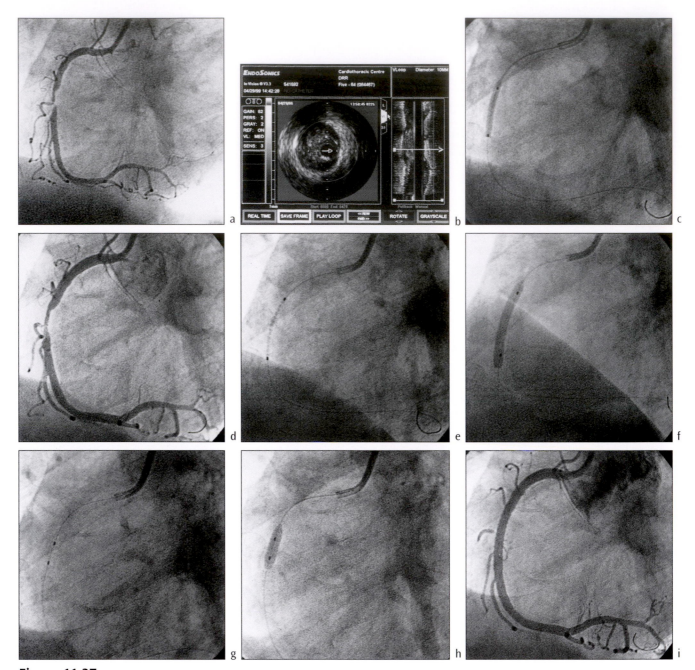

Figure 11.37

(a) A severe stenosis in the mid-third of the RCA of a 55-year-old man.
  The lesion was crossed with a 0.014-inch Floppy® guidewire.
  (b) IVUS performed with a Visions® FX™ catheter (Endosonics) showed a severe, complex, bulky stenosis. The longitudinal cross-section (shown on the right) is obtained by a slow pullback of the IVUS catheter into the proximal RCA. The arrow identifies the level at which the tangential section is taken (shown on the left).
  (c) The lesion was then pre-dilated with a 2.5mm, 20mm long Worldpass™ balloon.
  Because of residual stenosis (d), a 4.0mm, 26mm long JoStent® flex stent (e) was implanted (f) and the stent was post-dilated with a 4.0mm, 9mm long Maxxum™ balloon (g, h).
  (i) This gave an excellent angiographic result.

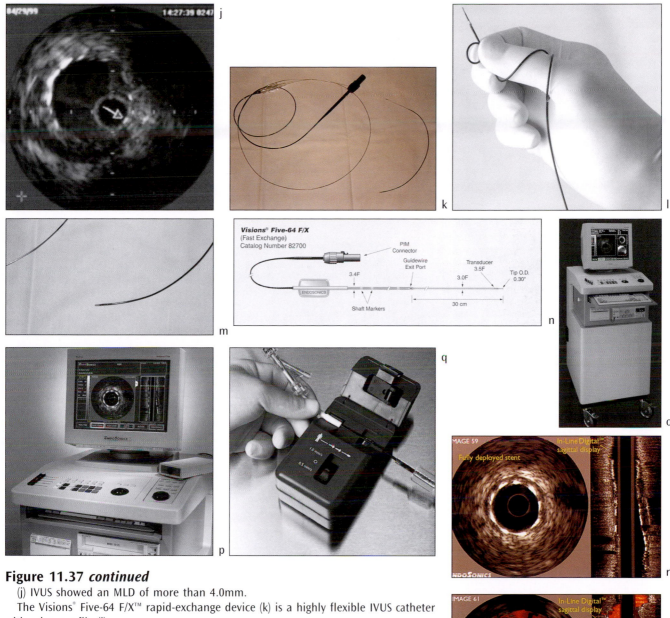

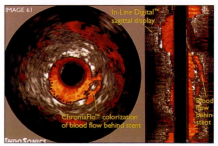

Figure 11.37 *continued*

(j) IVUS showed an MLD of more than 4.0mm.

The Visions® Five-64 F/X™ rapid-exchange device (k) is a highly flexible IVUS catheter with a low profile (l).

(m) Close-up view of the catheter tip.

(n) The catheter utilizes solid-state technology, which provides excellent handling performance. It is compatible with a 0.014-inch guidewire and its monorail length is 30cm. The distal-proximal shaft diameter is 3.0F-3.4F.

The catheter has 64 elements, a centre frequency of 20MHz and a system bandwidth of 10-40MHz. The Focus method is a dynamic aperture array.

(o) The catheter is used with the In-Vision™ IVUS imager (Endosonics). This state-of-the-art system provides patient data input, system parameter display, digital ultrasound and videoloop display, multiple screen formats, recordable CD-ROM archiving, measurement display area, digital image store, real-time display of external fluoroscopy, multiple screen menus, trackball and video cassette recorder operation controls. (p) Close-up of In-Vision™ IVUS imager.

(q) With the use of the disposable TrakBack™ automatic pullback device, the 'In-Line Digital' option provides a simultaneous longitudinal display as well as a 360° rotating image (r).

(s) With the use of the ChromaFlo™ option, the system provides real-time coloured blood flow imaging to the two-dimensional images.

Appearance of stents on IVUS

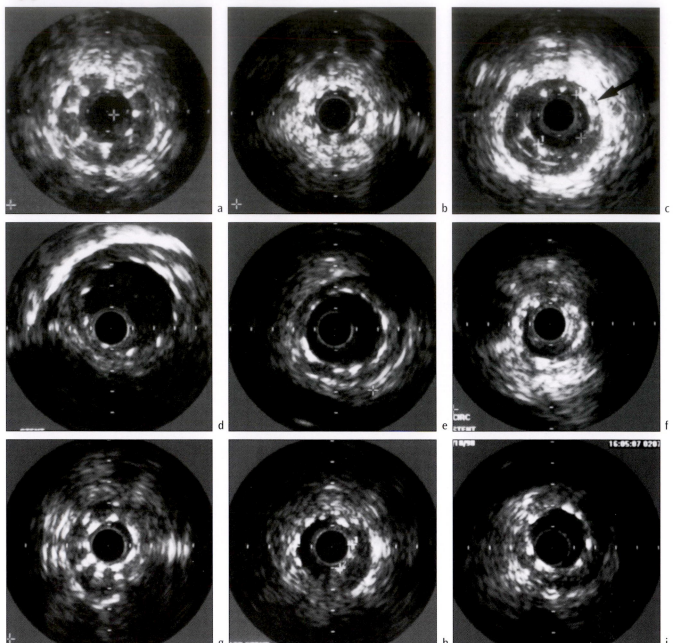

Figure 11.38
Some stents have a characteristic IVUS appearance that is dependent on factors such as strut geometry, strut thickness and echogenicity of the metal.
(a) The Microstent™ has eight brightly echogenic struts that are evenly arranged circumferentially.
(b) The smaller 2.5mm diameter Microstent shows the same characteristics when deployed in the distal RCA beyond an SVG.
(c) The BARD XT™ stent is less echogenic but the two struts fixed inside the 'junction unit' on the spine can be identified (arrow).
(d) The self-expanding 4.5mm Magic Wallstent™ has obliquely positioned struts.
(e) The Multilink Duet™ stent.
(f) The Wiktor-i™ coil stent has a non-uniform appearance on IVUS.
(g) The 2.5mm diameter beStent™.
(h) The Crossflex™ stent, also a coil stent, has an asymmetrical IVUS appearance.
(i) The original Multilink™ stent.

Preservation of side branches after stent deployment

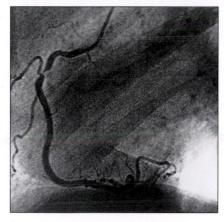

a

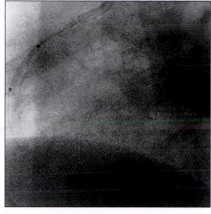

b

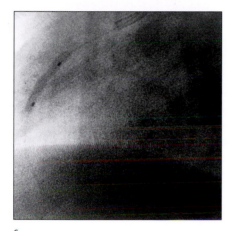

c

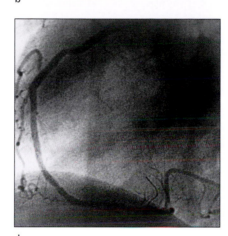

d

Figure 11.39

A 51-year-old typist with unstable angina was found to have (a) a severe eccentric stenosis in the proximal third of the RCA. Two branches exited the lesion site.

(b) A 2.5mm Rocket™ balloon was used to dilate the stenosis.

(c) Because of recoil, a 3.0mm, 15mm long Multilink™ stent was deployed.

(d) This gave an excellent angiographic result and preserved both side branches.

As with PTCA, side-branches that exit a stenosis and also have an ostial stenosis are more likely to occlude after the main lesion has been stented than those side-branches that appear to be free from significant ostial disease.

The EPISTENT trial showed that major complications after PTCA and stent implantation are significantly reduced by the use of the platelet glycoprotein IIb-IIIa inhibitor abciximab.

Reading

Beyar R, Leon MB. Functional design characteristics and clinical results with balloon-expandable and self-expanding stents. In: Beyar R, Keren G, Leon MB, Serruys PW. Frontiers in Interventional Cardiology. London: Martin Dunitz; 1997:69-81.

Blonder RD, Eastburn TE, Stark SS. Stent placement for coronary artery disease in a cardiac transplant patient. J Invas Cardiol 1996;8:266-8.

Chevalier B, Glatt B, Royer T, Guyon P. Placement of coronary stents in bifurcation lesions by the 'culotte' technique. Am J Cardiol 1998;82:943-9.

Columbo A, Hall P, Nakamura S, et al. Intracoronary stenting without anticoagulation accomplished with intravascular ultrasound guidance. Circulation 1995;91:1676-88.

Columbo A. The current practice of coronary stenting. In: Beyar R, Keren G, Leon MB, Serruys PW. Frontiers in Interventional Cardiology. London: Martin Dunitz; 1997:57-68.

de Jaegere P, Mudra H, Figulla H, et al. Intravascular ultrasound-guided optimized stent deployment. Immediate and 6 months clinical and angiographic results from the Multicenter Ultrasound Stenting In Coronaries study (MUSIC study). Eur Heart J 1998;19:1214-23.

Eeckhout E, Wijns W, Meier B, Goy JJ on behalf of the members of the Working Group on Coronary Circulation of the European Society of Cardiology. Indications for intracoronary stent placement: the European view. Working Group Report. Eur Heart J 1999;20:1014-19.

Fischman DL, Leon MB, Baim DS, et al for the Stent Restenosis Study Investigators. A randomized comparison of coronary stent placement and balloon angioplasty in the treatment of coronary artery disease. N Engl J Med 1994;331:496-501.

Fitzgerald PJ, Hayase M, Mintz GS, et al. CRUISE: Can Routine intravascular Ultrasound Influence Stent Expansion? Analysis of outcomes. J Am Coll Cardiol 1998;31:396A.

Frey AW, Roskamm H, Hodgson JM, et al. IVUS-guided stenting: does acute angiography predict long-term outcome? Insights from the Strategy of IVUS-guided PTCA and Stenting (SIPS) trial. Circulation 1997;96(Suppl I):I-222.

Garasic J, Rogers C, Edelman ER. Stent design and the biologic response. In: Beyar R, Keren G, Leon MB, Serruys PW. Frontiers in Interventional Cardiology. London: Martin Dunitz; 1997:95-100.

Gershlick AH. Stenting in acute coronary syndromes. Stent 1997;1:2-8.

Hodgson JM, Roskamm H, Frey AW, et al. Target lesion revascularization reduced after ultrasound guided interventions: findings after 6-month follow-up from the Strategy of ICUS-guided PTCA and Stenting (SIPS) trial. Circulation 1997;96(Suppl I):I-582.

Holmes DR Jr, Hirshfield J Jr, Faxon D, et al. ACC expert consensus document on coronary artery stents. Document of the American College of Cardiology. J Am Coll Cardiol 1998;32:1471-82.

Keren G. Intravascular ultrasound imaging: an update. In: Beyar R, Keren G, Leon MB, Serruys PW. Frontiers in Interventional Cardiology. London: Martin Dunitz; 1997:253-68.

Kutryk MJB, Serruys PW. Coronary Stenting. Current perspectives. A Companion to the Handbook of Coronary Stents. London: Martin Dunitz Ltd; 1999.

Lefèvre T, Louvard Y, Morice MC. Indexed management of bifurcation stenting. Stent 1999;2:34-43.

Lopez A, Heuser RR, Stoerger H, et al. Coronary artery perforation of an endoluminal polytetrafluoroethylene stent graft: two-center experience. Circulation 1998;98(Suppl I):I-855.

Mathew V, Hasdai D, Holmes DR Jr, et al. Clinical outcome of patients undergoing endoluminal coronary artery reconstruction with three or more stents. J Am Coll Cardiol 1997;30:676-81.

Mathew V, Rihal CS, et al. Clinical outcome of patients undergoing multivessel coronary stent implantation. Int J Cardiol 1998;64:1-7.

Morice MC, Louvard Y, Maillard L, et al. French registry of coronary stent grafts: acute and mid-term results. Circulation 1998;98(Suppl I):I-855.

Moussa I, Reimers B, Moses J, et al. Long-term angiographic and clinical outcome of patients undergoing multivessel coronary stenting. Circulation 1997;96:3873-9.

Mudra H, Henneke KH, Zeiher AM, et al. Acute and preliminary follow-up results of the 'OPTimization with ICUS to reduce stent restenosis' (OPTICUS) trial. J Am Coll Cardiol 1998;31:494A.

Mudra H. The role of intravascular ultrasound in coronary stenting. In: Beyar R, Keren G, Leon MB, Serruys PW. Frontiers in Interventional Cardiology. London: Martin Dunitz; 1997:297-304.

Peters RJ, Kok EM, Di Mario C, et al. for the PICTURE Study Group. Prediction of restenosis after coronary balloon angioplasty. Results of PICTURE (Post-IntraCoronary Treatment Ultrasound Result Evaluation), a prospective multicenter intracoronary ultrasound imaging study. Circulation 1997;95:2254-61.

Rombaut E, Urban P. Three vessel coronary revascularization as a single percutaneous procedure. J Invas Cardiol 1997;9:424-8.

Rozenman Y, Mereuta A, Mosseri M, et al. Initial experience with long coronary stents: the changing practice of coronary angioplasty. Am Heart J 1997;134:355-61.

Rozenman Y, Mereuta A, Schechter D, et al. Long-term outcome of patients with very long stents for treatment of diffuse coronary disease. Am Heart J 1999;138:441-445.

Savage MP, Fischman DL, Rake R, et al for the Stent Restenosis Study (STRESS) Investigators. Efficacy of coronary stenting versus balloon angioplasty in small coronary arteries. J Am Coll Cardiol 1998;31:307-11.

Serruys PW, de Jaegere P, Kiemeneij F, et al. for the Benestent Study Group. A comparison of balloon-expandable stent implantation with balloon angioplasty in patients with coronary artery disease. N Engl J Med 1994;331:489-495.

Serruys PW, Kutryk MJB, eds. Handbook of Coronary Stents, 2nd edn. London: Martin Dunitz; 1998.

The EPISTENT Investigators. Randomised placebo-controlled and balloon-angioplasty-controlled trial to assess safety of coronary stenting with use of platelet glycoprotein-IIb/IIIa blockade. Lancet 1998;352;87-92.

White CJ, Ramee SR. Coronary and saphenous vein graft stents. In: White CJ, Ramee SR, eds. Interventional Cardiology. New York: Marcel Dekker; 1995:157-74.

Windecker S, Meier B. Intervention in coronary artery disease. Heart 2000;83:481-90.

12

Catheter device synergy

As more difficult and complex coronary problems are addressed by interventional cardiologists, combinations of new devices are more frequently being employed to improve the acute result and the long-term outcome. Such lesions include:

- bulky calcified lesions;
- bulky lesions on acute bends;
- total occlusions with bulky atheromatous lesions;
- bifurcation lesions;
- restenosis within stents;
- ostial lesions; and
- SVG disease.

Combined procedures are more time consuming and more expensive and they need extra expertise from the interventional cardiologist. The operator is also exposed to more radiation, which requires careful attention to the dosage received and to appropriate protection. IVUS is playing an ever-increasing role in identifying which lesions may benefit from a combination of technologies.

DCA and Rotablator®

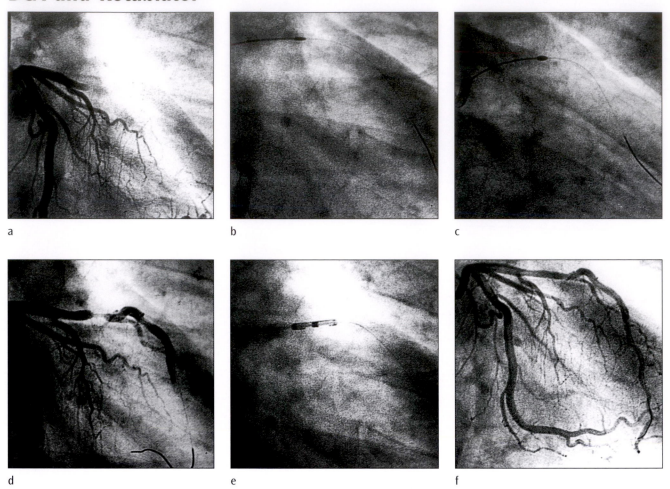

a

b

c

d

e

f

Figure 12.1

A 44-year-old farmer presented with a 2-month history of unstable angina.

(a) The proximal LAD was totally occluded.

It was possible to cross the occlusion with a 0.018-inch Intermediate® guidewire but not with a balloon catheter.

(b, c) The 0.009-inch Rotablator® C-wire was exchanged and positioned in the distal vessel and a 1.25mm Rotablator® burr followed by a 2.25mm Rotablator® burr were used to reopen the LAD.

(d, e) A 7F SCA-EX™ device was then used to debulk the remaining material.

(f) This produced an excellent result and abolished the symptoms. Restenosis did not occur.

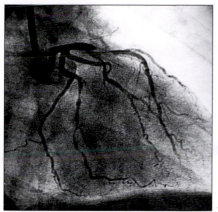
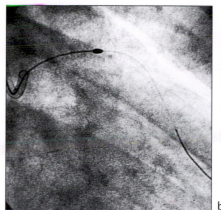
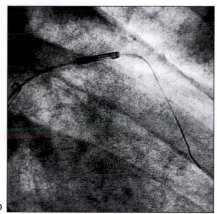

a   b   c

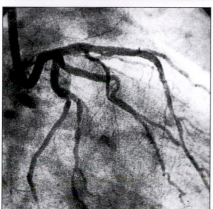

d

Figure 12.2

A 48-year-old media mogul with unstable angina had (a) a subtotally occluded LAD and a severe stenosis in an obtuse marginal branch of the LCx. The LAD appeared to be a large vessel.

(b) A 1.75mm Rotablator® burr was used over a 0.009-inch C-wire™ to ablate the plaque initially before finally debulking the lesion with a 7F SCA-EX™ device (c).

Nine pieces of atherosclerotic material were retrieved.

(d) A 3.5mm Olympix™ balloon was used for adjunctive PTCA with a good final result.

The OMCx lesion was also treated by a 1.5mm Rotablator® burr and a 2.0mm balloon.

a   b   d

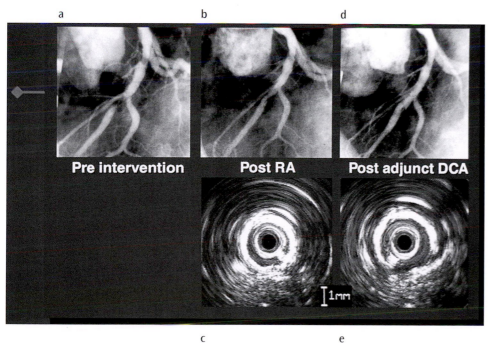

Pre intervention   Post RA   Post adjunct DCA

c   e

Figure 12.3

A 67-year-old man with angina pectoris had (a) a severe mid-LAD stenosis. A 6F Atherocath® could not cross the lesion and neither could an IVUS catheter. (b) Rotablator® atherectomy using a 2.0mm burr was performed with an improved angiographic result. (c) IVUS showed heavy concentric calcification.

A 6F Atherocath® was then used to perform DCA. Significant tissue retrieval resulted in an improved angiographic and IVUS appearance (d, e).

Courtesy of Dr KM Kent, Washington Heart Hospital Center, Washington, DC, USA.

DCA and stenting

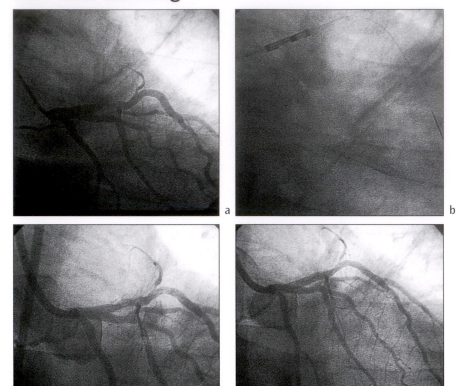

Figure 12.4
A 57-year-old bricklayer with uncontrolled angina had a severe eccentric proximal LAD stenosis (a).
(b) The lesion was debulked by DCA using a 7F SCA-EX™ device .
(c) This produced an improved but still suboptimal angiographic result.

After adjunctive PTCA with a 3.5mm Samba™ balloon catheter, a 15mm long Palmaz-Schatz™ stent was implanted on a 3.5/4.0mm CAT® balloon.
(d) This gave an excellent final result.

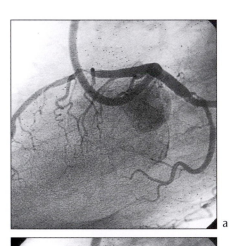
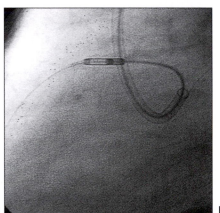
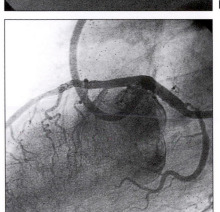

Figure 12.5
A 69-year-old man. (a) This bulky stenosis occurred on an angulated segment in the middle third of the LAD.

Such lesions are at increased risk of complications post-PTCA.
(b, c) The lesion was debulked by a 7F SCA-EX™ device.

It was then adjunctively dilated with a 3.5mm Samba™ balloon and then stented with a 3.5mm Wiktor® stent.

(d) This gave a good angiographic result.

The LCx was satisfactorily dilated with a 3.0mm Cheetah™ balloon.

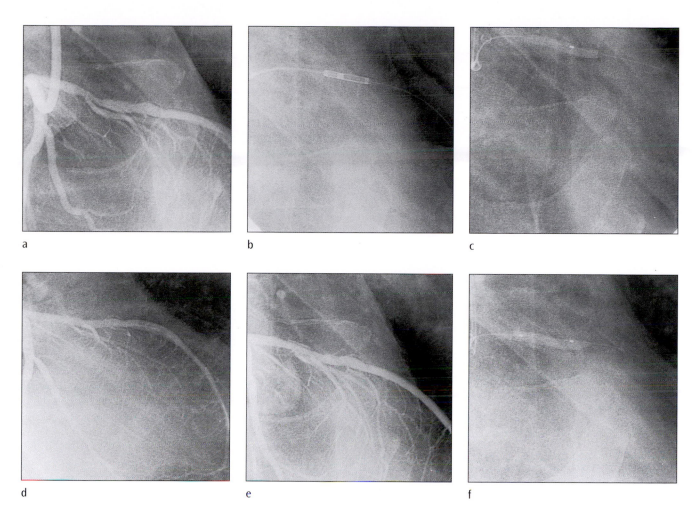

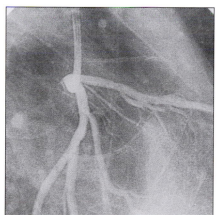

Figure 12.6

(a) A bulky, eccentric and partially calcified stenosis in the proximal LAD.

(b) The lesion was partially debulked by DCA using a 7F SCA-EX™ device.

(c) It was post-dilated (adjunctive PTCA) with a 3.5mm Express Supra™ balloon at low pressure (1.5 atmospheres).

(d) The initial result was probably acceptable.

(e) However, further PTCA at higher pressure caused a small intimal dissection.

(f, g) A 3.5mm, 15mm long Multilink™ stent was therefore implanted, which produced an excellent final result.

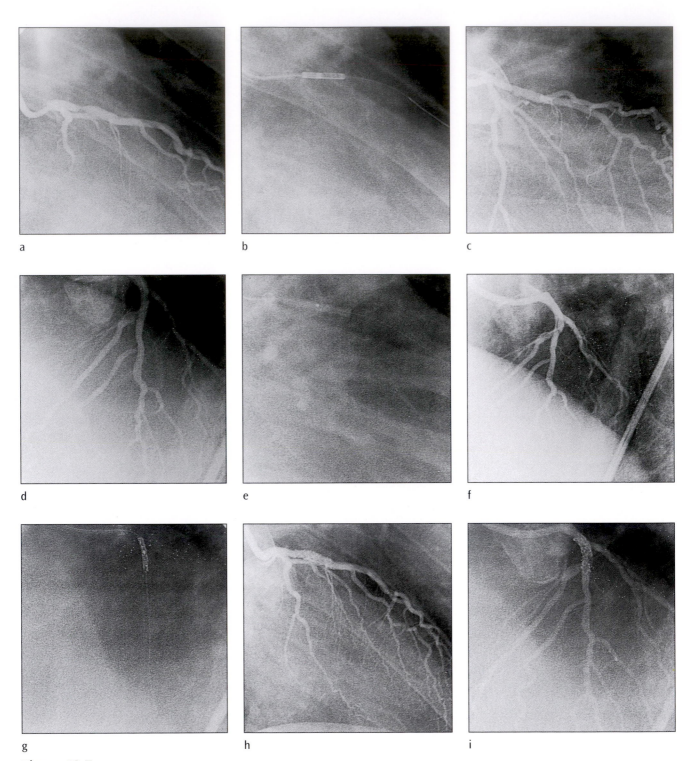

a

b

c

d

e

f

g

h

i

Figure 12.7

A 43-year-old man had poorly controlled angina due to (a) a significant, proximal LAD stenosis.

(b) DCA was performed using a 7F SCA-EX™ device.

(c, d) This left a residual 20% stenosis.

Adjunctive PTCA, using a 3.5mm balloon at low pressure (e) caused a loose intimal flap dissection (f) (LAO cranial projection).

(g-i) A 3.5mm Wiktor® stent was therefore deployed.

(i) However, part of the flap appeared to protrude through 'splayed' struts of the stent.

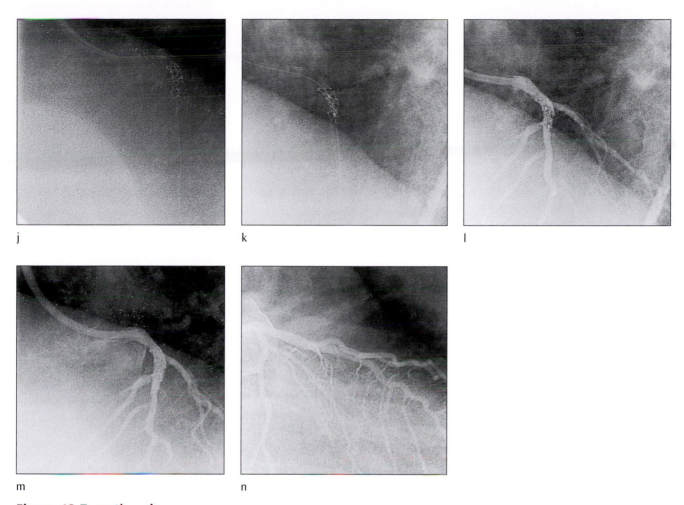

Figure 12.7 *continued*

(j) This can be seen in this view.

(k, l) A 12mm Microstent II™ was therefore positioned inside the Wiktor® stent and was fully deployed to yield a perfect angiographic result – (m) LAO projection; (n) RAO projection.

(This is the same patient as in Figs 7.23, 15.43 and 15.48.)

Primary atherostenting

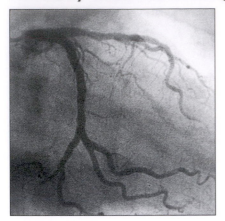

Figure 12.8
Debulking lesions may aid full stent deployment. A 60-year-old quarry worker with moderate angina had a severe, bulky, eccentric stenosis in a large LCx artery (see Fig. 6.16). DCA was initially performed with a 7F SCA-EX™ device and five pieces of tissue were removed. Although the angiographic result was markedly improved, a 3.5mm, 15mm long Multilink™ stent was deployed at 10 atmospheres with a good final result. This illustration shows the result at 6 months.

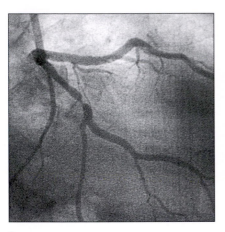
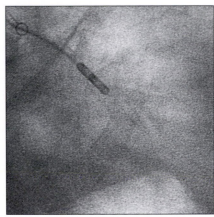
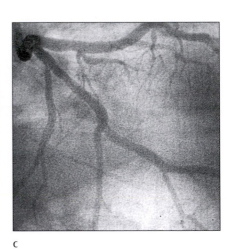

a   b   c

Figure 12.9
A 50-year-old funeral director had (a) a severe, bulky, eccentric lesion in the LCx.
(b) The lesion was first debulked with a 7F Atherocath GTO® device with a good result.
It was then stented with a 3.5mm, 15mm long Multilink™ stent with a good angiographic (c) and clinical result.

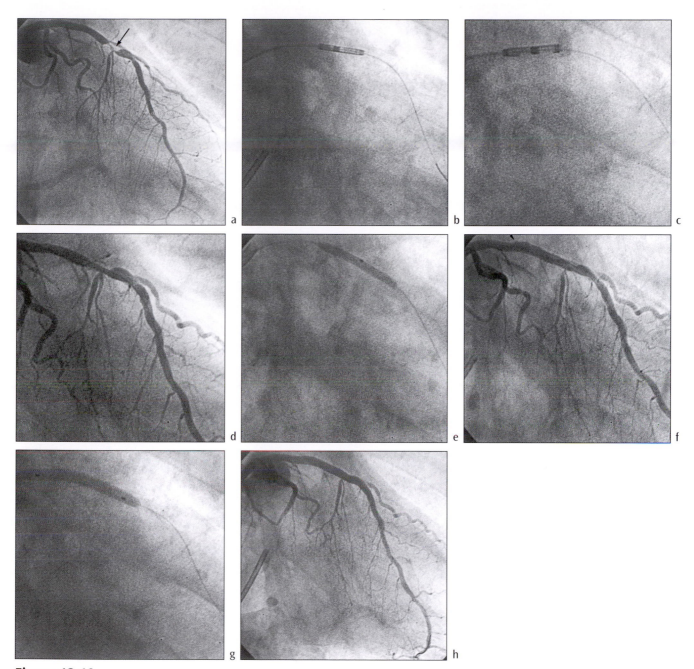

Figure 12.10

A 69-year-old retired telephone engineer with moderate angina, hypertension and hypercholesterolemia had (a) a severe bulky stenosis in the middle third of the LAD and a less severe stenosis just beyond.

The lesion was crossed with a 0.014-inch Floppy® guidewire via a 10F FL5 Medtronic guide catheter.

A 7F Bantam™ Atherocath (b) was used to remove nine pieces of atheromatous tissue from the proximal lesion. The window of the device is shown to be directed downwards in this view (c).

(d) Some improvement was obtained.

(e) Both lesions were adjunctively dilated with a 3.0mm, 30mm long Elipse™ balloon.

(f) They were then stented with a single 3.0mm, 25mm Multilink™ stent. There appeared to be a small dissection proximally (arrowhead) as a result of deep engagement of the guide catheter tip in order to deliver the Atherocath® from this dilated and unfolded ascending aorta.

(g) A 3.5mm, 25mm long Multilink™ stent was therefore placed in the proximal LAD to overlap the first stent.

(h) The junction was post dilated with the 3.5mm, 30mm balloon with an excellent final result.

The AMIGO randomized trial is comparing the long-term clinical outcome and angiographic restenosis rates in patients undergoing Multilink stent implantation with or without prior adjunctive DCA.

Rotablator® and stenting

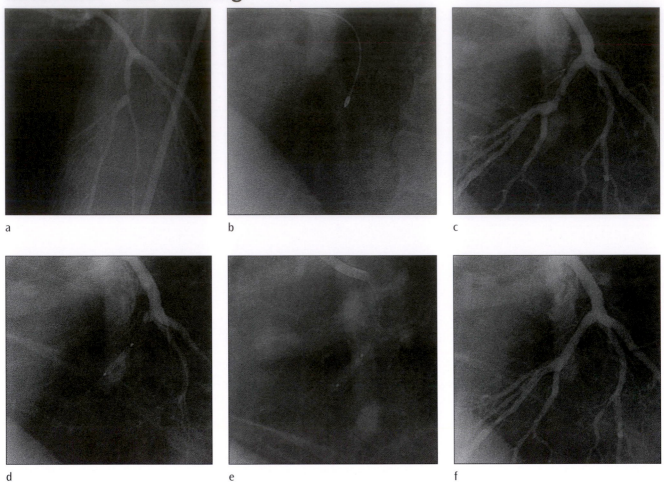

a

b

c

d

e

f

Figure 12.11

A 53-year-old professional hypnotist developed angina 2 weeks after a threatened anterior myocardial infarction and was found to have (a) a severe bulky stenosis in the proximal LAD.

The lesion was first debulked with a 1.5mm Rotablator® burr and then a 2.0mm Rotablator® burr (b), dilated with a 3.5mm Samba™ balloon (c) and then stented with a 3.5mm, 12mm long Microstent II™ (d, e).

(f) This gave an excellent angiographic result.

The principle of debulking a lesion prior to stenting (so-called Rotastenting) is thought to enhance full stent deployment and reduce recoil. The SPORT trial is currently examining whether rotational atherectomy plus NIR™ stenting is better than PTCA plus NIR™ stenting.

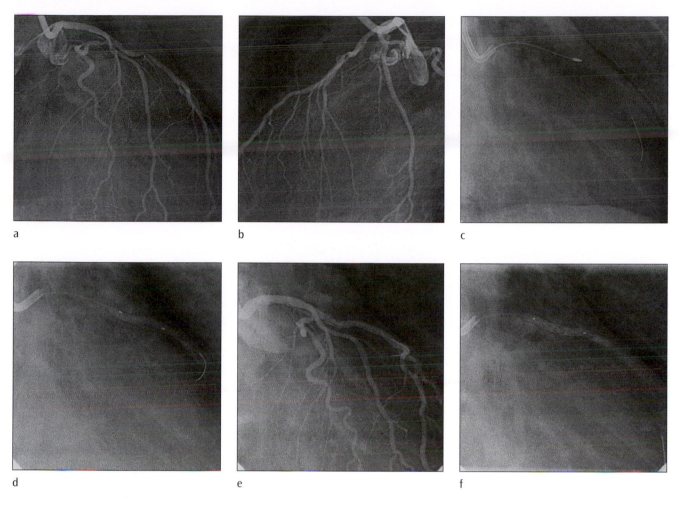

a

b

c

d

e

f

g

Figure 12.12

A 63-year-old man with hypertension and unstable angina had (a, b) a severe stenosis in the proximal LAD.

Rotablator® atherectomy with a 1.5mm burr and a 2.0mm burr (c) was followed by a 3.0mm, 15mm long Multilink™ stent (d).

(e) However, balloon dilatation at 10 atmospheres during stent deployment caused dissection proximal to the stent.

(f, g) This was treated by a further 3.0mm, 18mm long Microstent II™ implantation.

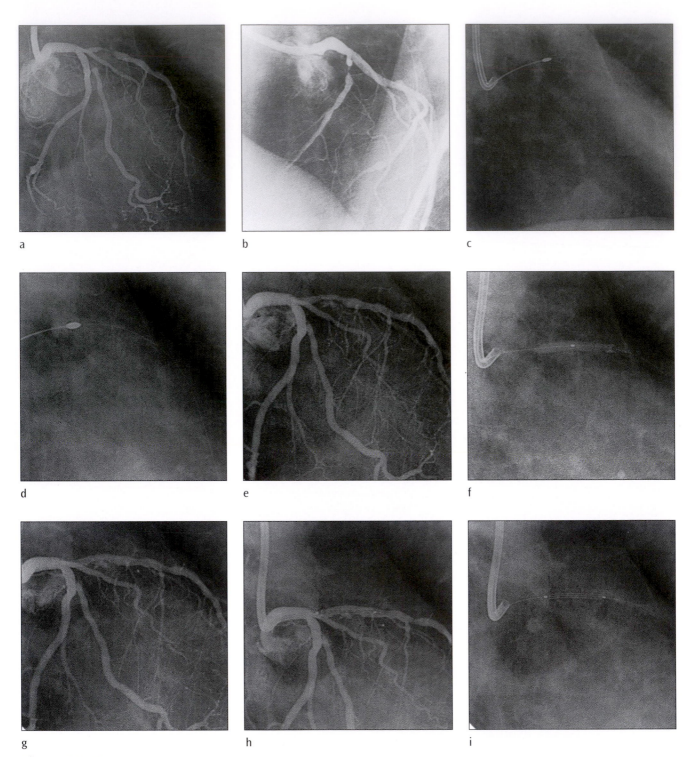

a

b

c

d

e

f

g

h

i

Figure 12.13

A 64-year-old business manager with severe limiting angina had (a, b) significant ostial and proximal LAD stenoses. Calcification was visible on fluoroscopy.

Both lesions were ablated with a 1.5mm Rotablator® burr (c) followed by a 2.25mm Rotablator® burr (d). Result (e).

Adjunctive PTCA with a 3.5mm Cheetah™ balloon at a pressure of 1.5 atmospheres was performed (f).

(g) However, PTCA produced a significant local dissection in the proximal lesion.

(h-j) This was stented with a 3.5mm Microstent™, which produced (k, l) an excellent angiographic result.

(m) The stent is radio-opaque.

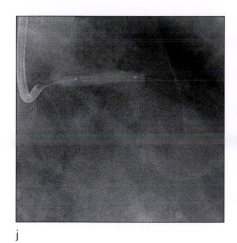

j

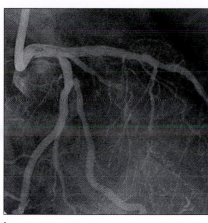

k

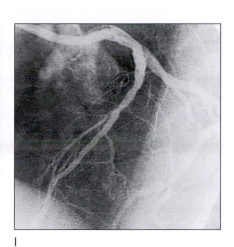

l

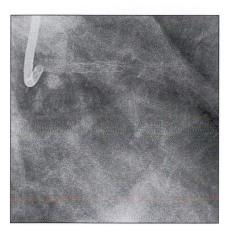

m

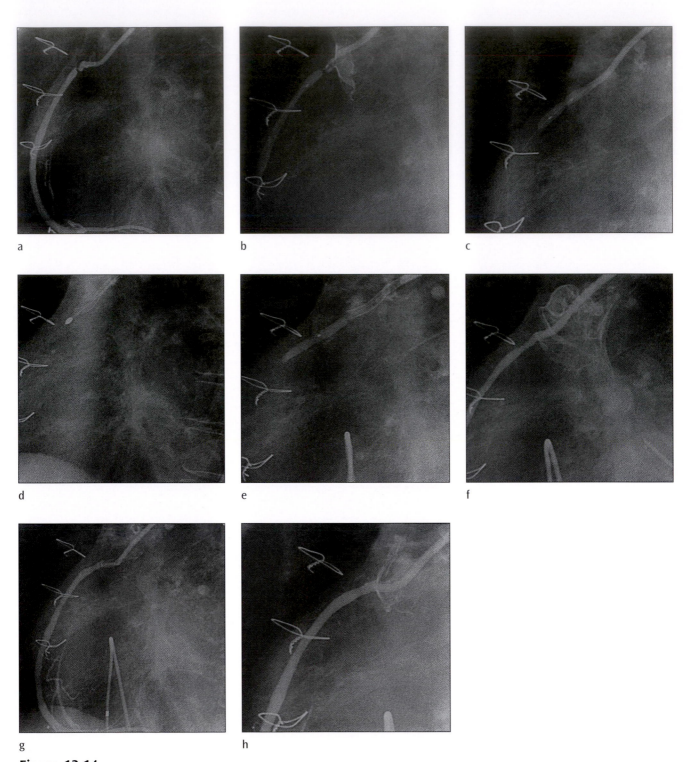

a

b

c

d

e

f

g

h

Figure 12.14

A 57-year-old woman presented with unstable angina 6 years after mitral valve replacement and SVG to the RCA and the OMCx. (a) The SVG in the RCA was found to have a severe eccentric stenosis in its proximal third.

(b, c) The lesion did not respond to 22 atmosphere inflation pressure with a 3.5mm Viva Primo™ balloon.

After Rotablator® atherectomy with a 2.5mm burr (d), the lesion was much improved and responded well to a 3.5/4.0mm CAT™ balloon up to 19 atmospheres (e, f) and a 9mm NIR™ stent implantation (g, h).

In dilatable lesions, there is some evidence that immediate procedural outcome and late clinical events are not substantially different in patients who undergo debulking before stenting in aorta-ostial SVG lesions from those in patients who undergo stenting alone.

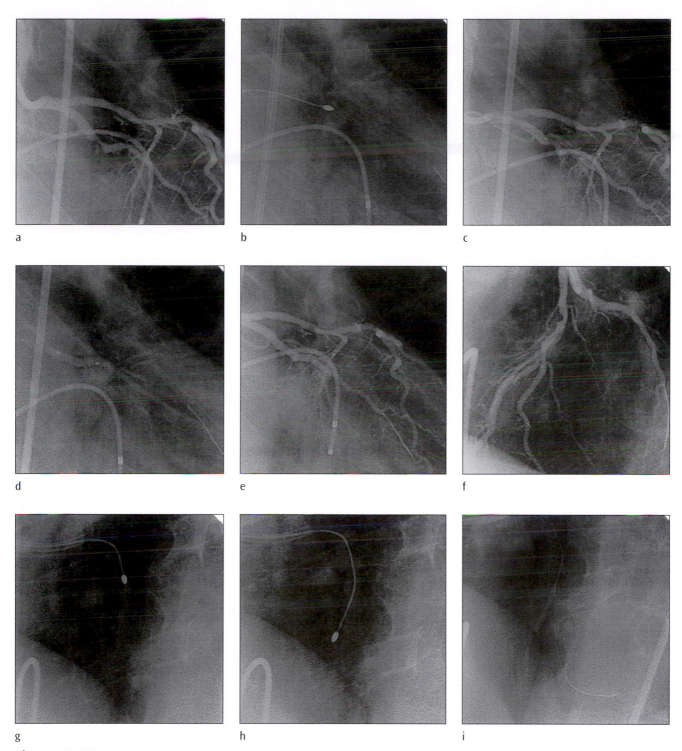

a

b

c

d

e

f

g

h

i

Figure 12.15

A 62-year-old general practitioner with recent unstable angina. Angiography showed severe calcified stenoses in both the LCx and LAD.

The stenosis in the tortuous LCx (a) was crossed with a 0.009-inch Rotablator® guidewire and ablated with a 2.0mm Rotablator® burr (b).

(c, d) A 3.0mm, 15mm long Multilink™ stent was then implanted.

(e) This gave a good result.

The LAD has an eccentric proximal stenosis as well as a bifurcation lesion involving the diagonal branch (e, f).

(g, h) The two LAD lesions were ablated with a 2.0mm Rotablator® burr.

(i) They were then adjunctively dilated with a 2.5mm Cheetah™ balloon.

continued

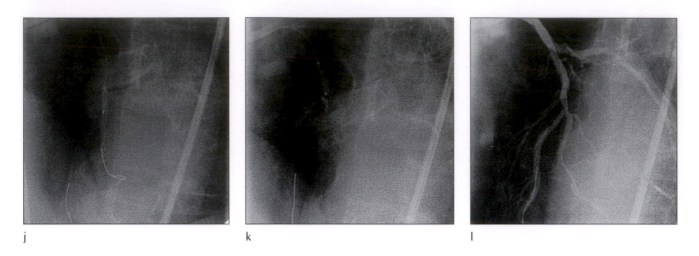

j   k   l

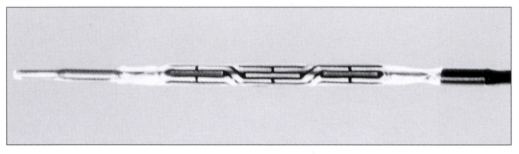

m

Figure 12.15 *continued*

(j) Once the DG had been 'wired' with a 0.014-inch Floppy® guidewire, the stenosis in the DG was also dilated with the 2.5mm balloon.

(k) The proximal LAD lesion then received a 3.0mm, 15mm Powergrip™ stent.

(l) This gave an excellent angiographic result.

(m) The Powergrip™ mounted Palmaz-Schatz™ stent. It has now been replaced by more flexible stents.

IVUS-assisted Rotablator® atherectomy and stenting

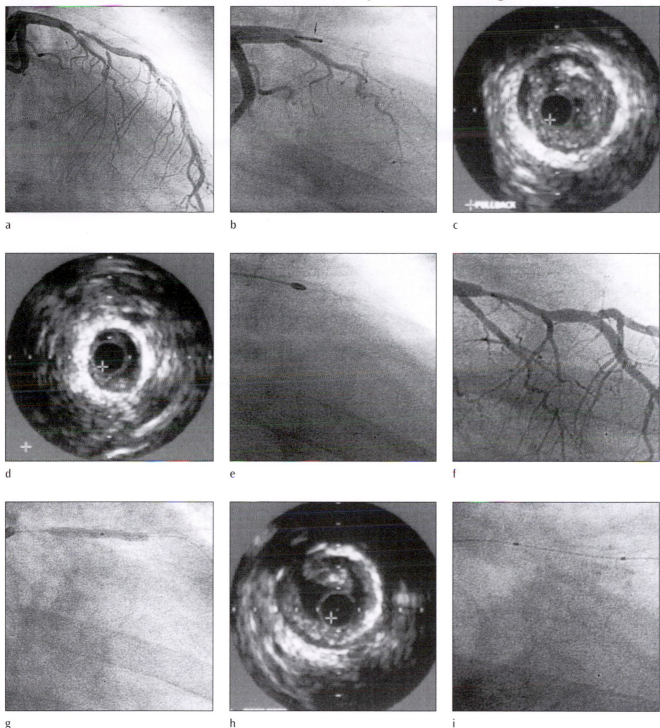

a

b

c

d

e

f

g

h

i

Figure 12.16

(a) A long segment of severe stenosis in the proximal LAD of a 58-year-old male transport manager with moderately severe angina. Mild LAD calcification was visible on fluoroscopy.

(b) IVUS using the Visions FX™ rapid-exchange catheter (Endosonics) (arrow) was performed.

(c) This revealed extensive dense intraluminal plaque with much calcification.

(d) In two areas, calcific plaque surrounded the entire circumference.

(e) Rotablator® atherectomy was performed using a 1.75mm burr followed by a 2.0mm burr and a 2.25mm burr.

Despite slow passage and careful upsizing of the burrs, distal embolization of debris resulted in severe hypotension (a systolic blood pressure of 50mmHg), which was promptly treated by intravenous adrenaline.

(f) Angiography showed improvement after rotational atherectomy.

However, even after PTCA with a 3.0mm, 30mm long Elipse™ balloon (g), IVUS still showed much intraluminal material protruding into the lumen of rote artery (h).

(i, j) The vessel was stented with two 3.5mm, 25mm long Multilink™ stents deployed at 10 atmospheres.   *continued*

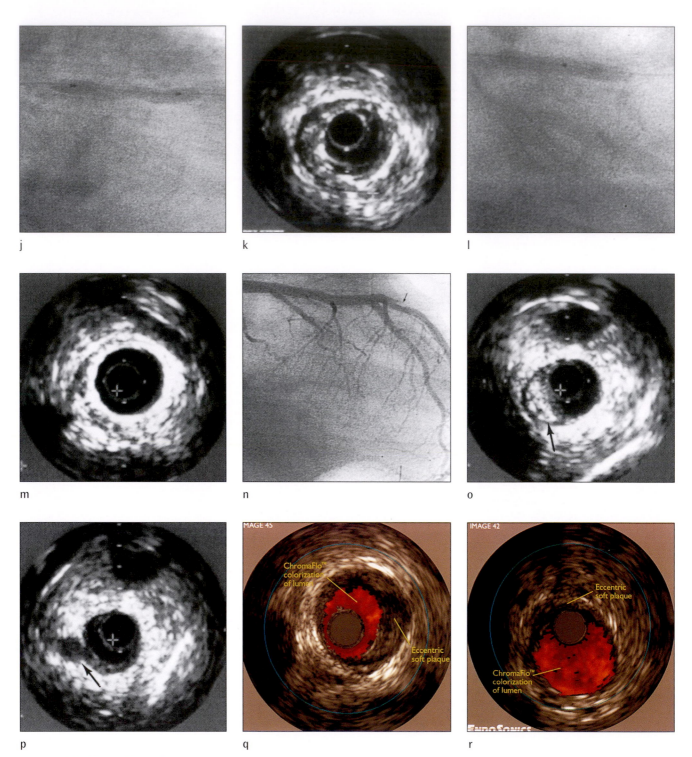

Figure 12.16 *continued*

(k) However IVUS showed uneven and incomplete stent expansion.

(l) A 4.0mm, 30mm long Elipse™ balloon was used to post-dilate the two stents up to 12 atmospheres.

(m) IVUS then showed better stent expansion and more plaque compression.

(n) The angiogram showed a good final result. However, distal to the more distally placed stent, a narrowed segment was visible angiographically (arrow), which suggested an 'edge-tear'.

(o) IVUS confirmed this to be an eccentric plaque (arrow).

(p) IVUS also showed a small side branch exiting from the proximal end of the plaque (arrow).

No further dilatations were performed and there were no complications.

(q, r) The In-Vision™ ChromaFlo™ option provides colour mapping of blood flow velocity on the IVUS image (Courtesy of Endosonics).

ELCA and stenting

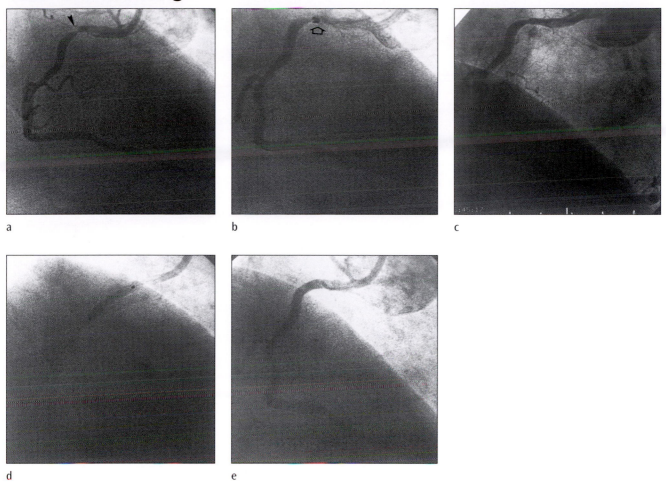

a   b   c

d   e

Figure 12.17

A 62-year-old gardener with angina on moderate effort had (a) a significant eccentric stenosis in the proximal RCA (arrow).
(b) A 1.7mm Vitesse® E ELCA catheter was used to ablate the plaque using 50mJ/mm² at a fluence rate of 25-40 pulses per second. The tip of the eccentric catheter can be seen (open arrow).
(c) After ELCA alone a modest improvement could be seen.

After dilatation with a 3.0mm Worldpass™ balloon, the lesion was stented with a 3.5mm, 15mm long Multilink™ stent (d) with an excellent final angiographic result (e). The patient remained free of angina at 12 months.

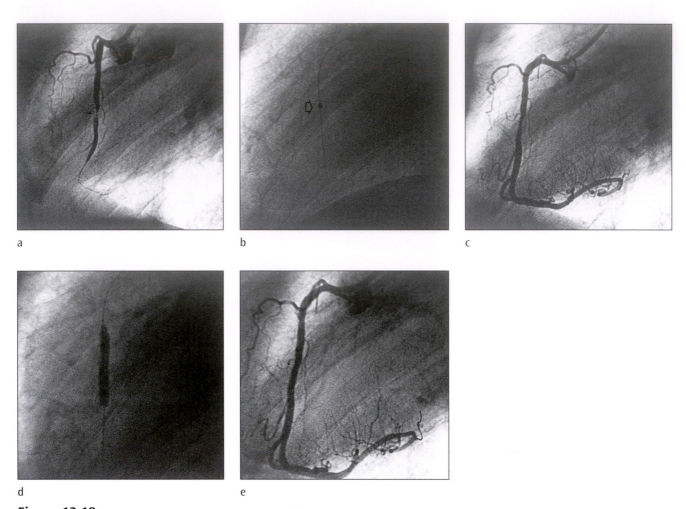

a

b

c

d

e

Figure 12.18
This 64-year-old man with moderately severe angina had (a) a severe concentric stenosis in the middle third of the RCA, which was causing a marked reduction in flow.
(b) A 2.0mm Vitesse® C ELCA catheter was used to deliver 50mJ/mm² at a repetition rate of 25-50 pulses per second. The tip of the catheter is radio-opaque (open arrow).
(c) The result after ELCA showed restoration of normal flow and little residual stenosis.
(d) A 3.0mm, 15mm long Multilink™ stent was then deployed.
(e) This gave an excellent final result. The patient was free of symptoms at 12 months.

TEC and DCA

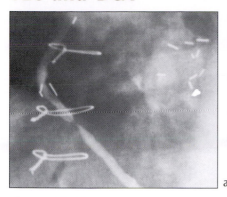

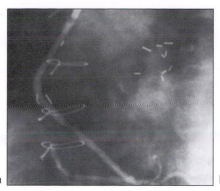

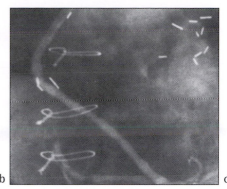

a   b   c

Figure 12.19

A 76-year-old woman with hypertension and end-stage renal disease presented with inferior myocardial infarction and post-infarction angina 3 years after CABG surgery. (a) Angiography revealed a high grade stenosis in the SVG to the PDA.
A multipurpose 10F TEC® guide catheter was used to deliver a 0.014-inch TEC® guidewire and a 7.5 F (2.5mm) TEC device.
(b) Several slow passes produced a marked improvement.
(c) DCA was performed to the residual stenosis, with good effect.
Courtesy of Dr ME McIvor, All Children's Hospital, St Petersburg, Florida, USA.

Therapeutic ultrasound-assisted PTCA

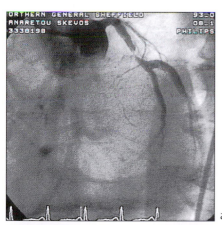

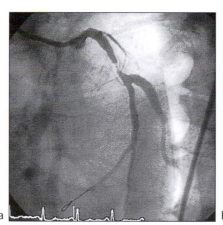

a   b

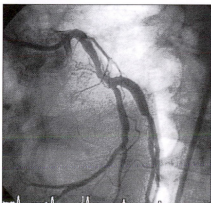

c

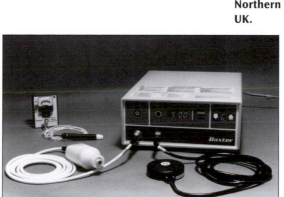

d

Figure 12.20

A previous attempt at PTCA of this severe LCx stenosis had failed because the stenosis failed to yield at 10 atmospheres. (a) Initial angiography showed the lesion to be unchanged.
(b) After 5 minutes of therapeutic ultrasound energy applied to the lesion, the stenosis showed only minor improvement.
(c) However, after PTCA at 5 atmospheres, the lesion was fully dilated and a satisfactory result was achieved.
(d) The therapeutic ultrasound device originally developed by Baxter®.
Courtesy of Dr D Cumberland, Northern General Hospital, Sheffield, UK.

Angiojet® thrombectomy and stent implantation

Figures 5.31 and 5.32 show examples of the combination of Angiojet® thrombectomy and stenting in the setting of an acute myocardial infarction.

Beta-irradiation for prevention of restenosis

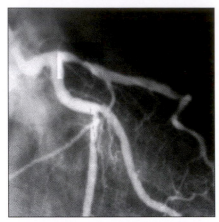

a

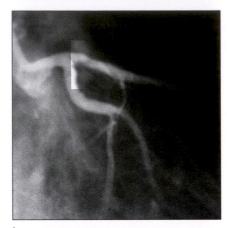

b

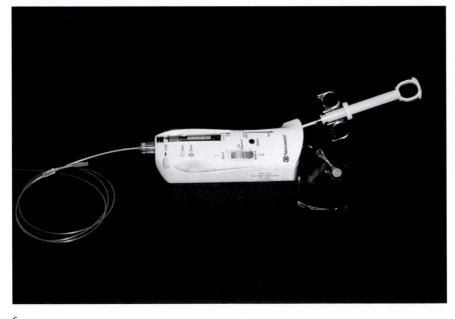

c

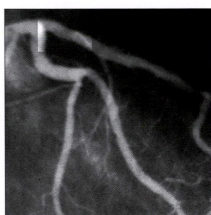

d

Figure 12.21

A 68-year-old man with a six month history of increasing angina had a large, reversible anterior defect on a stress thallium perfusion scan. (a) Angiography showed a significant, concentric stenosis in the proximal LAD.

(b) PTCA with a 3.5mm, 20mm long Bandit™ balloon at 12 atmospheres left a residual stenosis of 23%.

The dilated vessel segment was then treated with beta-irradiation therapy as part of the Beta Energy Restenosis Trial (BERT) using the Novoste™ radiation delivery catheter and transfer device (c).

At 3 months, a repeat stress thallium perfusion study was normal.

(d) At 6 months, angiography revealed a 7% stenosis at the PTCA site. The patient remains symptom free.

Courtesy of Drs ME Leimbach, NAF Chronos and SB King III, Andreas Gruentzig Cardiovascular Center, Emory University Hospital, Atlanta, Georgia, USA.

Reading

Al-Mubarak NA, Liu MW, Al-Saif SM, *et al.* Combined transluminal extraction Atherectomy (TEC) and Wallstents for treatment of saphenous vein graft disease. Circulation 1998;98(Suppl I):I-717.

Braden GA, Xenopoulos NP, Young T, *et al.* Transluminal extraction catheter atherectomy followed by immediate stenting in treatment of saphenous vein grafts. J Am Coll Cardiol 1997;30:657-63.

Dussaillant GR, Mintz GS, Pichard AD, *et al.* Mechanisms and immediate and long-term results of adjunct directional coronary atherectomy after rotational atherectomy. J Am Coll Cardiol 1996;27:1390-7.

Hoffmann R, Mintz GS, Kent KM, *et al.* Comparative early and nine-month results of rotational atherectomy, stents and the combination of both for calcified lesions in large coronary arteries. Am J Cardiol 1998;81:552-7.

Hong MK, Mintz GS, Popma JJ, *et al.* Safety and efficacy of elective stent implantation following rotational atherectomy in large calcified coronary arteries. Cathet Cardiovasc Diagn 1996;Suppl 3:50-4.

Kobayashi Y, Moussa I, De Gregorio J, *et al.* Low restenosis rate in lesions of the left anterior descending coronary artery with stenting following directional coronary atherectomy. J Am Coll Cardiol 1998;31:378A.

Moussa I, Di Mario C, Moses J, *et al.* Coronary stenting after rotational atherectomy in calcified and complex lesions. Angiographic and clinical follow-up results. Circulation 1997;96:128-36.

Nakagawa Y, Matsuo S, Yokoi H, *et al.* Stenting after thrombectomy with the Angiojet® catheter for acute myocardial infarction. Cathet Cardiovasc Diagn 1998;43:327-30.

Parks JM. TEC before stent implantation. J Invas Cardiol 1995;7(Suppl D):10D-13D.

Ramsdale DR, Chester MR. Rotastenting of a bifurcation lesion using the JoMed S side-branch stent. J Invas Cardiol 1998;10:220-2.

Rozenmann Y, Lotan C, Mosseri M, *et al.* Recent experience with percutaneous recanalization of 'protected' left main using new angioplasty devices. J Invas Cardiol 1997;9:475-8.

13

Intervention after CABG surgery

Recurrent angina after CABG surgery may be due to incomplete revascularization, new native vessel disease, stenoses in the grafts or graft occlusion.

Incomplete revascularization and acute thrombotic occlusion of the grafts or grafted native vessels may account for early recurrence of symptoms after surgery. Although distal graft stenoses also occur early after surgery (usually at 0-6 months), new native vessel disease, graft stenoses and graft occlusion generally tend to occur late (more than 3 years after surgery). However, there is considerable overlap.

Because PTCA in SVGs is associated with a higher post-procedural myocardial infarction rate and increased late major events, including death, myocardial infarction and higher restenosis rates (the rates in ostial and body lesions being greater than the rates in distal lesions), PTCA to native disease should always be considered first, especially if additional myocardium can be revascularized. Stent implantation may reduce the restenosis rates of lesions within SVGs, although very diffusely diseased grafts are not suitable for this.

Alternative technologies can be very useful. Rotablator® atherectomy may be appropriate for calcified lesions in native vessels, in balloon-resistant ostial SVG lesions and for in-stent restenosis. DCA may be indicated for focal, bulky lesions in large, non-tortuous SVGs, and TEC atherectomy may be of particular help in diffusely diseased SVGs, in ulcerated lesions associated with thrombus and in SVGs that have been recently occluded by thrombus.

Unfortunately, all techniques in SVGs are associated with significant rates of distal embolization and high restenosis rates. Abciximab does not appear to reduce major clinical events after percutaneous coronary intervention in SVGs. New mechanical devices may limit distal embolization.

Chronically occluded SVGs (i.e. SVGs that have been occluded for more than 3 months) are frequently impossible to open and should usually be left alone, since successful recanalization is often associated with poor long-term patency.

PTCA of SVGs

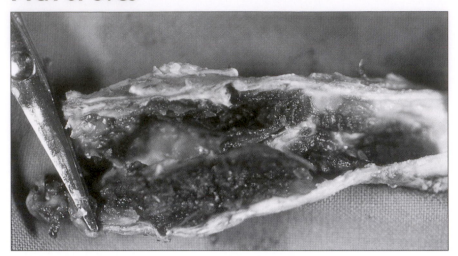

Figure 13.1
Old SVGs degenerate and become filled with much grumous atherosclerotic material and eventually with thrombus.

Distal lesions

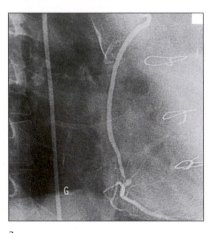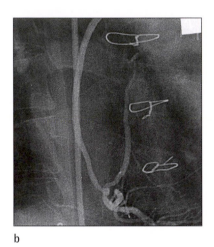

a   b

Figure 13.2
Distal stenoses respond well to PTCA and generally have lower restenosis rates than body or proximal lesions. This RCA SVG in a 56-year-old man occluded 6 years after CABG surgery. It was reopened by PTCA and intragraft thrombolytic therapy with rtPA. The distal stenosis was dilated successfully but the graft rethrombosed 9 weeks later despite treatment with warfarin. The SVG was reopened by PTCA and intragraft streptokinase, and a persistent lesion in the body of the graft was removed by DCA (see Fig. 13.14).

Five months after the original PTCA to the distal RCA SVG stenosis, the patient developed recurrent angina and was found to have (a) a severe distal anastomotic restenosis.

(b) Note the improved appearance after PTCA with a 3.0mm Europass™ balloon, which resulted in better filling of the RCA.

The patient developed a further restenosis 7 months later and was successfully treated by PTCA. Two years later, he developed recurrent angina and a further distal anastomotic restenosis. This was treated by stent implantation (see Fig. 13.45).

He remained well for a further 2 years, when his symptoms of angina returned. Angiography showed severe in-stent restenosis. He received a gastroepiploic arterial graft to the distal RCA and an SVG to an occluded OMCx. His left internal mammary artery (from his second CABG procedure) was still patent. Two years on, he remains symptom-free.

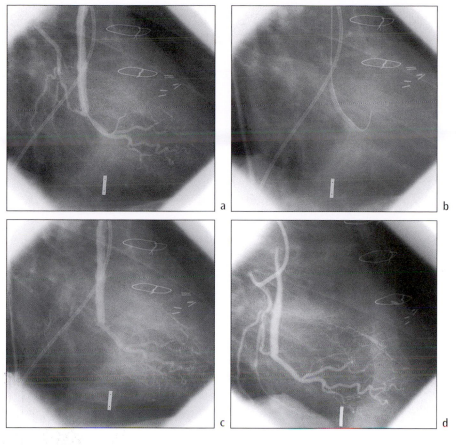

a

b

c

d

Figure 13.3
A 54-year-old man. (a) This distal OMCx SVG stenosis developed within 3 months after CABG surgery.
(b, c) It was successfully treated by PTCA with a Snake™ monorail balloon catheter (Schneider).
(d) The result remained unchanged angiographically over the next 9 years; the OMCx SVG can be seen filled via the native LCx.

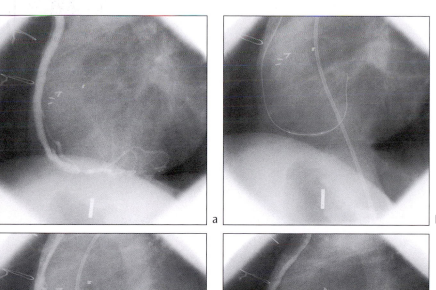

a

b

c

d

Figure 13.4
The same patient as in Fig. 13.3. (a) This distal RCA SVG stenosis developed at the same time after CABG surgery as the stenosis shown in Fig. 13.3a.
(b, c) It was successfully treated by PTCA with the same equipment.
(d) It too remained unchanged angiographically over the next 9 years.

Body lesions

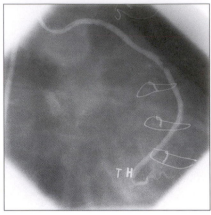
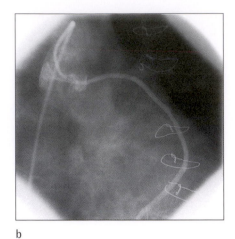

a b

Figure 13.5
This discrete stenosis in the body of an LCx SVG (7 years after CABG surgery) was thought to have associated thrombus. (a) However, 24 hours after intragraft urokinase, the appearance remained unchanged.
(b) The angiographic appearance after PTCA is much improved. Unfortunately, such lesions have high recurrence rates.

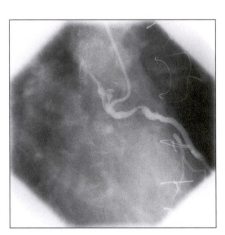

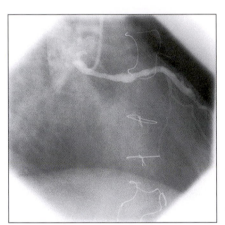

a b

Figure 13.6
(a) Stenosis in body of a 7-year-old LCx SVG.
(b) Result after PTCA.

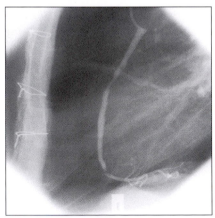
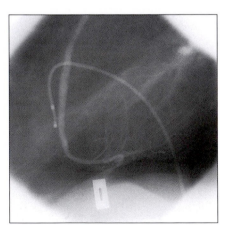

a b

Figure 13.7
A 9-year-old RCA SVG with body and distal stenoses (a) before and (b) after PTCA.

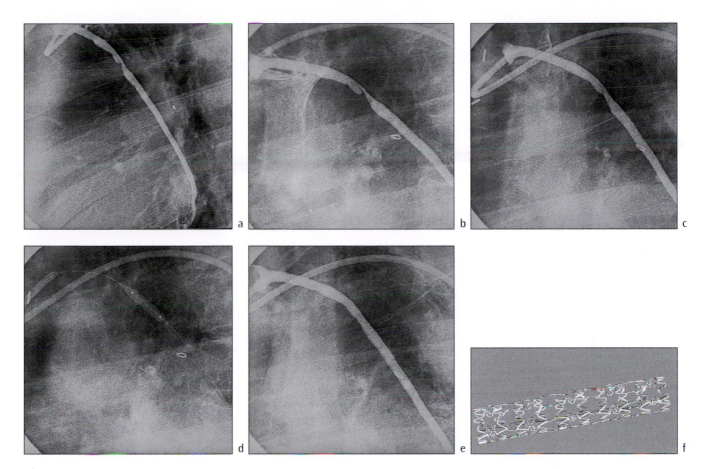

Figure 13.8

A 59-year-old man with moderate angina 6 years after CABG surgery. (a, b) The OMCx SVG had an eccentric, bulky stenosis in its mid-third.

(c) The stenosis was dilated with a 3.5mm Worldpass™ balloon, with improvement but significant recoil.

(d) A 3.5mm JoStent® flex stent was implanted with a good result (e), although perhaps the stent needed further dilatation at higher pressure.

(f) The JoStent® flex stent.

Proximal and ostial lesions

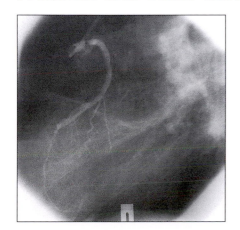

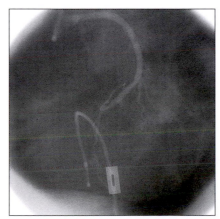

Figure 13.9

Proximal and ostial stenoses in SVGs have a relatively high recurrence rate.

(a) A tight stenosis in the proximal third of an LAD SVG.

(b) It responded well to PTCA and did not recur after 12 months.

PTCA of totally occluded SVGs

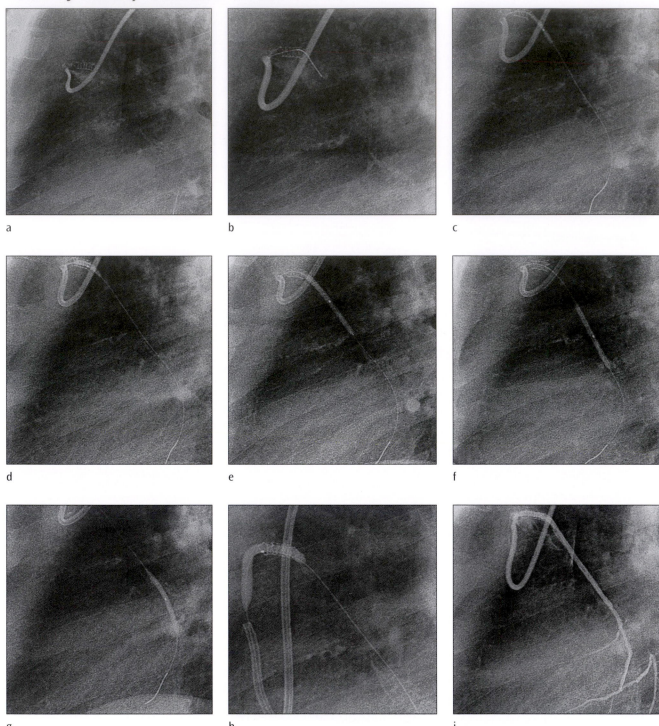

Figure 13.10
A 69-year-old diabetic man had had PTCA and Wiktor® stent implantation to the proximal third of an OMCx SVG 1 year earlier. He developed a recurrence of severe angina within 7 months of the procedure. (a) However, by the time of repeat angiography, the SVG was totally occluded at its origin.

Using a left Amplatz guide catheter, it proved possible to force a 0.014-inch Standard® guidewire through the occlusion, through the stent and down the SVG (a, b).

(c, d) A 2.0mm Passage® balloon was then forced along the graft and dilated sequentially from the distal end to the proximal end.

A 3.0mm, 40mm long Elipse™ balloon was then similarly inflated along the SVG (e-g) as well as at the ostium and within the Wiktor® stent (h).

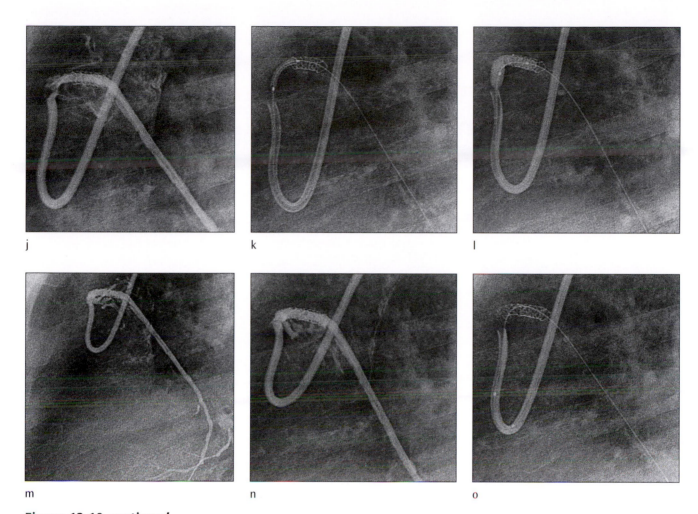

j

k

l

m

n

o

Figure 13.10 *continued*

(i, j) The result.

(k, l) A 4.0mm, 18mm long Microstent II™ was then implanted at the ostium of the SVG with a good angiographic result proximally and full patency.

(m, n) However, filling defects persist, owing to organized intraluminal thrombus and ulcerated plaque.

(o) The radio-opacity of the stent helps the operator to position the stent accurately.

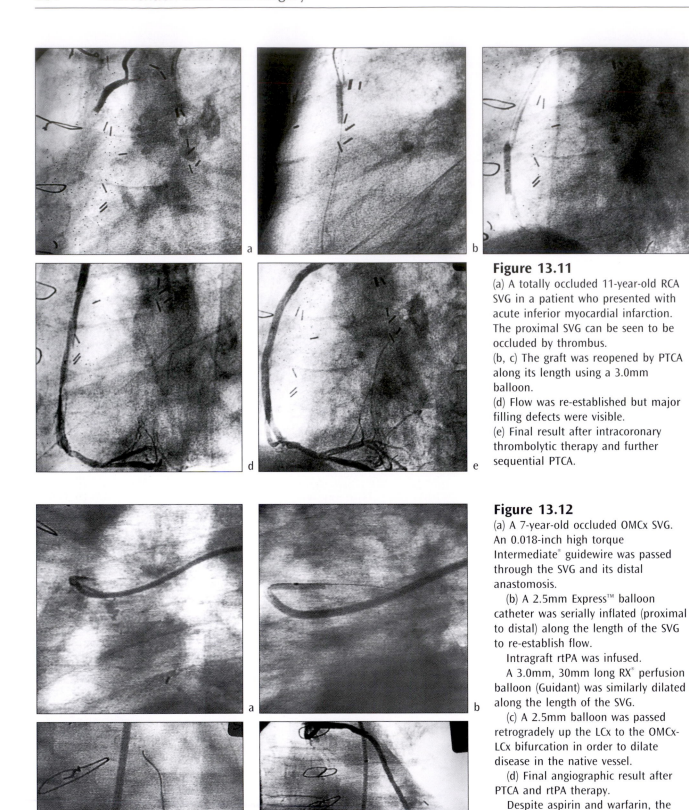

Figure 13.11
(a) A totally occluded 11-year-old RCA SVG in a patient who presented with acute inferior myocardial infarction. The proximal SVG can be seen to be occluded by thrombus.
(b, c) The graft was reopened by PTCA along its length using a 3.0mm balloon.
(d) Flow was re-established but major filling defects were visible.
(e) Final result after intracoronary thrombolytic therapy and further sequential PTCA.

Figure 13.12
(a) A 7-year-old occluded OMCx SVG. An 0.018-inch high torque Intermediate® guidewire was passed through the SVG and its distal anastomosis.
 (b) A 2.5mm Express™ balloon catheter was serially inflated (proximal to distal) along the length of the SVG to re-establish flow.
 Intragraft rtPA was infused.
 A 3.0mm, 30mm long RX® perfusion balloon (Guidant) was similarly dilated along the length of the SVG.
 (c) A 2.5mm balloon was passed retrogradely up the LCx to the OMCx-LCx bifurcation in order to dilate disease in the native vessel.
 (d) Final angiographic result after PTCA and rtPA therapy.
 Despite aspirin and warfarin, the SVG occluded 12 months later without clinical sequelae.

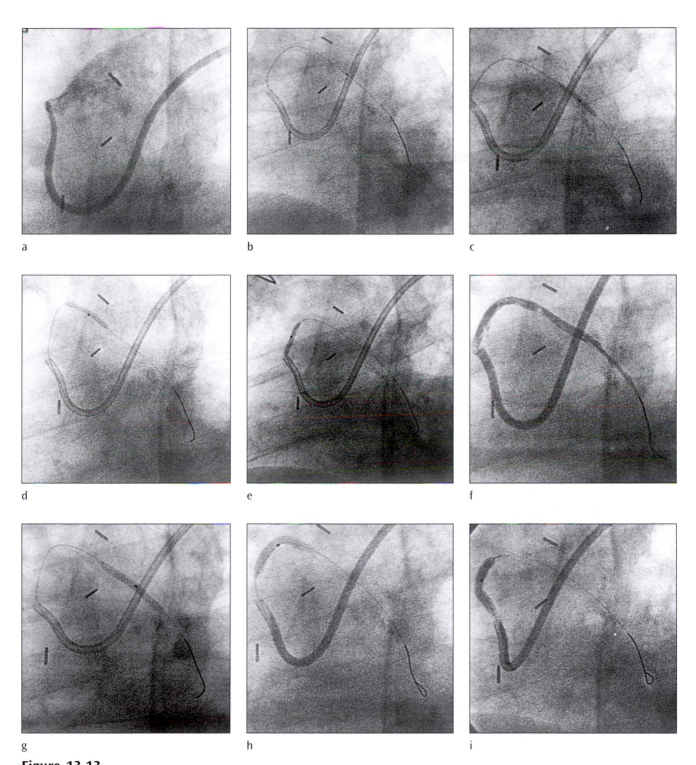

a
b
c

d
e
f

g
h
i

Figure 13.13

(a) This 11-year-old SVG to a diagonal artery became totally occluded by thrombus.

A mid-third stenosis had previously been stented 10 months earlier and subsequently treated by Rotablator® atherectomy because of in-stent restenosis after 5 months (see Figs 10.44 and 13.51). Recurrent angina had been present for 3 weeks before this restudy.

(b-e) The occlusion was crossed with a 0.014-inch Intermediate® guidewire and opened with a 2.0mm Worldpass™ balloon that was serially inflated along the length of the graft.

Much thrombus was visible within the graft and this was dilated with a 3.0mm, 30mm long Elipse™ balloon.

(f) However, thrombus was still visible.

The patient was treated with rtPA (up to 30mg over 30 minutes in 5mg boluses), which was injected down the graft in between inflations.

After further sequential dilatations with a 3.5mm, 40mm long Elipse™ balloon (g-i), obvious dissection and thrombus was still visible (j).

continued

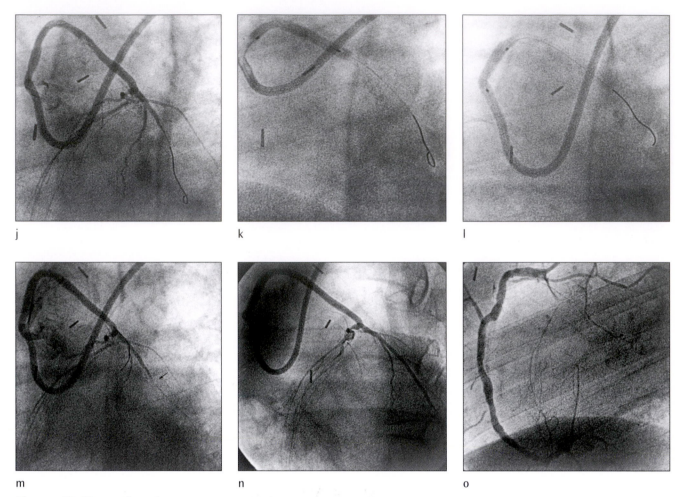

j   k   l

m   n   o

Figure 13.13 *continued*

Two stents (a 3.5mm, 35mm long Multilink™ stent in mid-graft (k) and a 3.5mm, 25mm long Multilink™ from this stent to the SVG ostium (l)) were placed end to end (overlapping) from the ostium to beyond the initial stent.

(m) The native vessel showed some intraluminal thrombus (arrow), which was treated by balloon dilatation with a 2.0mm Worldpass™ balloon.

(n) Overall, the angiographic result was acceptable and improved further after 24 hours.

The patient was rendered asymptomatic and commenced long-term warfarin in addition to aspirin. Ticlopidine was continued for 4 weeks.

(o) The occluded RCA that had been reopened 10 months earlier remained patent.

Long-term patency of occluded grafts, such as this DG SVG, is poor.

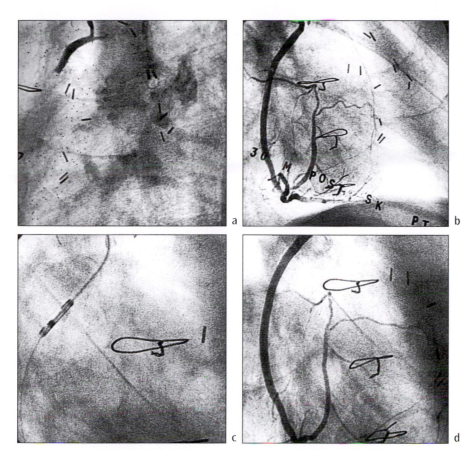

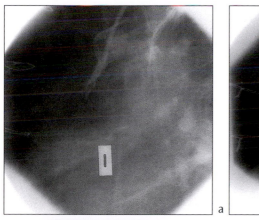

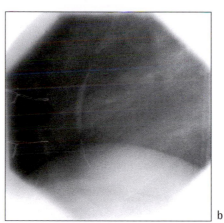

Figure 13.14
(a) Proximal reocclusion of a 6-year-old RCA SVG, 9 weeks after being reopened by PTCA and intragraft rtPA and dilatation of a distal anastomotic stenosis (see Fig. 13.2). Thrombus is evident at the point of occlusion.
(b) An angiogram 30 minutes after intragraft Streptokinase (300,000U) and sequential PTCA along the length of the SVG showed a good result but a persistent filling defect at the point of previous occlusion (arrow).
(c) DCA with a 7F SCA-EX™ device was performed to remove the intraluminal mass.
   Histological examination revealed that this mass was organized thrombus.
(d) An excellent angiographic result, showing absence of filling defects.

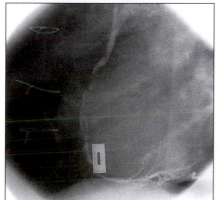

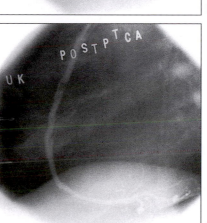

Figure 13.15
(a) Proximal occlusion of 12-year-old RCA SVG.
(b) A balloon catheter was advanced across the occlusion and inflated.
(c) The result was poor until inflations were made along length of graft and urokinase was infused. (d) Final result showed filling defects and a suboptimal result but it was clinically effective.

PTCA of native vessels via bypass grafts

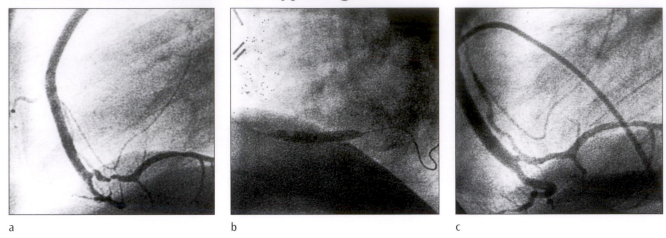

a   b   c

Figure 13.16
(a) A severe stenosis in the RCA just beyond the insertion of an SVG in a 62-year-old man with angina 8 years after CABG surgery.
(b) A guidewire and balloon were placed across the stenosis via the RCA SVG.
  Angiography after PTCA showed improved result (c) and produced relief of symptoms. This appearance persisted at 2 years.

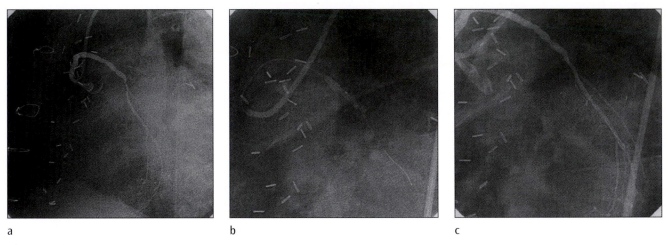

a   b   c

Figure 13.17
A 73-year-old man with unstable angina 12 years after CABG surgery. A patent left internal mammary artery showed no significant disease. (a) However, an OMCx SVG had a significant stenosis at its distal anastomosis site that involved the vessel itself.
(b) This stenosis was dilated with a 3.0mm Cheetah™ balloon with (c) a satisfactory result.

continued

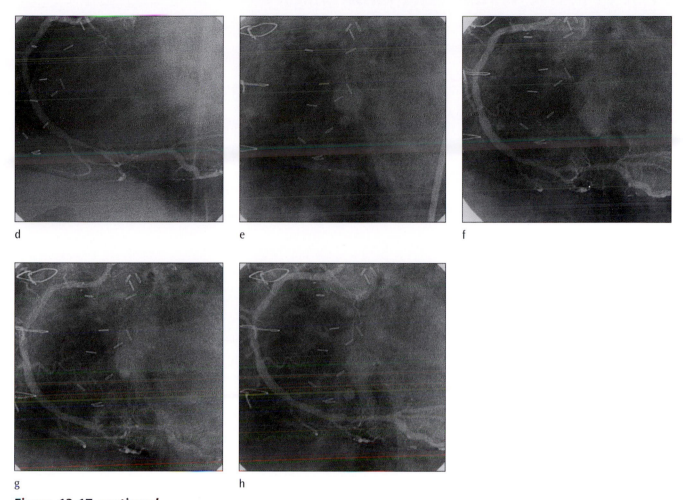

d   e   f

g   h

Figure 13.17 *continued*

(d) The RCA had developed a severe stenosis in its distal third.

(e) This was dilated with the same 3.0mm balloon, resulting in a local dissection (f).

(g) A 15mm Palmaz-Schatz™ stent was implanted using the same balloon (14 atmospheres) with a good result at the lesion site but it caused a dissection distal to the stent.

This was treated with a 3.0mm, 30mm long Elipse™ balloon at 8 atmospheres for 5 minutes.

(h) This gave a good final result.

PTCA of native vessels after CABG surgery

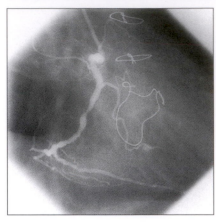

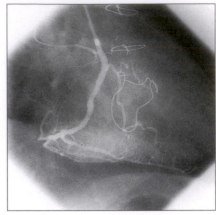

Figure 13.18
(a) Stenosis in middle third of the RCA in a patient with recurrent angina 10 years after CABG surgery.
(b) Angiogram showing good result after PTCA. This produced relief of symptoms for the patient.

a

b

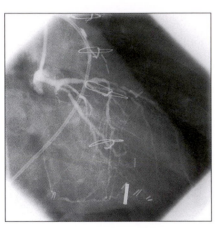

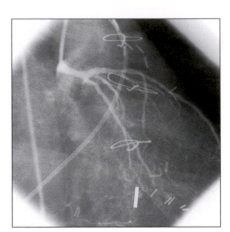

Figure 13.19
The LAD and the intermediate artery 5 years after CABG surgery (a) before and (b) after PTCA.

a

b

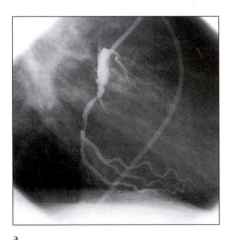

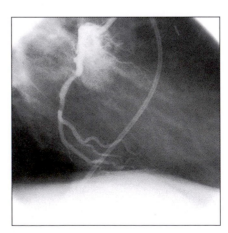

Figure 13.20
LCx stenoses 4 years after CABG surgery (a) before and (b) after PTCA.

a

b

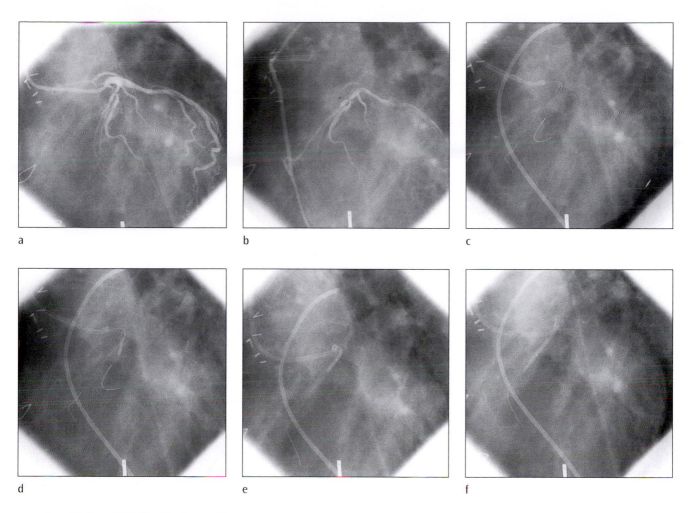

a

b

c

d

e

f

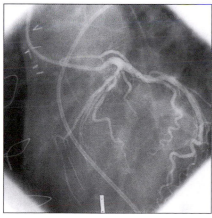

g

Figure 13.21

A 56-year-old man developed angina 7 years after CABG surgery. (a) Injection of the left coronary artery showed that there was a severe stenosis affecting the bifurcation of LAD and the DG, with no antegrade flow.

(b) The LAD was shown to be patent by a forceful injection down the patent LAD SVG.

(c) Two 0.014-inch Floppy® guidewires were negotiated across the stenosis; one was placed down the LAD and one was placed down the diagonal artery.

(d) A 2.0mm Datascope Compass® balloon catheter was used to dilate the DG lesion across the bifurcation.

A 2.5mm RX® balloon was used for PTCA to the LAD, again across the bifurcation (e) and along the segment between the stenosis and the insertion of the SVG (f).

(g) Final result, showing good antegrade flow.

This patient subsequently developed restenosis and required repeat PTCA (pre-stent era).

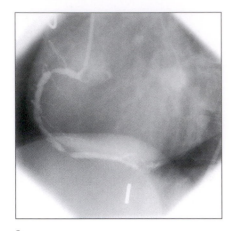

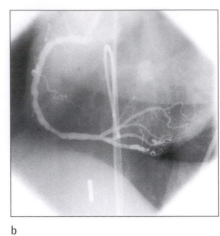

a

b

Figure 13.22
Proximal and distal RCA stenoses 8 years after SVG to the RCA (a) before and (b) after PTCA. The RCA SVG had occluded.

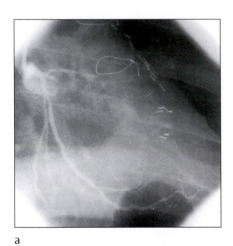

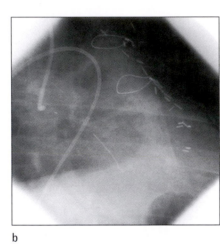

a

b

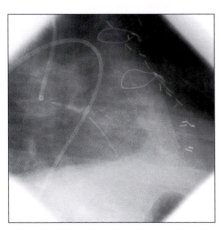

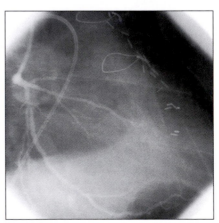

c

d

Figure 13.23
A 50-year-old boilermaker developed a sudden onset of severe chest pain 5 years after CABG surgery.
(a) Angiogram on presentation revealed acute occlusion of an intermediate coronary artery.
(b) Angiogram immediately on crossing occlusion with a 2.5mm fixed-wire balloon catheter and (c) during the balloon dilatation.
(d) Angiogram after PTCA, showing full recanalization of the intermediate artery.

PTCA and left internal mammary artery grafts

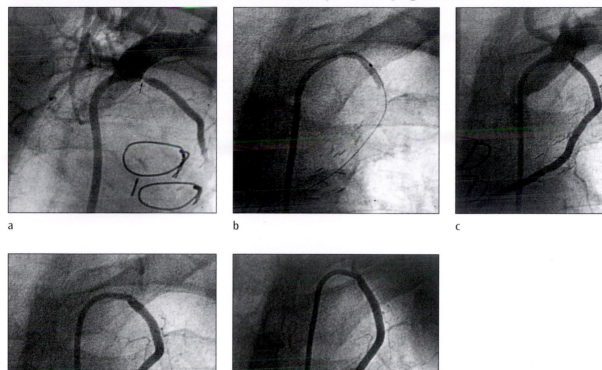

a   b   c

d   e

Figure 13.24

A 62-year-old retired draughtsman with moderate angina 7 years after CABG surgery was found to have (a) retrograde filling of the distal end of the left internal mammary artery on left coronary arteriography and a severe ostial stenosis in the left internal mammary artery itself (arrow).

A 6F right Judkins guiding catheter was used to cross the lesion with a 0.014-inch Floppy® guidewire.

(b) The stenosis was dilated with a 2.5mm Worldpass balloon.

This gave a satisfactory result (c, d), abolition of retrograde flow and relief of symptoms.

(e) Repeat angiography at 6 months showed no evidence of restenosis.

Ostial stenoses of the left internal mammary artery are rare. Great care is required with small-sized, soft-tipped guiding catheters and a correctly sized balloon in order to avoid dissection of the left internal mammary artery.

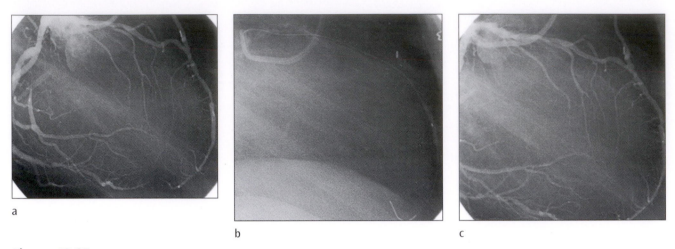

Figure 13.25

Two stenoses in the LAD beyond insertion of the left internal mammary artery (a) before, (b) during and (c) after PTCA with a 2.5mm balloon catheter via the patent native vessel.

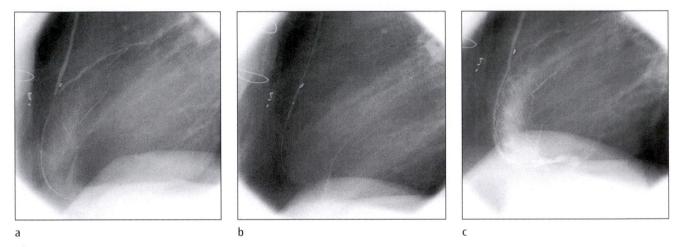

Figure 13.26

(a) Severe stenosis at the distal anastomosis of the left internal mammary artery and the LAD 10 months after CABG surgery in a 54-year-old man (left lateral projection).

(b) During balloon inflation of the stenosis with a 2.0mm Low Profile Plus® balloon catheter.

(c) After PTCA, there was a good result, with blushing of anterior wall and apex. This good result persisted 8 years later.

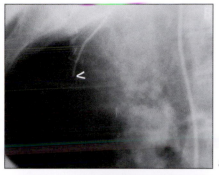
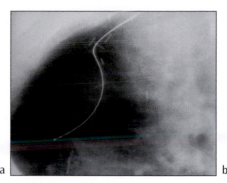
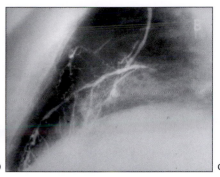

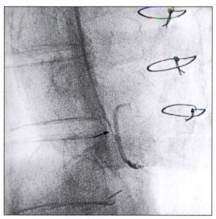

Figure 13.27

(a) The left internal mammary artery occluded in the middle segment (arrow).

(b) Recanalization with Magnum™ guidewire supported by a 2.5mm Magnarail™ balloon.

(c) Angiogram after passage of the Magnum™ wire, showing a recanalized left internal mammary artery with distal stenoses in the LAD.

(d) The final angiogram after PTCA with Magnarail™ balloon showed a recanalized left internal mammary artery with good run-off into a widely patent LAD.

Illustrations provided by B Meier and published with permission from Mehan VK, Meier B, Urban P. Balloon recanalisation of a chronically occluded left internal mammary artery graft. Br Heart J 1993;70:195-7.

PTCA in right internal mammary artery grafts

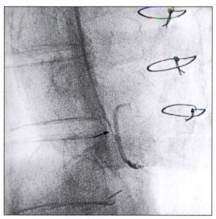
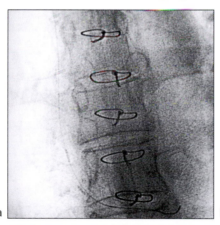
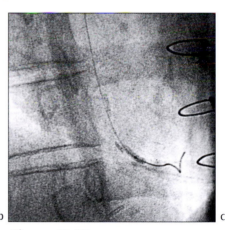

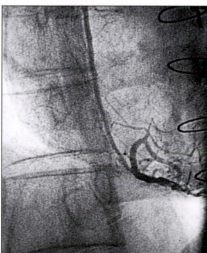
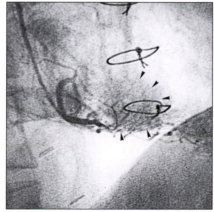

Figure 13.28

A 59-year-old woman had recurrent angina 6 months after undergoing right internal mammary artery grafting to the mid-RCA. (a) Angiography using a left internal mammary artery diagnostic catheter via a right brachial artery approach showed a severe stenosis at the distal anastomosis site (arrow).

(b) The catheter was exchanged for an 8F LIMA guiding catheter and the stenosis was easily crossed with a 0.014-inch Floppy® guidewire.

(c) PTCA was performed using a 2.0mm Adante™ balloon.

(d) This gave an excellent final result.

(e) Angiography showed much blushing of the inferior wall (arrowheads) once the stenosis had been dilated.

Access to the right internal mammary artery is easiest via a right brachial or radial artery approach.

PTCA in gastroepiploic artery grafts

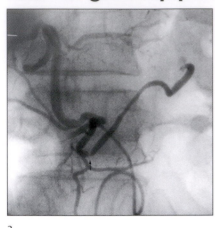
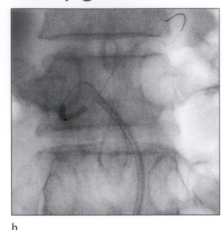
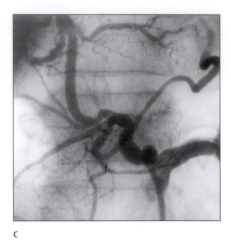

a   b   c

Figure 13.29
(a) A severe stenosis in a gastroepiploic artery inserted into the RCA (arrow) of a 51-year-old man.
(b) The lesion was dilated with a 2.5mm Viva™ balloon through an 8F Multipurpose guide catheter.
(c) The final result was excellent (arrow).
Courtesy of Dr N Komiyama, Department of Cardiovascular Medicine, Toranomon Hospital, Tokyo, Japan.

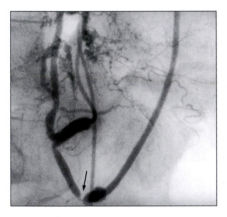
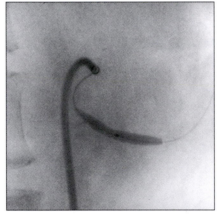
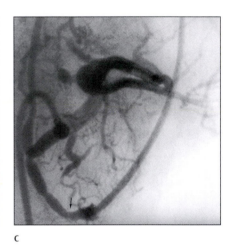

a   b   c

Figure 13.30
A 44-year-old woman with aortitis syndrome had (a) a stenosis just before an aneurysmal segment of the body of a gastroepiploic artery graft inserted into the RCA (arrow). This angiogram was taken only 3 weeks after surgery.
(b) The lesion was dilated with a 4.0mm Viva™ balloon over a 0.014-inch Traverse® (Guidant) guidewire and through an 8F El Gamal guide catheter.
(c) The result was satisfactory (arrow), but note the spasm proximal to the site of the lesion. Arterial spasm is a feature of PTCA in gastroepiploic arteries and nitrates and calcium antagonists should be used liberally.
Courtesy of Dr N Komiyama, Department of Cardiovascular Medicine, Toranomon Hospital, Tokyo, Japan.

Rotablator® atherectomy after CABG surgery

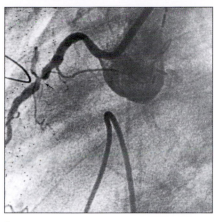
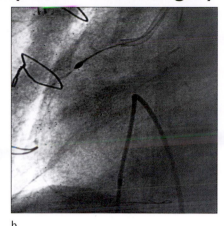
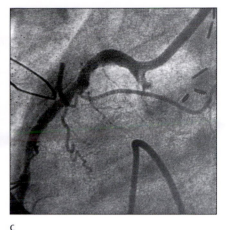

a   b   c

Figure 13.31

(a) Severe, hard, discrete stenosis in proximal RCA (arrow) in a man with recurrent angina 2 years after CABG surgery. Rotablator® atherectomy (b) and adjunctive PTCA produced a good angiographic result (c) and relief of symptoms.

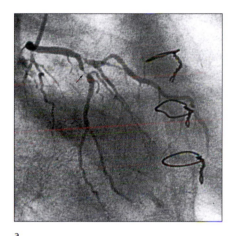
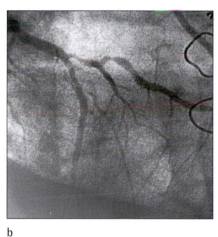

Figure 13.32

Severe stenosis in the first DG of the LAD (arrow) (a) before and (b) after Rotablator® atherectomy in this patient 8 months after CABG surgery. The SVG had been mistakenly placed on the small, occluded second DG2!

a   b

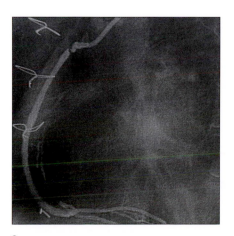
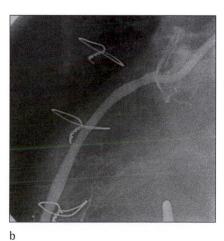

Figure 13.33

A 57-year-old lady presented with unstable angina 6 years after mitral valve replacement and SVG to the RCA and the OMCx. (a) The RCA SVG had a severe eccentric stenosis in its proximal third.

The lesion did not respond to 22 atmospheres inflation pressure with a 3.5mm Viva Primo™ balloon.

After Rotablator® atherectomy with a 2.5mm burr the lesion was much improved and responded well to a 9mm NIR™ stent on a 3.5mm/4.0mm CAT™ balloon inflated up to 19 atmospheres (b).

a   b

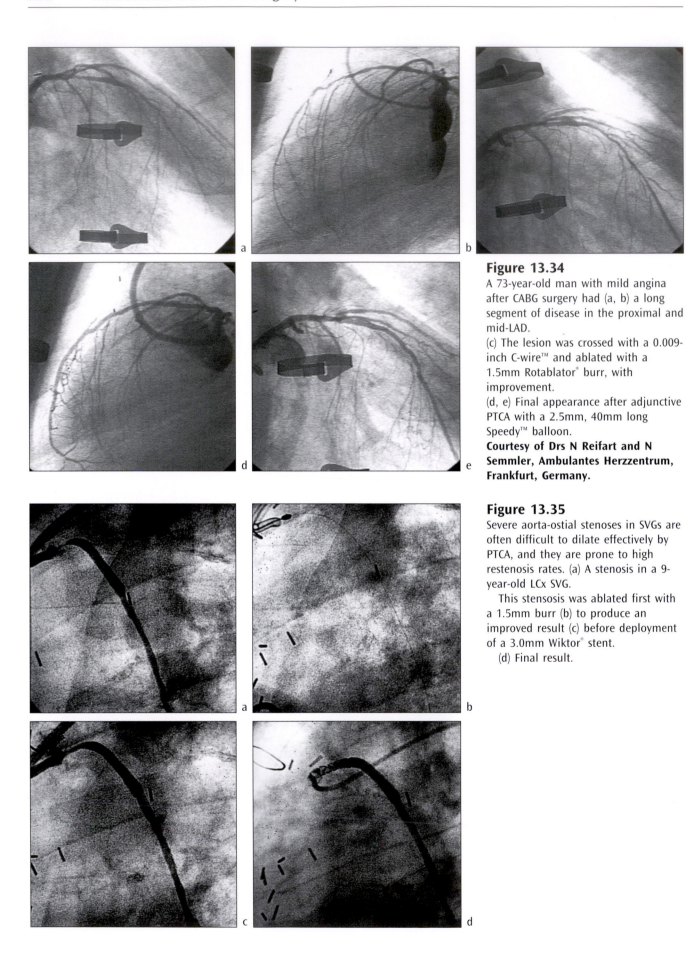

Figure 13.34
A 73-year-old man with mild angina after CABG surgery had (a, b) a long segment of disease in the proximal and mid-LAD.
(c) The lesion was crossed with a 0.009-inch C-wire™ and ablated with a 1.5mm Rotablator® burr, with improvement.
(d, e) Final appearance after adjunctive PTCA with a 2.5mm, 40mm long Speedy™ balloon.
Courtesy of Drs N Reifart and N Semmler, Ambulantes Herzzentrum, Frankfurt, Germany.

Figure 13.35
Severe aorta-ostial stenoses in SVGs are often difficult to dilate effectively by PTCA, and they are prone to high restenosis rates. (a) A stenosis in a 9-year-old LCx SVG.
This stensosis was ablated first with a 1.5mm burr (b) to produce an improved result (c) before deployment of a 3.0mm Wiktor® stent.
(d) Final result.

DCA after CABG surgery

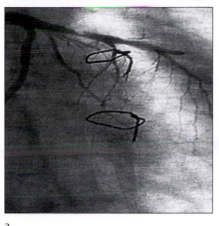

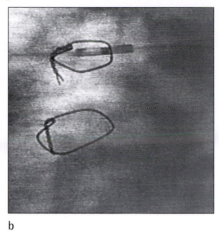

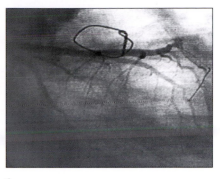

a

b

c

Figure 13.36

(a) RAO projection showing a bulky eccentric stenosis in the proximal LAD in a man 4 years after CABG surgery.

(b) A 7F Simpson Atherocath® excised atheromatous lesion (nine specimens).

(c) The result after DCA was satisfactory.

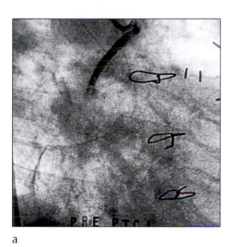

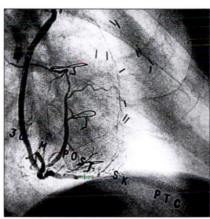

a

b

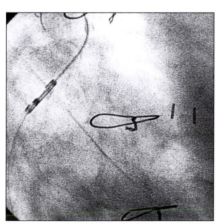

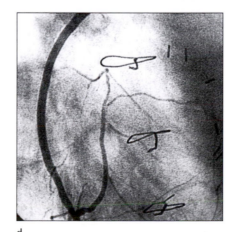

c

d

Figure 13.37

(a) This 6-year-old RCA SVG in a 56-year-old newspaper proprietor became occluded for the second time (see Figs 13.2 and 13.14).

He had undergone two previous CABG operations. The SVG was reopened by PTCA with a 3.5mm Gold-Ex™ balloon catheter and intracoronary streptokinase was infused to lyse visible thrombus within the graft.

(b) A persistent filling defect (arrow) was evident at the site of previous occlusion.

This filling defect remained despite PTCA at high pressure.

(c) DCA was performed with a 7F SCA-EX™ device.

(d) An excellent angiographic result was achieved.

Three specimens were retrieved; histologically these showed organized thrombus.

Transluminal extraction coronary atherectomy after CABG surgery

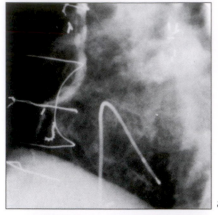

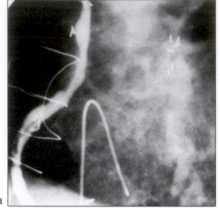

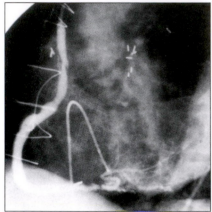

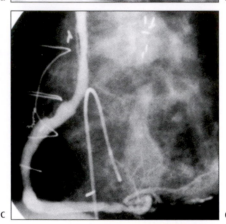

Figure 13.38

A 61-year-old man had undergone CABG surgery 3 years previously. After he had presented with acute inferior myocardial infarction, emergency catheterization showed that the RCA SVG was occluded in its middle third. Multiple filling defects were consistent with thrombus (a).

After 250,000U urokinase, filling defects were still present.

(b) These persisted despite an overnight urokinase infusion.

A 7.5F (2.5mm) TEC® device was advanced into the SVG and multiple passes were made.

(c) Post-TEC® angiography revealed a 50% residual stenosis and a 95% distal anastomotic stenosis with TIMI III flow.

(d) Final result after adjunctive PTCA with a 3.0mm balloon in the body of the SVG and a 2.5mm balloon in the anastomotic lesion.

Courtesy of Drs R Cain, J Work and JH Fleisher, Encino-Tarzana Medical Center, Encino, California, USA.

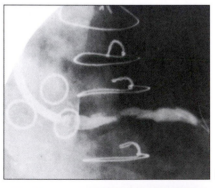

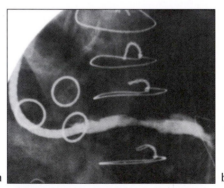

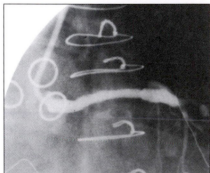

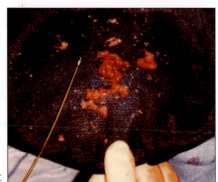

Figure 13.39

A 52-year-old man presented with severe ischaemic cardiomyopathy 10 years after CABG surgery. He had suffered multiple myocardial infarctions and had received an automatic implantable cardioverter defibrillator for treatment of a malignant ventricular tachycardia at 48 years of age. He was admitted with unstable angina. (a) Angiography showed degeneration of the SVG to the mid-LAD with a severe, proximal, ulcerated subtotal occlusion and large amounts of intraluminal debris.

A 10F TEC® guide catheter, a 0.014-inch TEC® guidewire and a 7.5F TEC® device were used to remove material from the SVG.

(b) The native LAD became opacified and flow improved although a significant residual stenosis remained.

(c) Adjunctive PTCA and stent implantation produced a successful final result.

(d) The vacuum bottles contained copious amounts of thrombus.

Courtesy of Dr J Quan, Riverside Community Hospital, Riverside, California, USA.

ELCA in SVGs

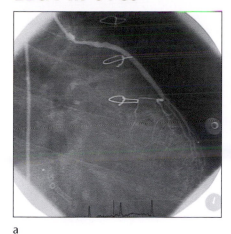

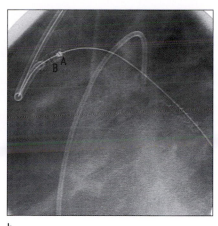

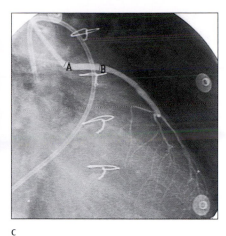

a   b   c

Figure 13.40

A 63-year-old lady had a 3.5mm Palmaz-Schatz™ stent deployed in the ostial portion of an SVG to LAD 12 years after CABG surgery. Four months later she developed (a) a 75% restenosis within the stent.

The LAD SVG was intubated with an 8F Multipurpose guide catheter with side holes and wired with a Standard® 0.014-inch guidewire.

(b) The lesion in the stent was treated with two passes of a 1.7mm diameter monorail laser catheter followed by a 2.0mm device (energy 50mJ, repetition rate 25Hz, saline flush during firing).

An improvement was seen. A 3.5mm Pronto Rely™ balloon was then used (up to 18 atmospheres) for adjunctive PTCA.

(c) The final result was good.

Courtesy of Dr M Webb-Peploe, St. Thomas's Hospital, London, UK.

Stents in SVGs

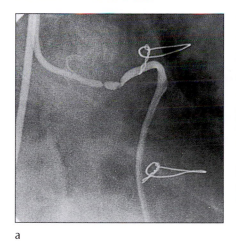

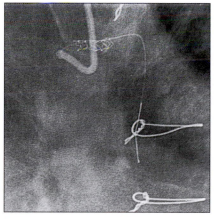

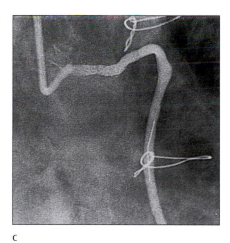

a   b   c

Figure 13.41

(a) Tandem stenoses in the proximal third of an 11-year-old RCA SVG.

(b) After PTCA, a 3.5mm Wiktor® stent was implanted.

(c) This produced a satisfactory result.

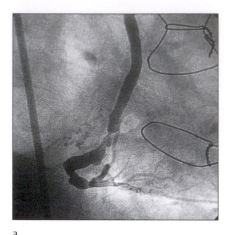
a

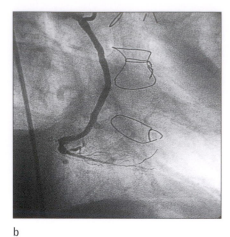
b

Figure 13.42
A 65-year-old man presented with recurrence of angina 13 years after CABG surgery. (a) A complex, ulcerated lesion in the distal third of the RCA SVG was found.
(b) Result after PTCA with a 3.5mm Elipse™ balloon catheter and 4.0mm Multilink™ stent implantation and post-dilatation with a 4.0/4.5mm CAT® balloon at 13 atmospheres.

The SAVED trial showed that stenting of focal SVG lesions results in an improved procedural success (92% versus 69%) and event-free survival at 6 months (rate of major adverse cardiac events 26% versus 39%) when compared with PTCA, despite similar angiographic restenosis rates (37% versus 46%).

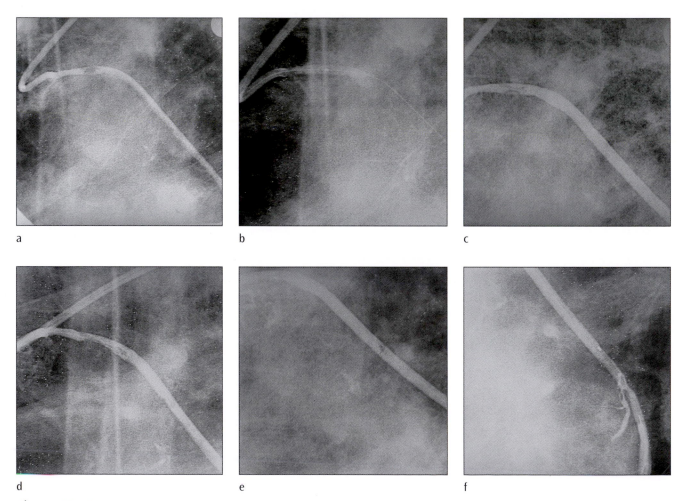
a   b   c

d   e   f

Figure 13.43
(a) A complex, bulky lesion, probably associated with thrombus, in the proximal third of a 10-year-old LCx SVG.
  PTCA with a 3.5mm balloon (b) caused plaque disruption and partial embolization of friable material (c).
  Free embolization occurs down the SVG (d, e), and thrombotic material lodges in small obtuse marginal branch (f).

continued

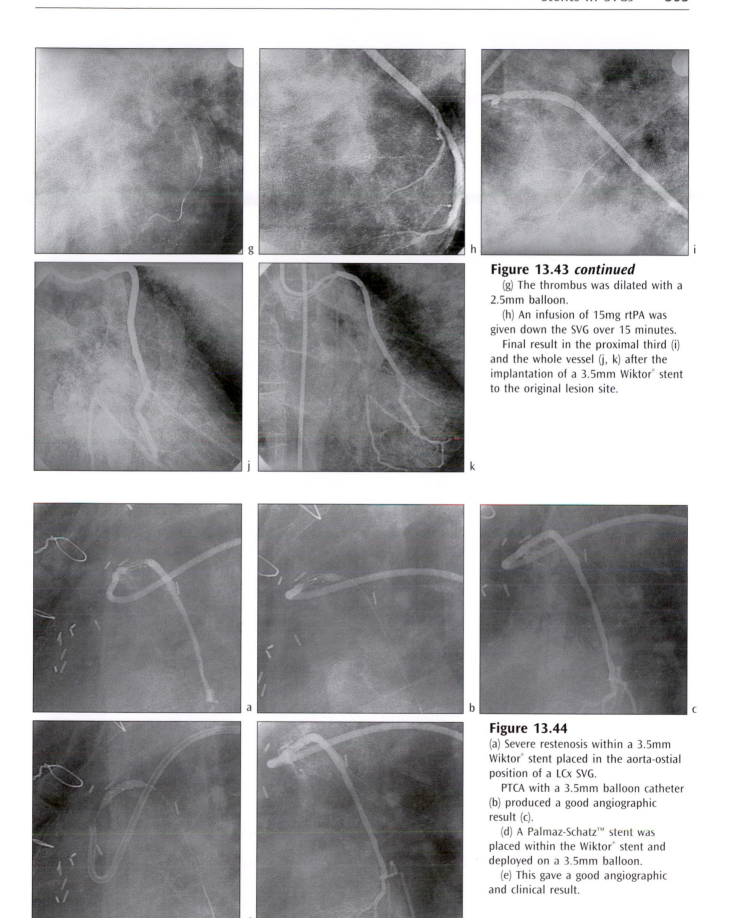

Figure 13.43 *continued*

(g) The thrombus was dilated with a 2.5mm balloon.

(h) An infusion of 15mg rtPA was given down the SVG over 15 minutes.

Final result in the proximal third (i) and the whole vessel (j, k) after the implantation of a 3.5mm Wiktor® stent to the original lesion site.

Figure 13.44

(a) Severe restenosis within a 3.5mm Wiktor® stent placed in the aorta-ostial position of a LCx SVG.

PTCA with a 3.5mm balloon catheter (b) produced a good angiographic result (c).

(d) A Palmaz-Schatz™ stent was placed within the Wiktor® stent and deployed on a 3.5mm balloon.

(e) This gave a good angiographic and clinical result.

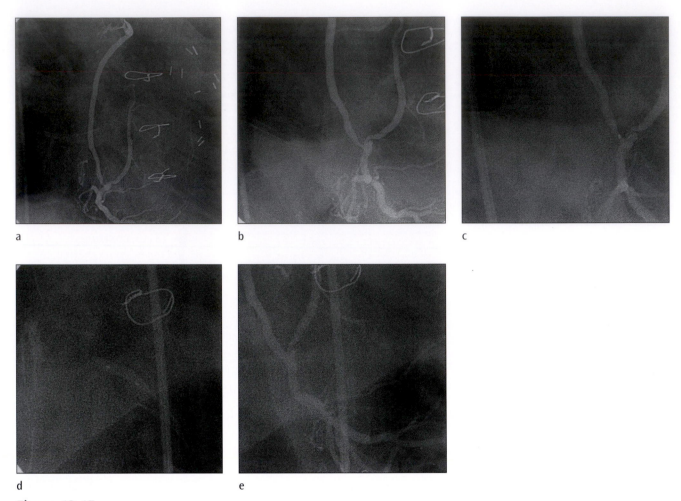

a

b

c

d

e

Figure 13.45

A 59-year-old man (the same patient as in Figs 13.2, 13.14 and 13.37) presented with recurrent angina 9 years after CABG surgery.

(a, b) An angiogram showed a third restenosis in the distal RCA SVG 3 years and 4 months after the first PTCA.

(c) A 15mm long Palmaz-Schatz™ stent was implanted using a 3.0/3.5mm CAT™ balloon, but this clearly left a residual stenosis at the 'bridge' point.

(d) A 9mm NIR™ stent was therefore positioned at this precise point and deployed by a 3.5mm Primo Viva™ (Scimed) at 14 atmospheres.

(e) Final result.

The subsequent outcome is described in Fig. 13.2.

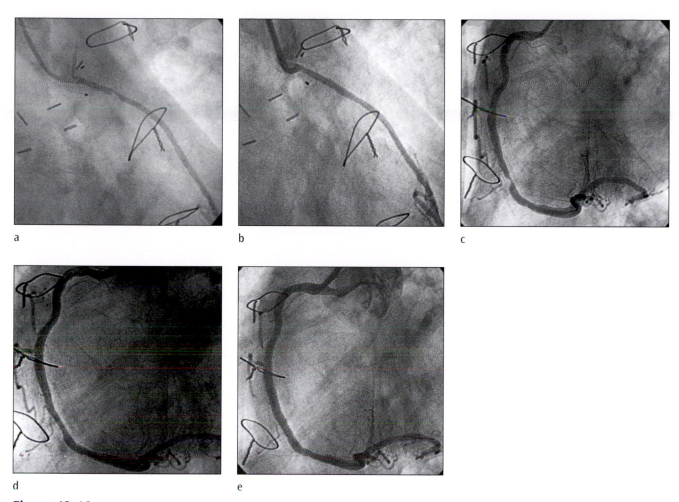

a   b   c

d   e

Figure 13.46

A 66-year-old man had unstable angina 12 years after CABG surgery and 4 years after PTCA and stent implantation to the LCx. Coronary arteriography showed a new severe stenosis in the LAD SVG body and a severe stenosis in the mid- and distal thirds of the RCA. The stenosis in the LAD SVG (a) was crossed with a 0.014-inch Floppy® guidewire and stented without pre-dilatation with a 3.0mm, 13mm long Duet™ stent.

(b) This gave a good angiographic result.

(c) The stenosis in the RCA can be seen in this view.

It was crossed with the same guidewire and pre-dilated with a 3.0mm Rocket™ balloon.

(d) This gave some improvement but there was residual stenosis.

The lesion was therefore stented with a 3.5mm, 18mm long Multilink Duet™ stent and post-dilated with a 4.0mm, 12mm long Seajet® balloon. There was obvious proximal edge spasm or dissection and so a second 4.0mm, 9mm long NIRoyal™ stent was placed at the proximal edge of the first stent, and both stents were dilated with the 4.0mm, 12mm long Seajet® balloon; care was taken to stay inside the two stents.

(e) The final result was excellent.

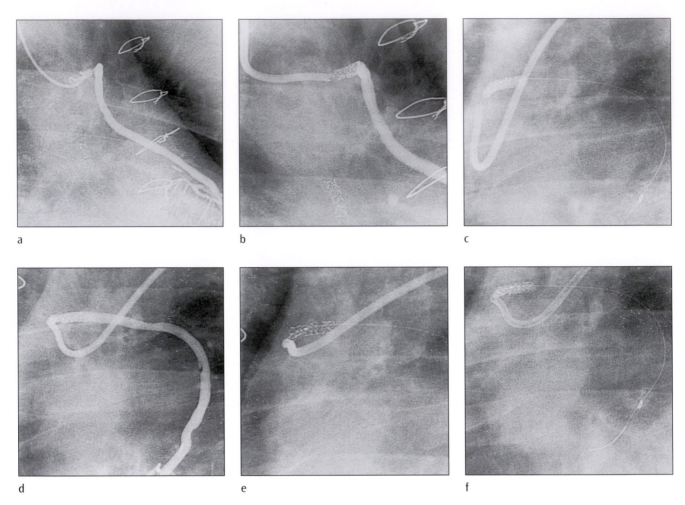

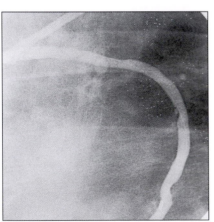

Figure 13.47

(a, b) This 8-year-old LAD SVG developed a severe restenosis inside a 3.5mm Wiktor®
stent that had been placed in the aorta-ostial position only 3 months earlier, causing
recurrence of severe angina.

Restenosis within a radio-opaque stent such as the Wiktor stent is often difficult to
see angiographically. In this case it appears as a lack of contrast during angiography
of the SVG.

(c) A 3.0/3.5mm CAT™ balloon was used to pre-dilate the restenosis.

(d) This produced a good result.

(e) A 15mm long Palmaz-Schatz™ stent on the CAT™ balloon was deployed within
the Wiktor® stent (f).

This produced an excellent result (g) and relief of symptoms.

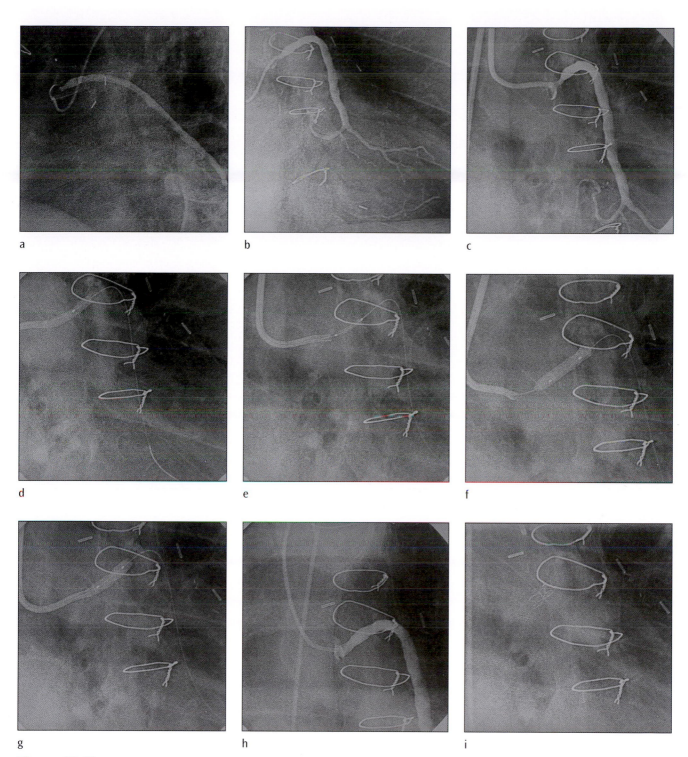

a   b   c

d   e   f

g   h   i

Figure 13.48

A 61-year-old retired bank manager was asymptomatic 6 years after multivessel CABG surgery. His ECG showed new T-wave inversion in leads V1-V3. (a-c) Angiography demonstrated that the RCA SVG and the second OMCx SVG were both occluded and that the first OMCx SVG had a significant stenosis at its ostium.

It was decided to dilate and stent this stenosis on prognostic grounds.

(d) A 3.5mm Express™ balloon was used to dilate the lesion.

(e, f) A 4.0mm, 12mm long Microstent II™ was deployed at 15 atmospheres.

Engagement of the guide catheter was troublesome and it had to be 'backed out' from the ostium for stent deployment.

Despite further dilatation with a 4.0 mm balloon (g), a residual stenosis was still evident (h).

However it was decided to accept this result rather than risk damaging the front end of the stent with the tip of the guide catheter or a 5.0mm balloon. The stent is radio-opaque and helps positioning (i).

This result was unchanged at 18 month angiography.

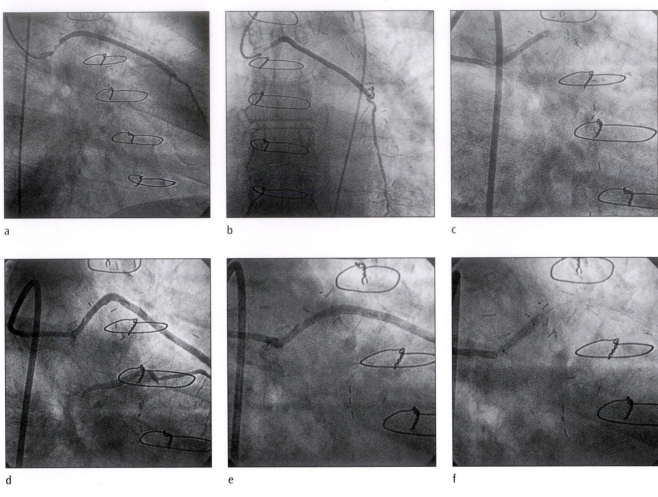

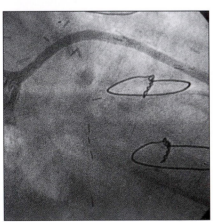

Figure 13.49

A 63-year-old diabetic man with hypercholesterolemia presented with a 4 week history of recurrent angina 6 years after CABG surgery. (a, b) The LAD SVG had a severe ostial stenosis that extended over a 10-12mm segment.

(c) The lesion was dilated with a 3.0mm Passage® balloon.

Because of residual stenosis (d), the lesion was stented with a 3.5mm, 15mm long Palmaz-Schatz™ stent (e, f).

This gave an excellent angiographic (g) and clinical result.

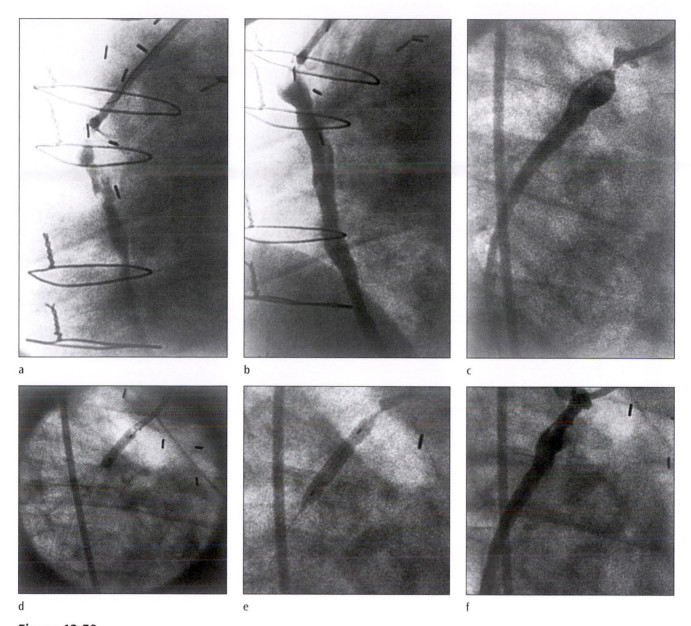

a   b   c

d   e   f

Figure 13.50

A 64-year-old man presented with recurrent angina 8 years after CABG surgery. The left main and right coronary arteries were occluded, as were grafts to the LCx, OMCx and diagonal arteries. The left internal mammary artery to the LAD was patent but the RCA SVG had a 95% stenosis at its ostium. Within 10 minutes of the diagnostic angiograms, the patient developed severe chest pain and ST-segment elevation in the inferior ECG leads. (a) Repeat angiography showed occlusion of the RCA SVG with much thrombus occluding the ostium and filling an ectatic segment just beyond it.

An intravenous bolus and infusion of abciximab was given.

(b, c) The occluded segment was crossed with a 0.014-inch Traverse® guidewire.

(d) The stenosis dilated with a 4.0mm, 20mm long Maxxum™ balloon.

This gave immediate pain relief and normalization of the ECG.

(e) A 4.0mm, 9mm long NIR™ stent was deployed at 16 atmospheres at the ostium of the RCA SVG.

This stent was post-dilated with a 5.0mm Bypass Speedy™ balloon.

(f) Final result.

There was no rise in cardiac enzymes, and the patient was discharged on antiplatelet therapy.

Courtesy of Dr S Ray and A Cooper, Wythenshawe Hospital, Manchester, UK.

SVG In-stent restenosis treated by Rotablator® atherectomy

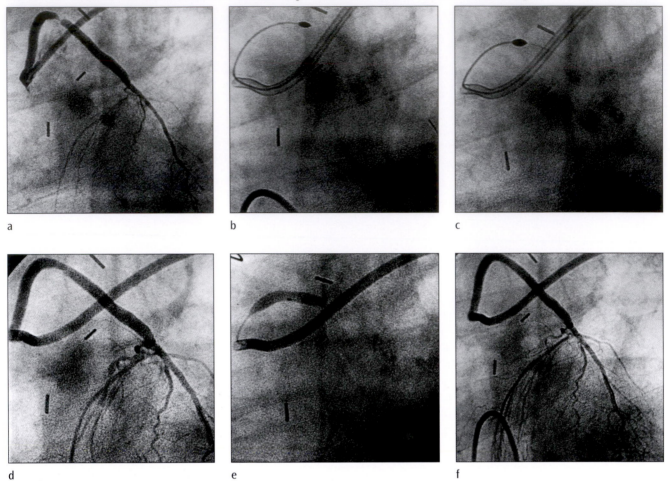

a   b   c

d   e   f

Figure 13.51

A 63-year-old ophthalmologist (see Figs 10.44 and 13.13) developed recurrence of angina 4 months after PTCA and Multilink™ stent implantation to a large first DG SVG. (a) Angiography showed a severe restenosis inside the stent.

IVUS showed full stent deployment, and the lesion was therefore ablated with a 1.75mm Rotablator® burr (b) and a 2.25mm Rotablator® burr (c).

(d) There was improvement but some residual stenosis remained.

(e) This was treated by PTCA with a 3.5mm Samba™ balloon.

(f) Final result.

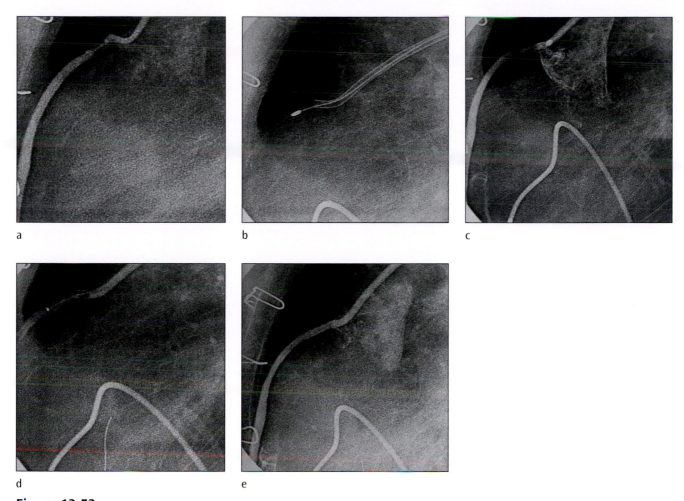

a   b   c

d   e

Figure 13.52
A 58-year-old woman (the same patient as in Fig. 13.33) developed recurrent angina 5 months after PTCA and NIR™ stenting to the aorta-ostial segment of her RCA SVG.
(a) Angiography showed a severe restenosis within the stent.
IVUS showed full stent deployment.
(b, c) Rotablator® atherectomy was performed using a 1.5mm and a 2.0mm Rotablator® burr.
(d) The residual lesion was post-dilated with a 3.0mm, 10mm long Finale balloon.
(e) This gave a good final result.

Biliary stents for large SVGs

Two examples of the use of biliary stents in large SVGs are presented in Figs 10.49 and Figure 10.50.

Wallstent for SVG disease

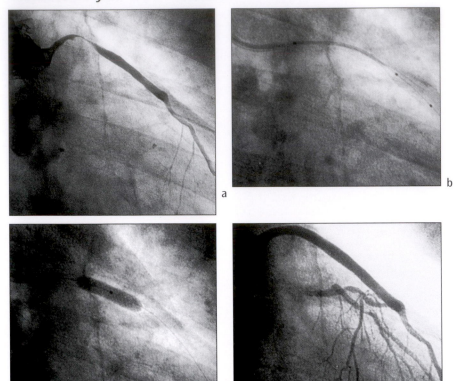

Figure 13.53

A 62-year-old man presented with a 2 week history of unstable angina 8 years after CABG surgery. His ECG showed new anterior T-wave inversion.

(a) Angiography showed a severe stenosis in the proximal segment of the LAD SVG.

After pre-dilatation with a 2.5mm Europass™ balloon, a 6 35mm long Wallstent™ was deployed (b) and finally expanded with a 4mm Speedy™ balloon inflated to 14 atmospheres (c).

(d) This gave an excellent angiographic and clinical result.

Courtesy of Dr MS Norell, Hull Royal Infirmary, Hull, UK.

Stents to native vessels after CABG surgery

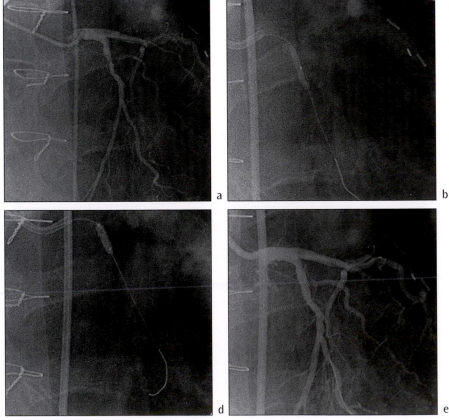
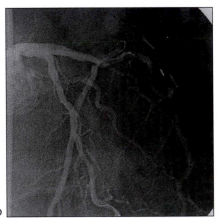

Figure 13.54

A 68-year-old retired plumber with moderate angina 5 years after CABG surgery had (a) a significant proximal stenosis in the LCx.

(b, c) The lesion was dilated with a 2.5mm Elipse™ balloon.

(d) A 3.0mm Palmaz-Schatz™ stent was implanted.

(e) This gave a satisfactory result. A septal branch of LAD was also dilated at the same sitting.

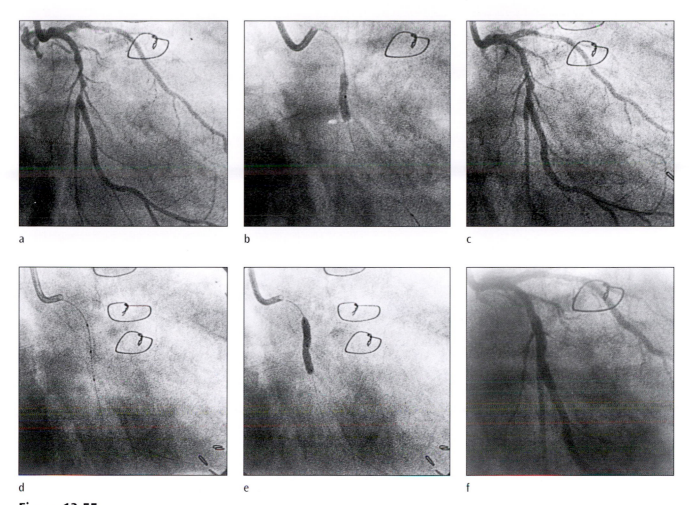

a   b   c

d   e   f

Figure 13.55

A 67-year-old man presented with angina 7 years after CABG surgery. (a) He was found to have severe disease in the proximal LCx.
(b) The lesions were dilated with a 3.0mm balloon but with a suboptimal result (c).
(d, e) The lesions were therefore stented with a 3.5mm, 26 mm long Joflex stent with (f) a good angiographic and clinical result.

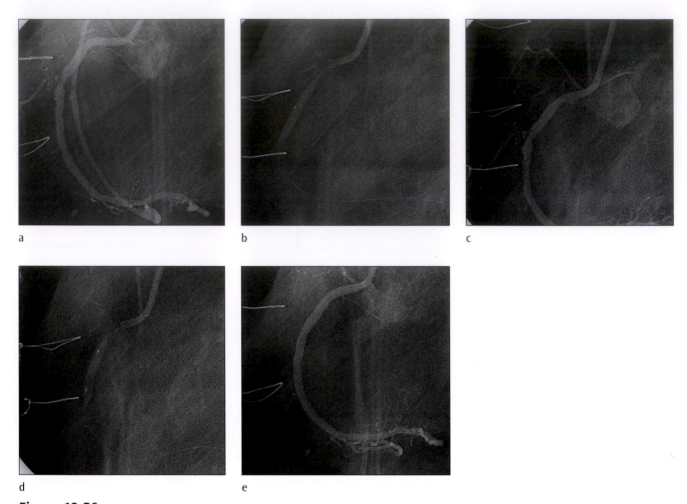

a

b

c

d

e

Figure 13.56

A 57-year-old man had persisting mild angina 18 months after CABG surgery. (a) His RCA SVG supplied the posterior descending branch of the RCA, but flow into the large posterolateral branch was compromised by the 75% stenosis in the proximal RCA.

(b, c) The lesion was dilated with a 3.5mm Comet™ balloon (Guidant).

(d) A 3.5mm, 15mm long Multilink™ stent was implanted.

(e) This gave an excellent angiographic result.

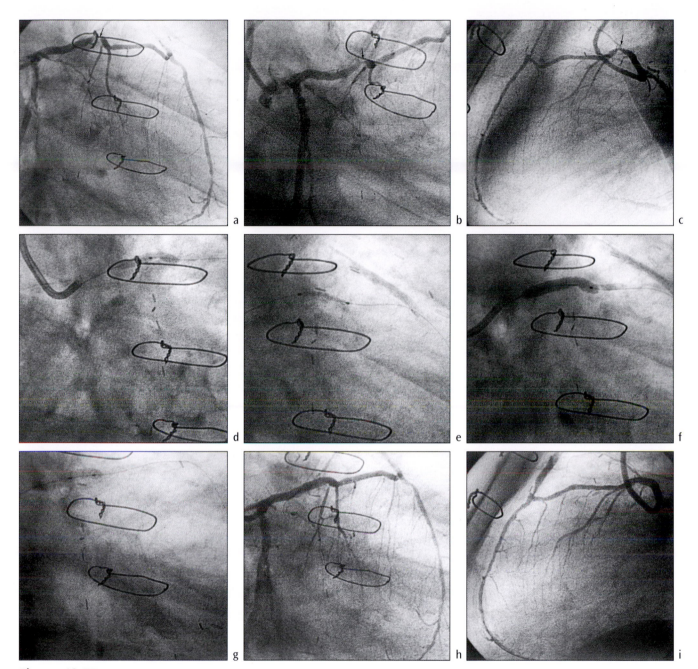

Figure 13.57

A 64-year-old entrepreneur (the same patient as in Fig. 13.49) had a 1-week history of unstable angina. He was found to have a totally occluded LAD SVG 10 months after a 3.5mm Palmaz-Schatz™ stent had been implanted to its ostium. The SVG appeared to be full of thrombus. Since the native LAD was still patent, it was decided to attempt PTCA and stent implantation to the severe, eccentric lesion in the proximal LAD – (a, b) RAO caudal projections; (c) left lateral projection.

In addition, there were two significant lesions in the distal LAD. All three lesions were dilated with a 2.0mm Worldpass™. A good angiographic result was obtained in the distal vessel but the balloon ruptured on the proximal lesion.

A 3.0mm LOGO™ balloon (JoMed) (d) also ruptured at 10 atmospheres.

(e, f) A 3.5mm, 16mm long Paragon™ stent was implanted.

The balloon ruptured at 12 atmospheres of pressure and the stent was further dilated with a 3.5mm, 12mm long Cruiser II® balloon (g) up to 18 atmospheres.

This gave an excellent angiographic result – (h) RAO caudal projection; (i) left lateral projection.

The patient was rendered free of angina and remained asymptomatic at 36 months. Balloon rupture at relatively low pressure may be due to calcified spicules in hard lesions. In retrospect, IVUS and Rotablator® atherectomy would perhaps have been most useful in this hard lesion.

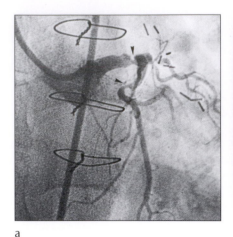
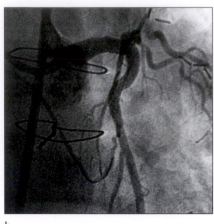
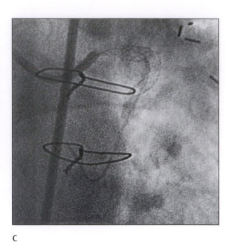

a   b   c

Figure 13.58

A 56-year-old man with angina 8 years after CABG surgery was found to have (a) a severe stenosis at the distal end of the left main coronary artery and in the tortuous proximal segment of the LCx (arrows).

It was possible to cross into the distal LCx with a 0.014-inch Floppy® guidewire and to dilate the left main and LCx lesions with a 3.0mm Freeway™ balloon. The LCx stenosis was stented with a 3.0mm, 18mm long GFX™ stent because of local dissection, and the left main coronary artery was stented with 4.0mm, 24mm long GFX™ stent from the mid-segment across the distal third and into the LCx (overlapping with the stent already placed in the LCx). A 4.0mm, 9mm long NIRoyal™ stent was placed in the proximal left main coronary artery (again overlapping with the previously deployed GFX™ stent). The stents were all post-dilated with a 4mm, 9mm long Chubby™ balloon up to 16 atmospheres.

This gave an excellent angiographic (b) and clinical result.

The GFX™ stents were chosen in this case because of their flexibility in negotiating tortuous bends and the NIRoyal™ stent was chosen because of its extra radio-opacity for helping in accurate positioning of the stent.

(c) The radio-opaque stents illustrate how they have conformed to the bends that were present in this case.

PTCA and stent implantation for left subclavian artery stenosis after left internal mammary artery CABG surgery

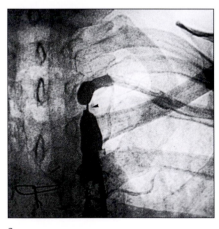
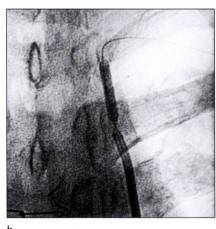
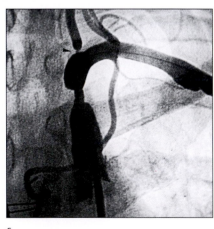

a   b   c

Figure 13.59

A 58-year-old man had severe angina 6 years after CABG surgery and noticed that his left hand and arm felt cold. (a) Cardiac catheterization showed a severe stenosis in the left subclavian artery shortly after its origin (arrowhead). The vertebral artery was not visible and the left internal mammary artery and rest of the subclavian artery only filled faintly.

(b) The stenosis was crossed with a 0.014-inch Floppy® guidewire and dilated with a 4.0mm Freeway™ balloon.

(c) This produced significant improvement. The vertebral artery was then visualized and shown to have a severe ostial stenosis (arrowhead) and the left internal mammary artery looked normal with fast antegrade flow. The patient noticed immediate warming of his left hand.

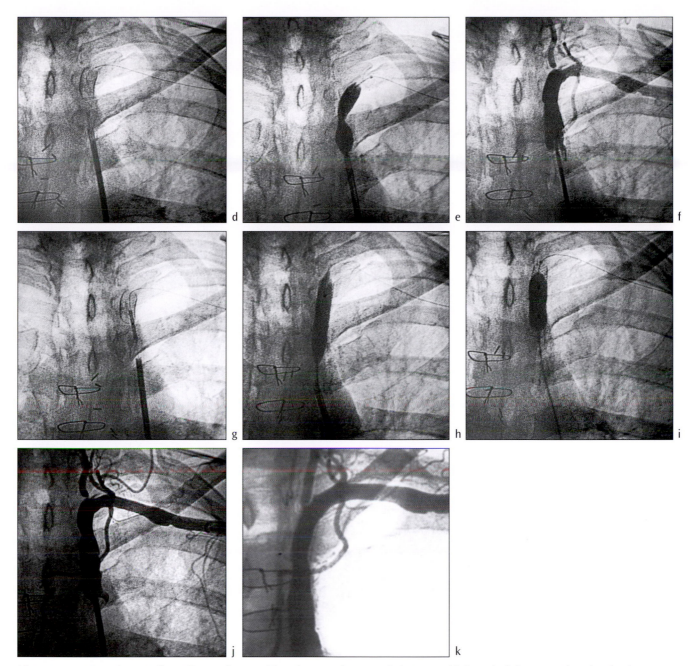

(d) A 10mm, 20mm long Wallstent™ was then positioned across the stenosis but, on withdrawal of the protective sheath, the shortening self-expanding stent 'melon-seeded' forwards so that it only partially covered the stenosis.

An 8mm, 30mm long Powerflex Plus (Cordis/Johnson and Johnson) balloon was then used to further dilate the stent. It was then apparent that the stenosis was very hard and resistant to dilatation (e) and presumably this had been the reason for the forward displacement of the Wallstent™ .

(f) Local dissection was visible beginning just after the origin of the vertebral artery with associated spasm in the subclavian artery itself.

(g) A 17mm long JoStent Flex™ stent was then crimped on to a 6mm, 20mm long Bypass Speedy™ balloon and deployed over the stenosis and overlapping the stents.

(h) An 8mm, 30mm long Blue Max balloon was used to post-dilate the two stents.

(i) This was followed with a 10mm, 20mm long Powerflex Plus balloon at 14 atmospheres.

(j) This final result was accepted.

The patient's angina improved dramatically and there were no sequelae as a result of the dissection or of the ostial stenosis in the vertebral artery. The decision was made not to stent this non-occlusive tear since this would have resulted in the ostium of the left internal mammary artery being covered.

(k) At 4 months the dissection was shown to have healed angiographically. The patient remained asymptomatic.

Prevention of distal embolization during intervention in SVGs
The Percusurge Guardwire™ System

The PercuSurge Guard Wire™ temporary occlusion and aspiration system (PercuSurge, Sunnyvale, California) consists of 3 components:

(1) The GuardWire™, a 210cm 0.014" hollow, nitinol guidewire with a central lumen connected to a compliant distal occlusion balloon (5.5mm long) available in sizes from 3mm to 6mm (nominal size is reached at an inflation pressure of < 2 atmospheres). The guidewire-balloon catheter has a distal, shapeable radiopaque 3.5cm tip to facilitate lesion crossing. Regular balloon catheters and stent delivery systems can be advanced over this wire to perform percutaneous interventions.

(2) A proprietary valve sealing system at the proximal end of the guidewire maintains distal balloon inflation despite disconnection of the inflation device. The detachable MicroSeal™ Adapter accesses the hypotube lumen by displacing a small seal, allowing inflation and deflation of the distal balloon.

(3) The Export™ Aspiration Catheter. This 135cm long, 5F monorail catheter has an internal lumen diameter of 0.040" and allows removal of particulate debris before deflation of the occlusive balloon. The catheter is connected to a 20m1 syringe providing a low-pressure vacuum to remove debris and thrombus from the SVG.

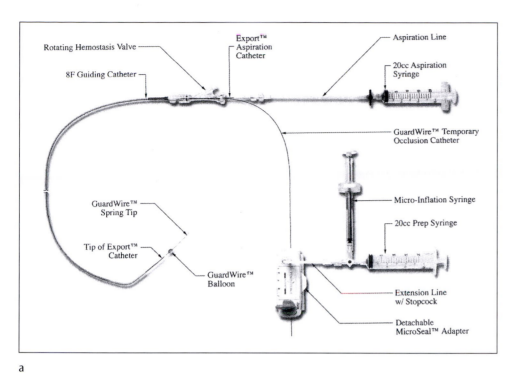

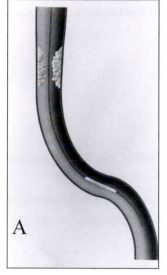
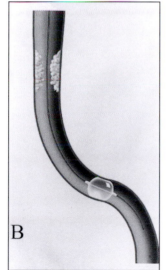
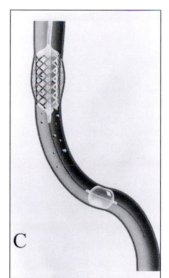
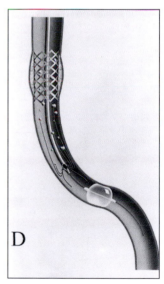

A

B

C

D

b

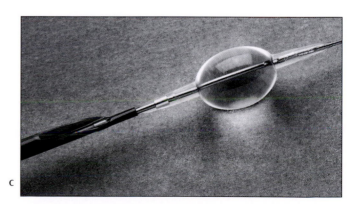

c

Figure 13.60
(a) Schematic of the particulate retrieval system. (b) The mechanism of particulate containment and retrieval with the PercuSurge™ emboli containment system. A. The GuardWire™ is advanced across the stenosis. B. The distal occlusion balloon is inflated. C. Routine stenting is performed. D. Particulate debris is aspirated and removed via the Export™ aspiration catheter. (c) The distal occlusion balloon and aspiration catheter. **(Courtesy of Dr J Webb, St Paul's Hospital, Vancouver, British Columbia, Canada)**

a

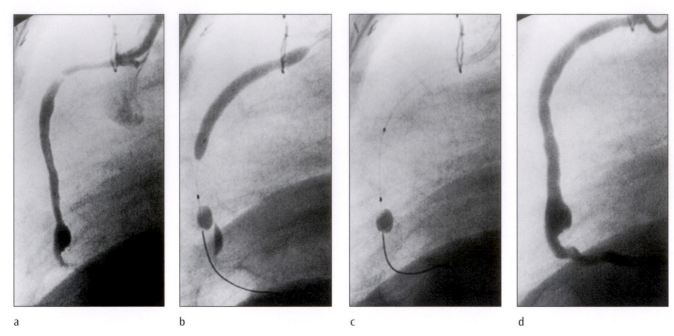

a   b   c   d

Figure 13.61

A 59 year old man presented with unstable angina 13 years after CABG surgery. Angiography revealed proximal occlusions of all native coronary arteries, a patent LIMA to LAD and patent SVG to LCx. The SVG to the dominant RCA was found to have a severe ulcerated stenosis with poor distal filling (a). To protect against distal embolization at the time of intervention, a GuardWire™ was placed distal to the stenosis. The distal vessel was poorly visualized so the occlusive balloon was inflated to an unexpected diameter of 4.5mm immediately proximal to an ectatic segment (b). The visible hold-up of contrast in the distal segment confirms adequate balloon occlusion and the absence of distal flow. Without pre-dilatation a 4.0mm 32mm long NiRoyal™ stent was advanced across the stenosis and deployed at 12 atmospheres (b).

After withdrawal of the stent delivery balloon, the Export™ catheter was advanced into the graft and 20 ml of blood was forcefully aspirated. The radiopaque marker of the catheter can be seen proximal to the occlusion balloon and its marker (c). Particulate debris was grossly visible in the aspirate. Following removal of the guidewire, the SVG was widely patent with no evidence of distal embolization or no reflow (d).

(Courtesy of Dr J Webb, St Paul's Hospital, Vancouver, British Columbia, Canada)

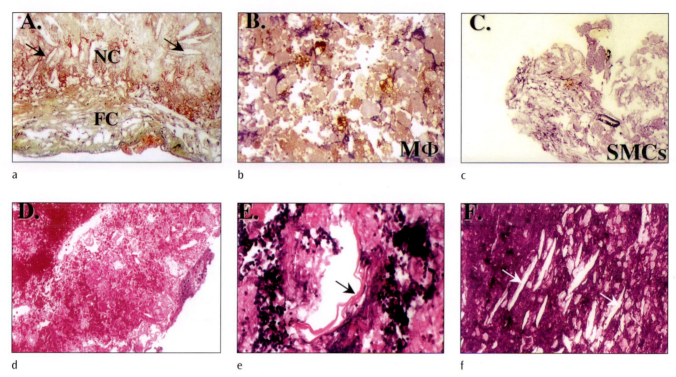

a

b

c

d

e

f

Figure 13.62

Micrographs of plaque material from SVG aspirates show:

(a) Fibrous cap (FC) overlying a lipid-rich core (NC) containing numerous cholesterol clefts (arrows).

(b) Section stained for resident macrophages (dark brown).

(c) Section stained to recognize smooth muscle cells (brown); note the paucity of brown staining.

(d) Necrotic core with plaque haemorrhage.

(e) Aspirate material showing strands of collagen (arrow).

(f) Lipid-rich core area with cholesterol clefts (arrows).

Event rates, including CK elevations (11.1%) and non-Q MI (3.7%) are perhaps lower than after PTCA without such protection.

(Courtesy of Dr J Webb, St Paul's Hospital, Vancouver, British Columbia, Canada)

The Angioguard™ emboli capture guidewire system

The Angioguard™ emboli capture guidewire system (Cordis/Johnson & Johnson) consists of a 300cm long 0.014" diameter guidewire with a 3.5cm shapeable radiopaque tip and a retractable polyurethane filter basket towards its distal end. The basket (currently available in 4mm, 5mm and 6mm diameters; 7mm and 8mm in development) is supported by self-expanding nitinol struts which are contained within a deployment sheath (4.5–5.5F). Once the device is across the lesion, the sheath is removed and the umbrella-shaped filter basket is deployed for the duration of the intervention.

The numerous (390 in a 4mm filter) 100 micron diameter pores allow continuous perfusion while ensuring capture of microemboli and preventing showering of debris into the distal native circulation. After the interventional procedure is completed, insertion of a 5F capture sheath closes the nitinol struts and the basket capturing the debris for removal from the SVG. The system is compatible with an 8F guiding catheter.

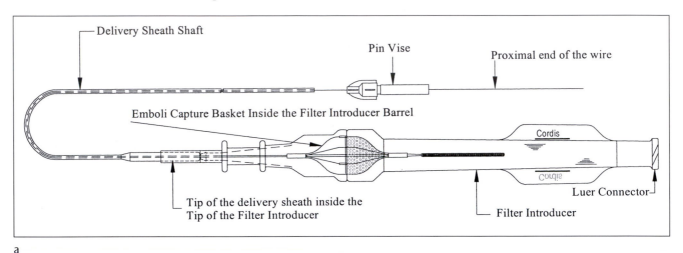

a

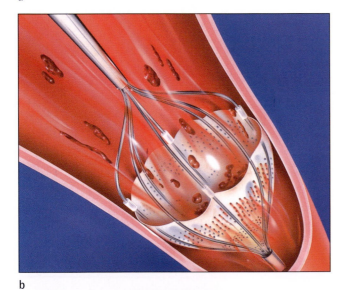

b

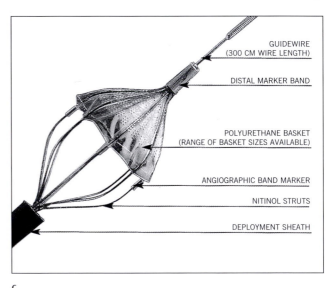

c

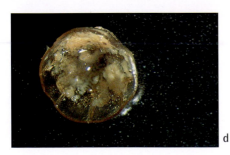

d

Figure 13.63.
(a) Schematic diagram of Angioguard™ emboli capture guidewire system.
(b) Illustration of polyurethane basket deployed in a SVG showing capture of embolizing debris but blood perfusion through the micropores.
(c) Close-up of features of the Angioguard™ basket.
(d) Filter shown containing much captured debris from an SVG. Histology shows non-homogeneous, eosinophilic, hypocellular matrix consistent with chronic thrombus.

continued

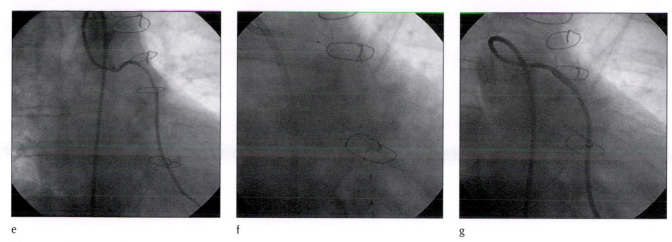

e   f   g

Figure 13.63 continued
(e) Severe proximal disease in an old SVG.
(f) Angioguard™ deployed in distal part of SVG during stent deployment. Note the radiopaque markers and distal guidewire.
(g) SVG post-stent implantation.
(Courtesy of Donna Hatcher, Cordis/Johnson & Johnson, Warren, NJ, USA)

Reading

Brener SJ, Ellis SG, Apperson-Hansen C, *et al.* Comparison of stenting and balloon angioplasty for narrowings in aortocoronary saphenous vein conduits in place for more than five years. Am J Cardiol 1997;79:13-18.

de Feyter PJ, van Suylen RJ, de Jaegere PPT, *et al.* Balloon angioplasty for the treatment of lesions in saphenous vein bypass grafts. J Am Coll Cardiol 1993;21:1539-49.

de Jaegere PPT, van Domburg RT, de Feyter PJ, *et al.* Long-term clinical outcome after stent implantation in saphenous vein grafts. J Am Coll Cardiol 1996;28:89-96.

de Scheerder IR, Strauss BH, de Feyter PJ, *et al.* Stenting of venous bypass grafts: a new treatment modality for patients who are poor candidates for reintervention. Am Heart J 1992;123:1046-54.

Douglas JS Jr. Interventional approaches in the postbypass patient. In: Faxon DP, ed. Practical angioplasty. New York: Raven Press; 1994:121-33.

Grube E, Webb J, Prpic R *et al.* Clinical safety and efficiency of the PercuSurge Guardwire in the Saphenous Vein Graft Angioplasty Free of Emboli (SAFE) Study. J Am Coll Cardiol 2000;35:41A.

Hartmann JR. Thrombolysis of occluded vein grafts. In: White CJ, Ramee SR, eds. Interventional Cardiology. New York: Marcel Dekker; 1995:201-26.

Hearne SE, Davidson CJ, *et al.* Internal mammary artery graft angioplasty: acute and long-term outcome. Cathet Cardiovasc Diagn 1998;44:153-8.

Hong MH, Leon MB, Kent KM. Treatment for saphenous vein grafts. In: Beyar R, Keren G, Leon MB, Serruys PW. Frontiers in Interventional cardiology. London: Martin Dunitz; 1997;29-39.

Komiyama N, Nakanishi S, Yanagishita Y, *et al.* Percutaneous transluminal angioplasty of gastroepiploic artery graft. Cathet Cardiovasc Diagn 1990;21:177-9.

Mathew V, Grill DE, Scott CG, *et al.* The influence of abciximab use on clinical outcome after aortocoronary vein graft interventions. J Am Coll Cardiol 1999;34:1163-9.

Meany TB, Leon MB, *et al.* Transluminal extraction catheter for the treatment of diseased saphenous vein grafts: a multicenter experience. Cathet Cardiovasc Diagn 1995;34:112-20.

Ramee SR, White CJ. Saphenous vein bypass graft angioplasty. In: White CJ, Ramee SR, eds. Interventional Cardiology. New York: Marcel Dekker; 1995:299-316.

Ramsdale DR, Morris JL. Treatment of in-stent restenosis in saphenous vein grafts by Rotablator® atherectomy. J Invas Cardiol 1998;10:89-91.

Ramsdale DR. Intervention after coronary artery bypass surgery. In: Grech ED, Ramsdale DR, eds. Practical Interventional Cardiology. London: Martin Dunitz; 1997:83-122.

Savage M, Douglas J, Fischman D, *et al.* Stent placement compared with balloon angioplasty for obstructed coronary bypass grafts. N Engl J Med 1997;337:740-7.

Waksman R, Weintraub WS, Ghazzal Z, *et al.* Short and long-term outcome of narrowed saphenous vein bypass graft: a comparison of Palmaz-Schatz™ stent, directional coronary atherectomy and balloon angioplasty. Am Heart J 1997;134:274-81.

Webb JG, Carere RG, Virmani R *et al.* Retrieval and analysis of particulate debris after Saphenous Vein Graft Intervention. J Am Coll Cardiol 1999;34:468–75.

White CJ, Ramee SR, Collins TJ, *et al.* Placement of 'biliary' stents in saphenous vein coronary bypass grafts. Cathet Cardiovasc Diagn 1993;30:91-5.

14

Coronary artery intervention with special balloons or devices

A variety of balloon catheters is available for addressing specific coronary anatomical problems. Short, long, tapered and angulated balloons are (or have been) available, as are compliant, non-compliant and semicompliant balloons. High-pressure balloons can be used for dilating hard or calcific lesions and stent deployment, and perfu- sion balloons allow prolonged inflations without produc- ing too much myocardial ischaemia. Balloons are available with various numbers of radio-opaque markers (one, two or three); these markers are useful not only for position- ing the balloon at the lesion and identifying the tip of the catheter but also for precise stent placement.

Long balloons

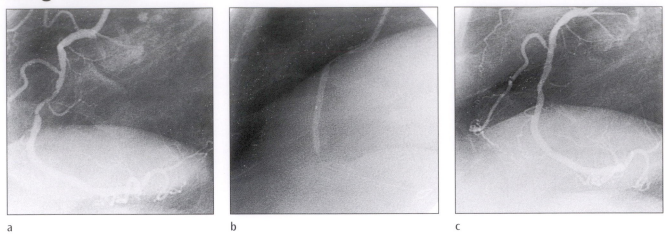

a   b   c

Figure 14.1
(a–c) 30mm long Elipse™ balloon used to dilate a long segment of disease in the mid-third of an RCA.

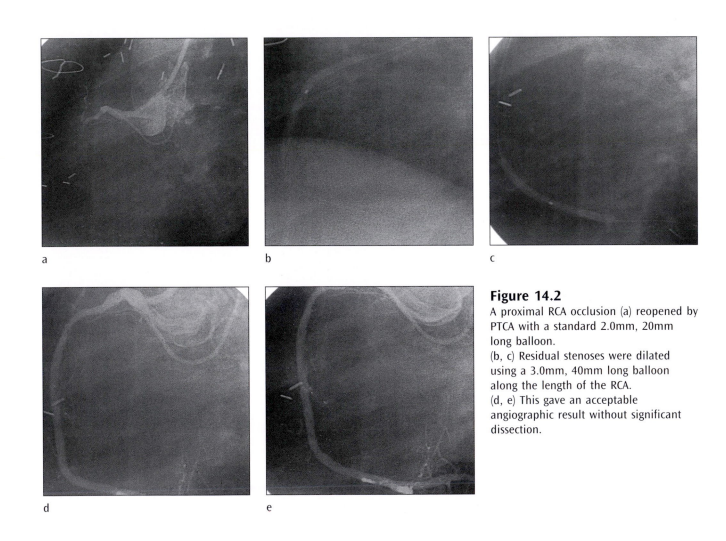

a   b   c

d   e

Figure 14.2
A proximal RCA occlusion (a) reopened by PTCA with a standard 2.0mm, 20mm long balloon.
(b, c) Residual stenoses were dilated using a 3.0mm, 40mm long balloon along the length of the RCA.
(d, e) This gave an acceptable angiographic result without significant dissection.

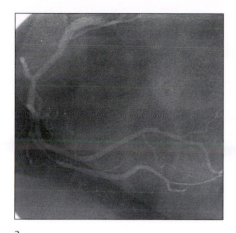
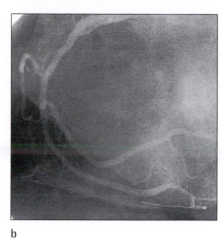

a   b

Figure 14.3
(a, b) A long RCA stenosis treated by a 3.0mm, 30mm long balloon.

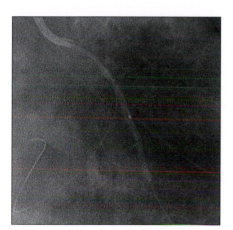

Figure 14.4
A long segment of disease in LCx treated by a 3.0mm, 30mm long balloon with a single central marker.

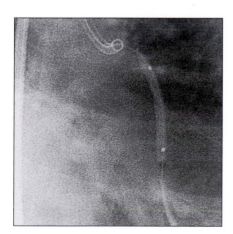

Figure 14.5
A long balloon with double markers used to deploy a 39mm long Microstent™ .

Short balloon

Figure 14.6
This 4mm, 13mm long Viva Primo™ balloon was used to post-dilate this 3.5mm, 18mm long Microstent™ with good effect.

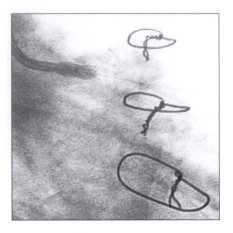

Figure 14.7
After deployment of a 12mm GFX™ stent in this left main coronary artery, the stent was further dilated with a 4.0mm, 10mm long Finale™ balloon.

Perfusion balloons

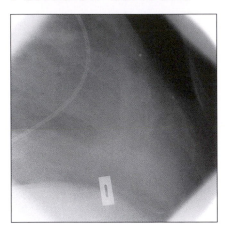

a

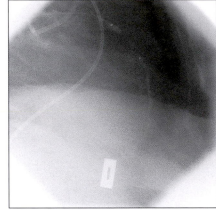

b

Figure 14.8
(a) A proximal LAD stenosis with local dissection being treated by PTCA with a 3.0mm RX® perfusion balloon.
(b) Contrast agent reached the distal vessel via perfusion holes during balloon inflation.
(c) The RX Lifestream™ dilatation catheter (Guidant), which takes a 0.014-inch guidewire, is a rapid-exchange catheter and is available with balloon diameters of 2.0mm, 2.5mm, 3.0mm, 3.5mm and 4.0mm.

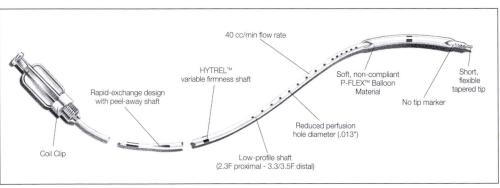

c

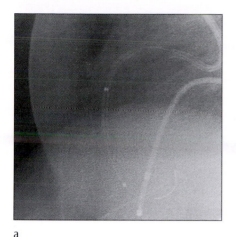

a

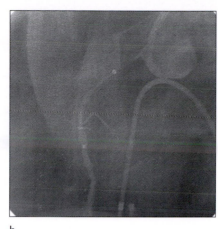

b

Figure 14.9
(a) An RCA treated by PTCA with a 3.0mm RX® perfusion balloon.
(b) The distal vessel filled with contrast via the perfusion holes in the catheter.

Perfusion balloons are rarely used now for sealing occlusive dissections after PTCA by prolonged balloon inflation. This 'rescue role' has been taken over by coronary stenting.

Tapered balloons

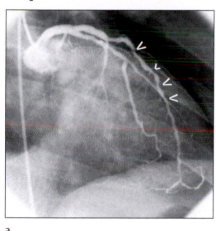

a

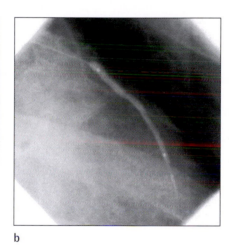

b

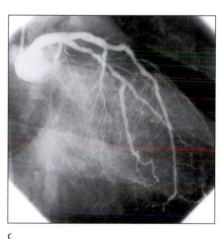

c

Figure 14.10
A 41-year-old unemployed Asian man with severe limiting angina had (a) a long segment of significant disease in the mid-LAD (arrows).
(b) A 6cm long, tapered Malvina™ balloon (Schneider) was used to dilate this long segment of disease. Proximally, the balloon is 3.2mm diameter but it tapers to 2.0mm diameter distally.
(c) Result after PTCA.
Courtesy of Dr O Ormerod, Cardiac Department, John Radcliffe Hospital, Oxford, UK.

Fixed-wire balloons

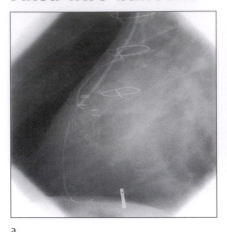
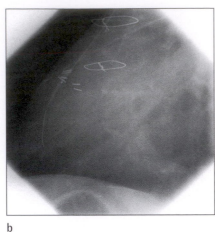
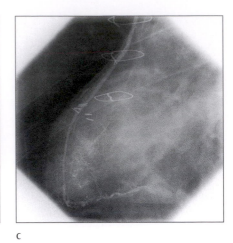

a   b   c

Figure 14.11
(a) Severe stenosis at the distal anastomosis site of the left internal mammary artery to the LAD.
(b) A 2.0mm Fixed-wire ACE™ balloon catheter (Scimed, Boston Scientific) was used to dilate the stenosis.
(c) The result was good.
This type of catheter has a very low profile but limited manoeuvrability. With the advent of modern, low-profile, rapid-exchange balloon catheters, their use has become unnecessary and they have all been discontinued.

Double-marker balloons

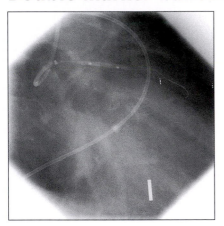

Figure 14.12
Some balloon catheters with radio-opaque markers at either end of the balloon can be useful for accurate positioning of the balloon during PTCA and for precise stent deployment. Note the radio-opaque tip of this particular guiding catheter.

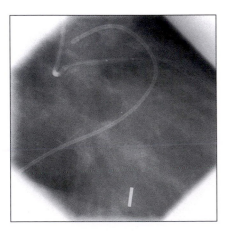

Figure 14.13
Some balloon catheters had a marker in the centre of the balloon as well as a marker at the catheter's tip.

Central marker balloons   Cutting balloon

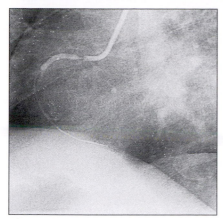

Figure 14.14
Balloons with central markers are also available for PTCA.

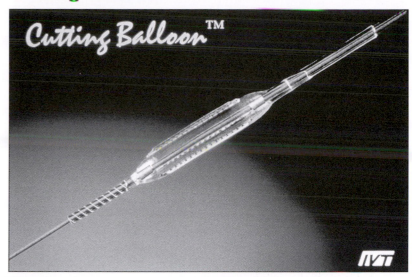

a

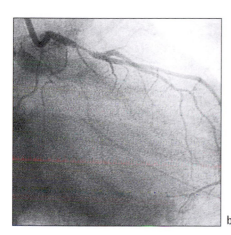

b

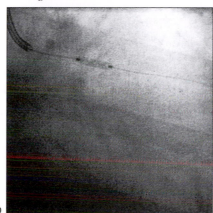

c

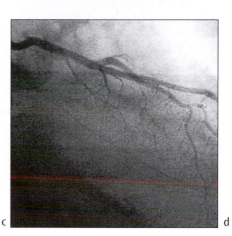

d

Figure 14.15
The Barath™ 'Cutting Balloon™' has been developed to produce a controlled splitting of atheromatous plaque during PTCA. This is achieved by the balloon's three microsurgical blades, which are arranged lengthwise at 120° radial intervals. The blades have a total height of 0.010 inches, of which the working height is 0.005 inches. The width is 0.003 inches (a).

The blades are protected before and theoretically after inflation by the folds of the balloon. Unfortunately, the blades limit flexibility of the balloon, and it is difficult to pass the balloon around sharp bends. The Cutting Balloon™ catheter is manufactured in shorter lengths (10-15mm), which helps somewhat in this respect.

The device is useful in tough lesions that are resistant to conventional PTCA (e.g. ostial stenoses), but its role in calcified lesions, long lesions and in-stent restenosis is still under investigation.

A 46-year-old lady with unstable angina was found to have (b) a severe concentric, tubular stenosis in the proximal LAD.

(c) A 3.0mm Barath™ Cutting Balloon™ was inflated to 6 atmospheres.

(d) This produced a good angiographic result.

The three stainless steel cutting blades attached to the balloon cannot be seen on fluoroscopy.

Recently, the Cutting Balloon Ultra™ has been introduced which has an hydrophilic balloon coating and a 2.9F catheter shaft to improve trackability and crossability. Balloons of diameter 2.0 mm–4.0 mm (0.25 mm increments) are available in 10–15 mm lengths. The 2.0 mm–3.25 mm balloons have three microsurgical blades while balloons of 3.5 mm–4.0 mm have four microblades.

The CAPAS and CUBA studies suggested similar acute angiographic and in-hospital clinical outcomes but a moderate decrease in 3- and 6-month angiographic restenosis respectively (due to late loss) in patients treated with the Cutting Balloon™ versus conventional PTCA. A much larger randomized clinical trial with the Cutting Balloon™ will compare clinical and angiographic outcomes at 6 months.

The Japanese REDUCE trial showed that Cutting Balloon™ angioplasty results in a similar improvement of acute luminal dimensions to that from PTCA, but that Cutting Balloon™ angioplasty has a lower incidence of angiographic dissections.

The CBBEST study is evaluating the effect of Cutting Balloon™ angioplasty as a pre-dilatation method before stenting to reduce vascular trauma.

IVUS/balloon catheters

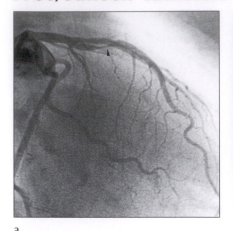

a

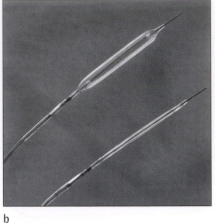

b

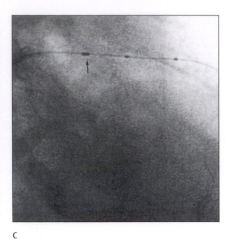

c

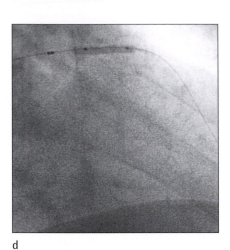

d

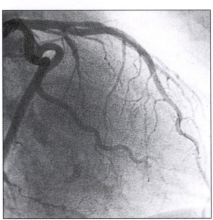

e

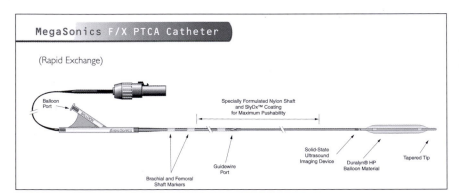

f

Figure 14.16

(a) A severe bulky lesion in the proximal LAD (arrowhead) of a 55-year-old man.
(b) Before planned DCA, IVUS was performed using the rapid exchange Megasonics F/X™ catheter (Endosonics).
(c) This catheter has a balloon with two markers distal to the transducer (arrow).

In this case IVUS showed heavy calcification in the bulky lesion, and so DCA was not performed.

After pre-dilatation with the IVUS 3.0mm balloon (d), a 3.5mm, 25mm long Multilink™ stent was implanted.

(e) This produced an excellent angiographic result.

However, repeat IVUS examination showed eccentric stent deployment because of the bulk of the calcified plaque. A 3.5mm, 20mm long Viva Primo™ balloon was used to dilate the stent more fully and to compress the plaque further. One of the limitations of this combined device is that the lesion has to be crossed by the balloon-section before IVUS can be performed and again on every subsequent occasion (e.g. after stenting).

(f) The Megasonics F/X™ has a proximal-distal shaft diameter of 3.5F-3.0F and is compatible with a 0.014-inch guidewire. Balloon diameters (length 20mm) of 2.5mm, 3.0mm, 3.5mm and 4.0mm are available. The transducer is 4mm long and has a diameter of 3.5F.

IVUS/stent/balloon catheters

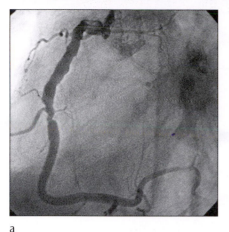

a

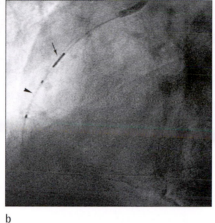

b

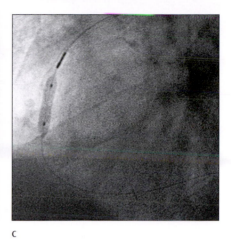

c

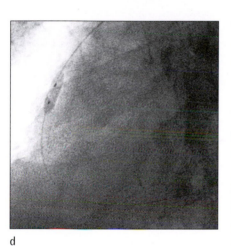

d

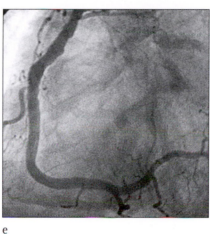

e

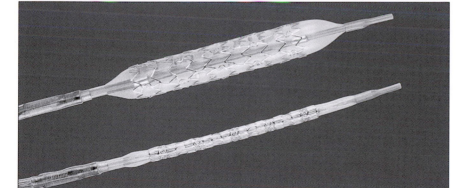

f

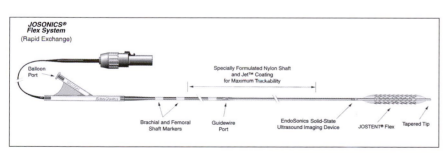

g

Figure 14.17

A 59-year-old man developed moderately severe angina 7 years after successful DCA to the LAD. (a) Angiography showed no significant restenosis in the LAD but a significant lesion in the mid-third of the RCA.

(b, c) The lesion was crossed with a 0.014-inch Floppy® guidewire and a 4.0mm, 16mm long JoStent® Flex stent on the rapid-exchange Endosonics Ultrasound Guided Delivery System (JoSonics® Flex System) was deployed at 15 atmospheres. In (b), the ultrasound transducer (arrow) can be seen proximal to the stent (arrowhead) mounted between its balloon markers.

IVUS showed good stent deployment, but the stent was further dilated with a 4.0mm, 9mm long Maxxum™ balloon up to 19 atmospheres (d).

(e) This gave an excellent angiographic result.

Repeat IVUS showed a diameter of 4.1mm at the end of the procedure.

(f) This device combines solid-state ultrasound with low-profile stent technology. It is very flexible, tracks well and the stent provides good radial strength.

Ultrasound imaging guides optimal deployment.

(g) The catheter is available with balloon/stent diameters of 3.0, 3.5 and 4.0mm with lengths of 9.0, 16 and 26mm.

One of the drawbacks of this device is that the stent has to be advanced beyond the lesion in order to image the lesion before stent deployment. Moreover after stent deployment or after post-dilatation with a high-pressure balloon, the 'poorly rewrapped' balloon has to be advanced across the stent again if an IVUS image is to be obtained.

Marker guidewires

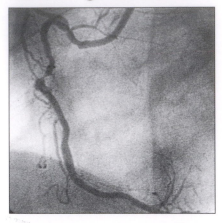

a

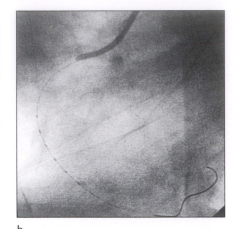

b

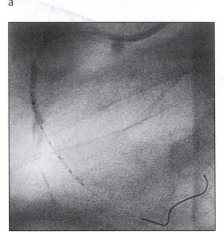

c

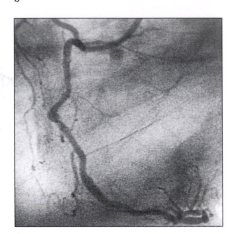

d

Figure 14.18

The Ruler™ guidewire (Guidant) has nine radio-opaque markers, each separated by 5mm. This can be useful for estimating the length of lesions and the length of stent required. The 'marker section' of the guidewire is stiff, although the radio-opaque 3cm section is floppy. Such a device is more useful in a straight section of artery; it is more difficult to place in a tortuous vessel, where it tends to straighten it as in this RCA. (a) Severe stenosis in the middle third of an RCA in a 70-year-old diabetic woman. (b) A Ruler™ guidewire in place straightens the vessel. The markers can be easily seen.

Balloon dilatation with a 2.0mm Worldpass™ balloon (c) through a 6F guide catheter.

(d) Final result after the guidewire was removed and the RCA has resumed its normal shape.

Doppler flow wires

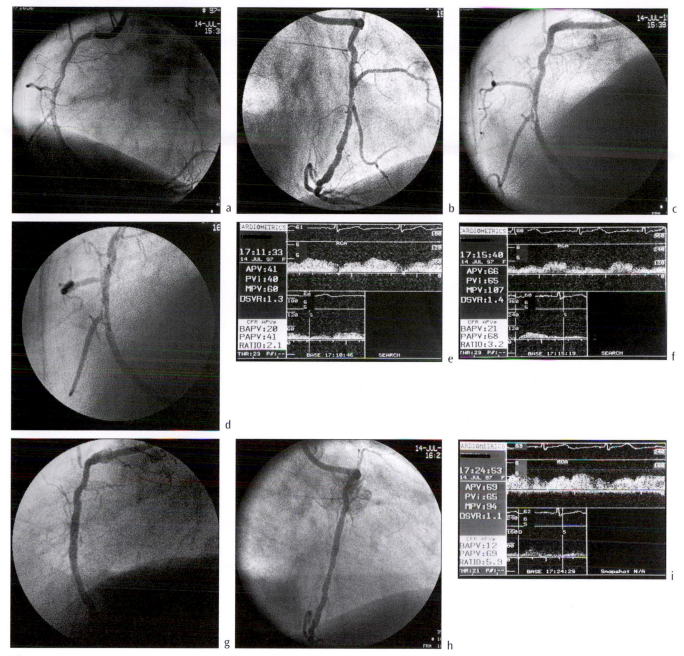

Figure 14.19

A 66-year-old man with unstable angina had (a) a long complex lesion in the middle third of the RCA. The RAO (b) and LLAT (c) projections suggested a local dissection flap on this 'ridged' lesion.

A hockey-stick guide catheter was used to pass a Doppler-tipped guidewire into the distal RCA, but no signal could be obtained in the distal vessel.

(d, e) With an uninflated 3.0mm balloon catheter positioned at the site of the 'flap', a good quality flow velocity signal appeared.

The CFR was 2.1. It was deemed that the lesion was haemodynamically significant and that PTCA was necessary.

(f) The lesion was dilated to 7 atmospheres and the CFR increased to 3.2.

However, the 'flap' appeared to persist.

(g, h) A 3.0mm, 15mm long NIR™ stent was deployed at 12 atmospheres.

(i) The CFR increased to 5.9.

The final angiographic appearance was satisfactory.

Courtesy of Dr C Ilsley and Dr M Mason, Royal Brompton and Harefield Hospital, Middlesex, UK.

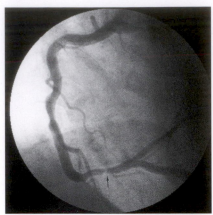
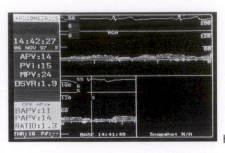
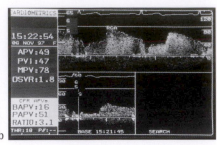
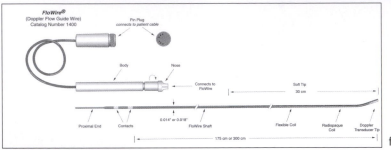
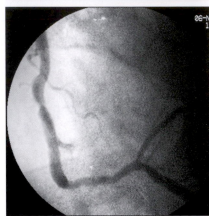
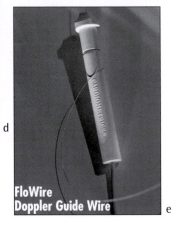
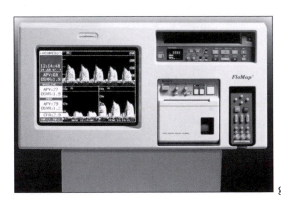

Figure 14.20

A 49-year-old man with unstable angina and an abnormal exercise stress test had (a) a severe, discrete stenosis in the RCA (arrow). (b) A hockey-stick guide catheter was used to pass a 0.014-inch Doppler-tipped guidewire (Flowire®) (Cardiometrics, California, USA) beyond the lesion. A CFR was measured as 1.3.

(c) A 3.0mm balloon was dilated up to 7 atmospheres and the CFR improved to 3.1.

(d) The angiographic appearance of the RCA was markedly improved, and stenting not performed.

Courtesy of Dr C Ilsley and Dr M Mason, Royal Brompton and Harefield Hospital, Middlesex, UK.

(e, f) The FloWire® (Cardiometrics-Endosonics) is a 0.014-inch or 0.018-inch Doppler guidewire with a piezoelectric transducer integrated into its tip.

(g) It connects to the FloMap® ultrasound instrument, which features a video screen, a video cassette recorder and a thermal printer.

This solid-state digital technology automatically calculates CFR (a measure of a lesion's functional severity).

The 0.014-inch Flowire® is available in straight and 'J'-tip shapes and with floppy, flex and firm tips.

Courtesy of Cardiometrics-Endosonics.

The DEBATE I trial evaluated whether Doppler flow velocity measurements were predictive of early or late clinical outcome after PTCA. CFR combined with diameter stenosis after PTCA was predictive of angina, target-vessel revascularization and angiographic restenosis at 6 months. It also suggested that CFR might help identify patients undergoing PTCA who would benefit from stenting.

The DEBATE II trial compared a strategy of primary elective stenting to Doppler-guided PTCA with secondary randomization to stenting or PTCA for patients who met optimal Doppler criteria.

The DESTINI trial will determine whether optimal PTCA (when CFR is over 2.0 and stenosis is less than 35%) using the Doppler flow wire guidance is preferable to stenting (if CFR is less than 2.0 and stenosis is more than 35%) in patients with native vessel disease.

Distal coronary artery pressure guidewires

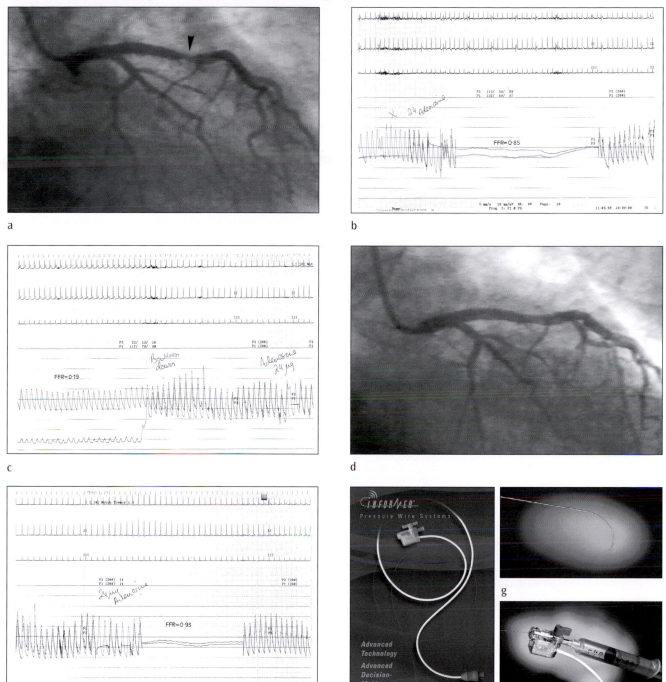

a

b

c

d

e

f

g

h

Figure 14.21

A 58-year-old man with a 6 month history of angina had ST-segment depression of 1mm on his ECG after 4 minutes of the Bruce protocol exercise stress test. (a) Quantitative coronary arteriography showed a 45% diameter stenosis in the mid-LAD (arrow).
(b) Functional assessment of the lesion using a 0.014-inch Informer® (Boston Scientific) coronary pressure guidewire confirmed an FFR – distal/proximal coronary pressure at maximal hyperaemia with intracoronary adenosine – of 78/92 (which gives a value of 0.85).

   PTCA was performed, although the lesion did not meet the criteria for functional significance (FFR of less than 0.75).

   (c) A 3.5mm Viva Primo™ balloon was used. During balloon inflation, the collateral FFR dropped to 17/90 (0.19), confirming a poorly collateralized territory.

   After PTCA, no residual stenosis was noted on orthogonal views (d), with an FFR of 82/88 (0.93) (e).

   This indicated successful dilatation and a statistical restenosis rate of 12% at 6 months follow-up. Given the satisfactory FFR value, no stent was deployed.

   (f, g) The Informer® pressure guidewire. (h) The Informer™ (SCIMED) pressure guidewire interface.

Courtesy of Dr N Uren, The Royal Infirmary Edinburgh, UK.

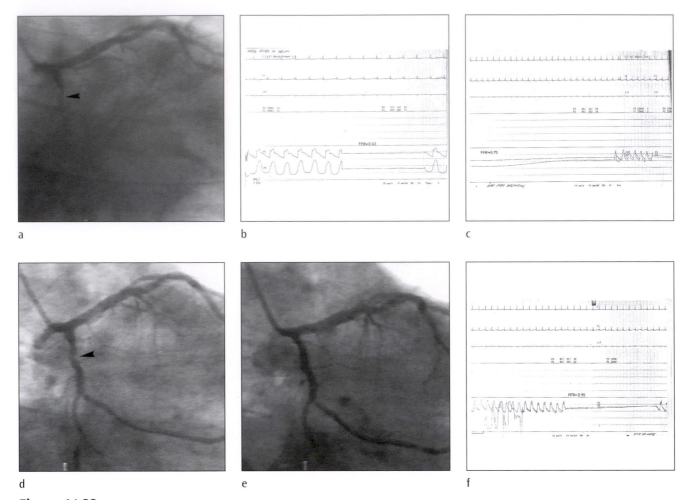

a   b   c

d   e   f

Figure 14.22

A 53-year-old man presented with severe chest pain caused by an acute myocardial infarction (his peak creatine phosphokinase level was 2203 IU per litre) and T-wave inversion in the anterolateral leads. A diagnosis of non-Q wave myocardial infarction was made and he was randomized to the invasive arm of the RITA-3 study. Coronary arteriography showed a normal LAD, proximal occlusion of the LCx (arrow) (a) and a 95% stenosis in the proximal segment of a dominant RCA.

The occluded LCx was crossed with a 0.014-inch floppy tip Informer® coronary pressure guidewire, resulting in TIMI I flow. The FFR was measured after intracoronary adenosine at a value of 32/77 (0.42) (b).

The occlusion was dilated using first a 2.0mm Viva Primo™ balloon followed by a 3.5mm Viva Primo™ balloon leading to restoration of TIMI III flow. The FFR was 48/64 (0.75) (c).

(d) There was also a residual lesion.

On the basis of the FFR and the residual lesion, a 9 cell 16mm long NIR™ stent was deployed on a 3.5mm balloon at 10 atmospheres.

(e) The final result was excellent.

(f) The FFR was measured at 69/73 (0.95).

Two months later the proximal stenosis in the RCA was successfully dilated and stented.

Courtesy of Dr N Uren, The Royal Infirmary Edinburgh, UK.

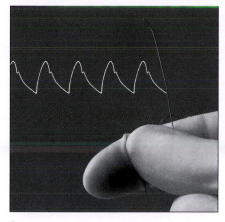

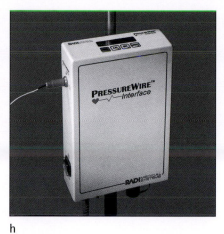

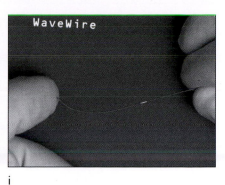

g

h

i

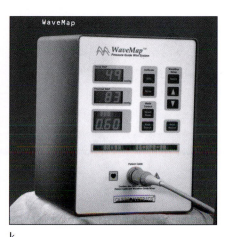

WaveWire Pressure Guidewire	Catalog Number 8400 & 8400J
Length	175 cm
Diameter	0.014"
Radiopaque segment	Distal 3 cm tip
Soft tip	30 cm

j

k

Figure 14.22 *continued*

(g) The Pressure Wire™ Sensor (Radi Medical Systems) is a 0.014-inch guidewire with a high fidelity pressure sensor near the tip. The transducer is a piezo resistive pressure sensor coupled in a wheatstone bridge.

Distal coronary pressure measured during hyperaemia is used to compute the FFR of the myocardium, a new concept for the determination of coronary blood flow. The FFR is defined as the ratio of maximal hyperaemic flow in the stenotic artery to the theoretical maximal hyperaemic flow in the same artery without a stenosis. FFR is computed as the ratio of distal mean coronary pressure and mean aortic pressure during maximal hyperaemia; it is thought to be a specific index of the coronary stenosis that is independent of the microvascular flow status.

The Pressure Wire™ is connected via the Pressure Wire Interface™ (h), which calibrates the pressure wire sensors to the catheter laboratory monitor.

Courtesy of Radi Medical Systems.

(i, j) The WaveWire® is a 175cm long, 0.014-inch diameter angioplasty guidewire with a floppy distal 30cm tip and a radio-opaque distal 3cm tip. The WaveWire® is available with a straight or 'J' tip.

The pressure sensor is positioned 3cm from its distal tip and the proximal end connects to a plug and cable and then to the WaveMap® console (k), on which the proximal and distal pressures and the Fractional Flow Reserve data are displayed.

Courtesy of Cardiometrics-Endosonics.

Intracoronary beta-irradiation after PTCA using a centred ^{90}yttrium source

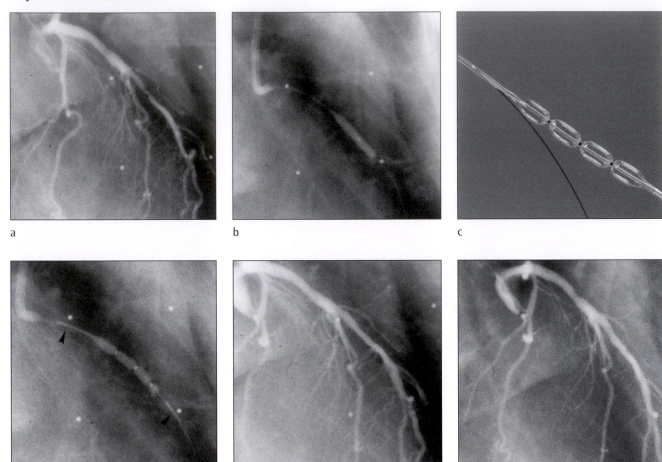

a b c

d e f

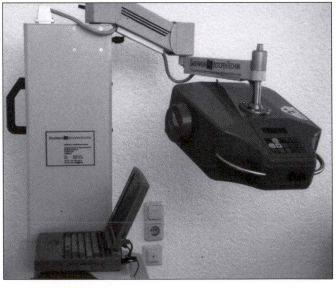

g

Figure 14.23

A 67-year-old woman had moderately severe angina, a positive exercise stress test and (a) a severe mid-third LAD stenosis.

(b) PTCA was performed using a 3.0mm balloon via a 7F guiding catheter.

(c) The Schneider® centring balloon has three constrictions to give four interconnecting compartments in order to provide a more homogeneous dose of irradiation to the wall of the artery.

(d) It was positioned and inflated at the lesion site. An air bubble can be seen within the distal segment. The ^{90}yttrium wire is positioned within the centring balloon and is visible on fluoroscopy owing to the two tungsten markers at either end (arrows).

(e) The post-PTCA/irradiation angiogram shows a satisfactory result.

(f) Six months later, there was no evidence of restenosis.

(g) The afterloading console is built by Sauerwein Isotopen Technik®.

The portable computer allows calculation of dwell time based on source activity and centring balloon diameter.

Courtesy of Dr P Urban, Cardiology Center, University Hospital, Geneva, Switzerland.

Intracoronary beta-irradiation for prevention of restenosis using the Novoste™ BETA-CATH™ system

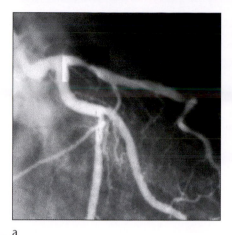

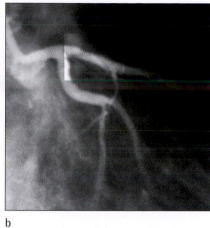

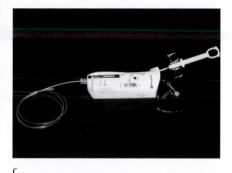

a   b   c

Figure 14.24

A 68-year-old man with a 6-month history of increasing angina was found to have a large, reversible anterior defect on a stress-thallium perfusion scan.

(a) Angiography showed a significant, concentric stenosis in the proximal LAD.

(b) PTCA with a 3.5mm Bandit™ balloon at 12 atmospheres left a residual stenosis of 23%.

(c) The dilated vessel segment was then treated with beta-irradiation therapy as part of the Beta Energy Restenosis Trial (BERT) using the Novoste™ radiation delivery catheter and transfer device.

Beta-irradiation is emitted from a 'train' of several miniature, cylindrical, sealed sources that contain the isotope ^{90}strontium, which is transported hydraulically down the delivery catheter.

At 3 months, a repeat stress-thallium study was normal.

(d) At 6 months, angiography revealed a 7% stenosis at the PTCA site. The patient remains symptom free.

Courtesy of Drs ME Leimbach, NAF Chronos and SB King III, Andreas Gruentzig Cardiovascular Center, Emory University Hospital, Atlanta, Georgia, USA.

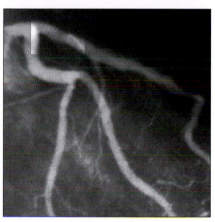

d

Several clinical trials have been designed to study whether beta-irradiation or gamma-irradiation can prevent restenosis in native coronary arteries or SVGs after PTCA or after coronary stent implantation. Others are attempting to determine whether irradiation can also prevent recurrent in-stent restenosis.

The small BERT trial showed that beta-irradiation administered after PTCA was safe and feasible and resulted in a lower than expected rate of restenosis (15%) at 6 months, owing to a substantial alteration in post-PTCA late lumen loss.

The larger BETA-CATH™ trial is attempting to compare the reduction in restenosis obtained by beta-irradiation (using ^{90}strontium) after either PTCA or stenting.

The BETA-WRIST trial is evaluating the efficacy and safety of beta-irradiation (using ^{90}yttrium) for the prevention of a recurrence of in-stent restenosis in patients with in-stent restenosis in native vessels.

The INHIBIT trial is evaluating the efficacy of vascular brachytherapy using the Nucletron afterloader (using ^{32}phosphorus as the source of radiation) in patients with in-stent restenosis

The PREVENT trial is evaluating the clinical safety and angiographic efficacy of a ^{32}phosphorus centring catheter and afterloader for the prevention of restenosis in de novo or restenotic lesions with or without a stent.

Other clinical trials have assessed and are currently evaluating the use of gamma-irradiation for the prevention of restenosis after PTCA and stent implantation.

The SCRIPPS trial showed that catheter-based intracoronary radiotherapy using gamma-irradiation (using ^{192}iridium as the source of radiation) after stenting in patients with restenosis in native vessels or SVGs reduced angiographic and IVUS restenosis rates and adverse clinical events at 6 months – the restenosis rate was 17% with ^{192}iridium versus 54% with placebo.

The GAMMA-1, WRIST and SVG-WRIST trials are assessing whether gamma-irradiation (using ^{192}iridium) can reduce the incidence of further in-stent restenosis in patients undergoing successful treatment for restenosis by PTCA or stenting in both native vessels and SVGs. The LONG WRIST trial is examining a similar strategy for treating long (45–80mm) in-stent restenosis lesions.

The ARREST and ARTISTIC trials are assessing the safety and efficacy of intravascular radiation therapy using the Angiorad system in patients undergoing PTCA or provisional stenting (ARREST) in de novo unstented lesions and in those with in-stent restenosis (ARTISTIC) in native vessels.

Therapeutic ultrasound thrombolysis

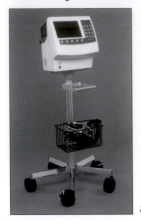
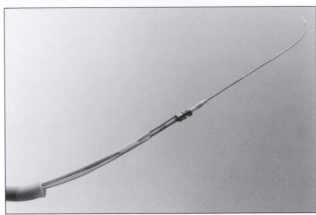
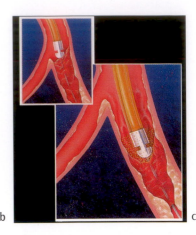

Figure 14.25

(a) The Acolysis™ ultrasound thrombolysis device (Angiosonics) consists of a controller, which is an electric signal generator with sophisticated computer controls and safety circuitry.

The controller software monitors output power to ensure that the appropriate level of ultrasonic energy is delivered to the thrombus throughout the procedure. An external transducer converts electrical energy into ultrasonic energy, which is delivered to the Acolysis Probe™ tip.

(b) The coronary ultrasound angioplasty probe has a 1.6mm tip and can be inserted in a 7F guide catheter in a monorail fashion over a 0.014-inch high-torque guidewire.

The distal segment of the probe trifurcates into three micro-thin wires, which allow for maximum energy delivery while maintaining excellent flexibility in tortuous coronary anatomy. The Acolysis™ system uses high-energy, low-frequency ultrasound to lyse clot rapidly and with minimized local heating.

(c) When activated, the probe tip produces cavitation and a resulting vortex which pulls the thrombus toward the distal tip of the probe.

Unlike mechanical thrombectomy devices, Acolysis™ liquifies fibrin-containing clots of various ages into basic blood components.

The ACUTE trial evaluated the feasibility of percutaneous transluminal coronary ultrasound thrombolysis in acute myocardial infarction.

Courtesy of Dr U Rosenschein, Tel Aviv Medical Center, Tel Aviv, Israel.

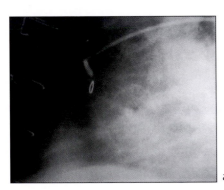
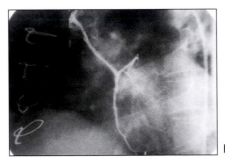
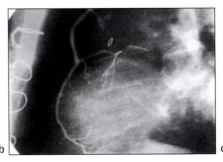

Figure 14.26

A 62-year-old patient had had CABG surgery 10 years earlier, with a single SVG to the LAD. One year ago, two stents had been deployed in the SVG because of diffuse narrowing and angina. The patient presented with a 2-week history of unstable angina. (a) Coronary arteriography revealed total occlusion of the SVG.

After sonification (41.9KHz, 18W for 3 minutes), (b) normal flow was restored to the artery with no embolization.

IVUS imaging showed in-stent tissue growth proximally, and the SVG was restented. Final result (c).

Courtesy of Dr U Rosenschein, Tel Aviv Medical Center, Tel Aviv, Israel.

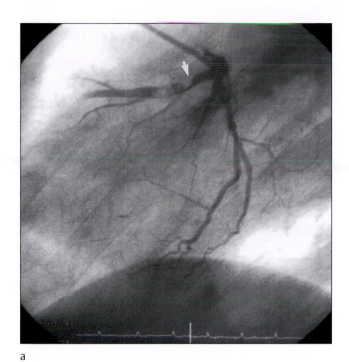
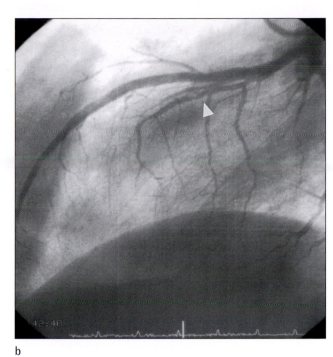

a   b

Figure 14.27

A patient with an acute myocardial infarction was found to have (a) large filling defects in the proximal LAD with TIMI I flow. The most proximal lesion was sharply scalloped, which is suggestive of a ruptured plaque (arrow), while the more distal lesion had the appearance of thrombus propagating distally from the ruptured plaque.

After sonification (41.9KHz, 18W for 3 minutes), the thrombus was lysed and TIMI III flow was restored.

(b) After adjunctive stenting of the proximal LAD lesion, there was full restoration of the vessel dimensions and morphology. A previously occluded diagonal branch reappeared (arrowhead).

Typically, there was no evidence of dissection, embolization, side-branch occlusion, spasm or perforation.

Courtesy of Dr U Rosenschein, Tel Aviv Medical Center, Tel Aviv, Israel.

The ATLAS trial is evaluating Acolysis™ versus abciximab followed by a definitive interventional treatment in SVGs with thrombus in patients who have acute coronary syndromes.

Therapeutic ultrasound to recanalize a chronic total occlusion using the Sonicross® device

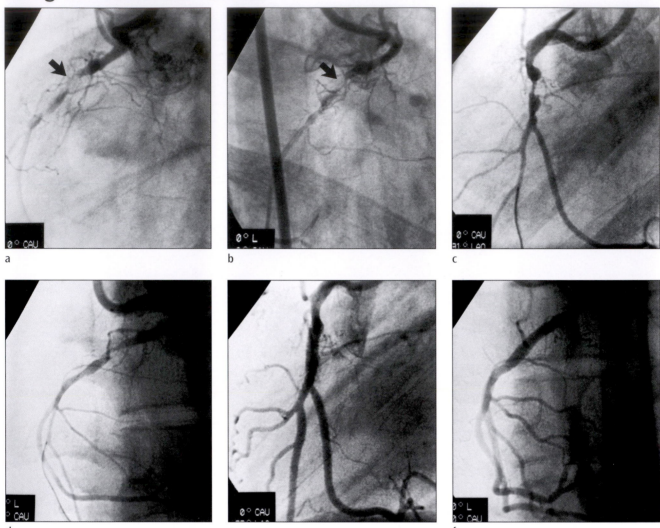

a b c

d e f

Figure 14.28

A 31-year-old man was found to have an occluded RCA of 15 weeks' duration. PTCA failed to reopen the vessel. (a, b) The coronary angiogram demonstrates a proximal occlusion of the RCA with bridging collaterals that antegradely fill the distal RCA.

An 8FR Amplatz guiding catheter was used. However, a 0.014-inch guidewire (HiTorque Super Sport™, ACS) failed to cross the occlusion despite support with a 1.5mm balloon catheter. The balloon catheter was then exchanged for the therapeutic ultrasound catheter, which was placed gently at the beginning of the occlusion.

(c, d) After the first treatment of 30 seconds, the guidewire easily passed the occlusion, and the vessel reopened with PTCA using the 1.5mm balloon catheter.

After additional ultrasound treatment, PTCA and stent deployment with a 3.0mm Multilink™ stent was performed.

(e, f) The angiographic result appeared excellent, with full recanalization. There was minimal residual stenosis and good distal run-off.

IVUS imaging confirmed the successful angiographic result and showed a well-expanded stent, no dissection and no thrombus in the RCA.

Courtesy of Drs T Nagai, N Eigler, H Luo, S Atar and RJ Siegel, Cedars-Sinai Medical Center, Los Angeles, California, USA.

Thrombectomy with the Angiojet® catheter

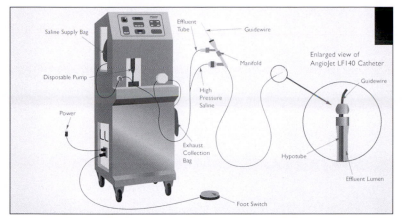

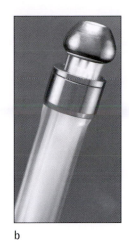

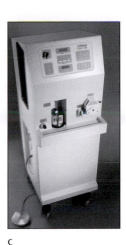

a

b

c

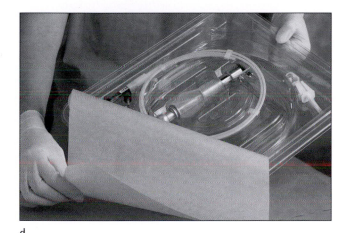

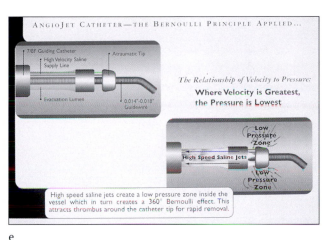

d

e

Figure 14.29

The AngioJet® (Possis Medical Inc) is a thrombectomy catheter that uses hydrodynamic forces created by a drive unit that develops pressures of up to 8,000-13,000 psi. This force is used to produce saline jets directed backwards towards the lumen of a 140cm long, steerable, 5F, over-the-wire catheter tip. This creates a Venturi effect that results in fragmentation and aspiration of the thrombus (rheolysis).

The AngioJet® LF140 is a catheter for coronary use. It is compatible with a guidewire of diameter 0.014-0.018 inches and an 8F guiding catheter.

(a) Diagrammatic representation of the AngioJet® rheolytic thrombectomy system.

(b) Close up view of distal tip of an AngioJet® LF140 catheter.

(c) The drive unit.

(d) The pump set and catheter. The single-use, pulsatile pump set pressurizes and delivers sterile saline to the catheter and provides a pathway for the removal of the thrombus mixture from the catheter to the collection bag.

(e) Explanation of the mechanism of action.

See also Figs 5.31 and 5.32.

Courtesy of Possis Medical Inc, Minneapolis, Minnesota, USA.

'X-SIZER™' helical atherectomy catheter

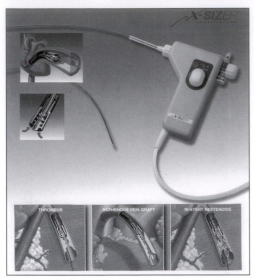

a

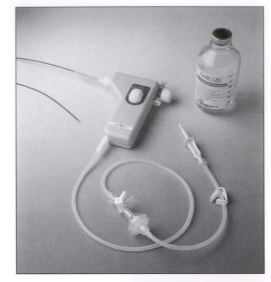

c

Figure 14.30

The X-SIZER™ (EndiCOR Medical Inc) is a catheter system that consists of a simple, hand-held control unit attached to a catheter with a helix cutter at its tip. The combination of the helix cutter (which rotates at approximately 2000 rpm) and the vacuum removes occlusive tissue from the diseased coronary vessel (a).

The system may be useful for debulking lesions before stenting, for the removal of thrombus and in the treatment of SVGs and in-stent restenosis. It is not suitable for calcified lesions.

The catheter is available in 6F size, requires an 8F guiding catheter, has a 2.0mm cutter and requires a 300cm guidewire.

(b) Close-up view of the distal end of the catheter.

(c) The X-SIZER™'s attachment to the vacuum bottle.

Courtesy of Endicor Medical Inc, San Clemente, California, USA.

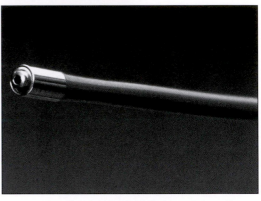

b

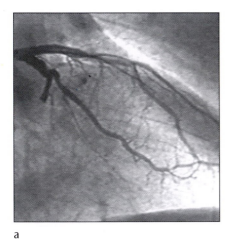

a

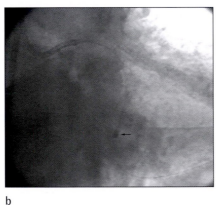

b

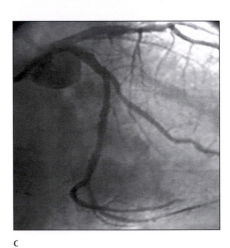

c

Figure 14.31

A 54-year-old man presented with an acute myocardial infarction caused by (a) an occluded LCx.

The X-SIZER™ catheter was selected to remove the fresh thrombus. An 8F AL2 guiding catheter was used to deliver a 0.014-inch Hannibal™ guidewire, with no improvement in TIMI flow.

(b) The X-SIZER™ was advanced through the lesion with slow back-and-forth movement (arrow).

The occlusive thrombus was removed and the LCx was significantly improved with a residual stenosis of 41%. PTCA was performed and a 4.0mm, 8mm long stent was deployed.

(c) The final result was good.

Courtesy of Dr T Ischinger, Klinik-Bogenhausen, Munich, Germany.

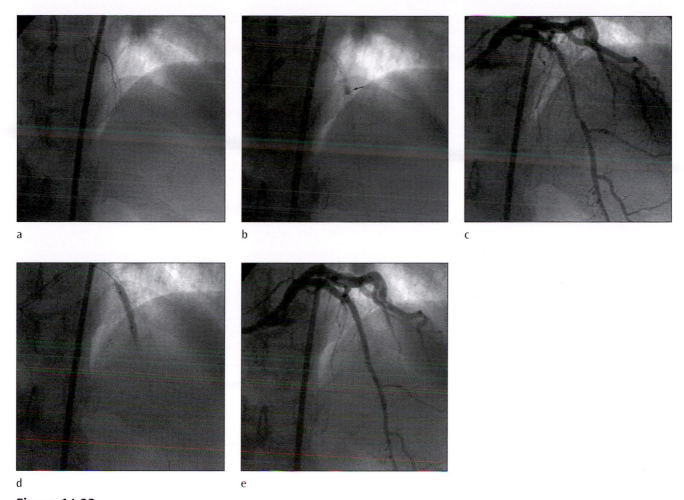

a   b   c

d   e

Figure 14.32

A 48-year-old woman had recurrent in-stent restenosis covering tandem lesions in the LAD. Four months earlier, rotational atherectomy had been performed for in-stent restenosis. (a) The LAD was virtually occluded and it was difficult to cross the lesion with a guidewire (a).

(b) A 5.5F/6F 2.0mm X-SIZER™ catheter made one pass through the occluded segment (arrow).

(c) This produced marked improvement and TIMI III flow.

(d) Adjunctive PTCA was then used.

(e) This produced a very satisfactory angiographic result.

Courtesy of Dr J Gaspar, Instituto Nacional de Cardiologia, Mexico City, Mexico.

Reading

Cannon L, Siegel R, Greenberg J *et al*. Recanalization of total coronary occlusions using the Sonicross low frequency ultrasound catheter. J Am Coll Cardiol 2000;35:41A.

Challenges in interventional cardiology: cutting balloon workshop. J Invas Cardiol 1996;8 (Special Suppl):1A-32A.

Davidson CJ, Gershony G, Lo S *et al*. Helixcision atherectomy for in-stent stenosis: initial in vivo experience. J Am Coll Cardiol 2000;35:41A.

de Franco AC, Tuzcu EM, Nissen SE. Interventional applications of coronary intravascular ultrasound. In: Topol EJ, Serruys PW, eds. Current review of interventional cardiology, 2nd ed. Philadelphia: Current Medicine; 1995:173-91.

di Mario C, Di Francesco L, Kobayashi Y, *et al*. Intracoronary Doppler: the technique and clinical applications. In: Beyar R, Keren G, Leon MB, Serruys PW, Frontiers in interventional cardiology. London: Martin Dunitz; 1997:339-52.

Ergene O, Seyithanoglu BY, Tastan A, *et al*. Comparison of angiographic and clinical outcome after cutting balloon and conventional balloon angioplasty in vessels smaller than 3mm in diameter: a randomized trial. J Invas Cardiol 1998;10:70-75.

Fitzgerald PJ, Yock PG, Hausmann D, Friedrich GF. Intravascular ultrasound imaging. In: White CJ, Ramee SR, eds. Interventional cardiology. New York: Marcel Dekker; 1995:1-23.

Funamoto M, Tsuchikane E, Moriguchi K, *et al*. Cutting balloon angioplasty vs plain old balloon angioplasty randomized study in type B/C lesions (CAPAS). J Am Coll Cardiol 1997;28:458A.

Hamburger J, Brekke M, di Mario C, *et al*. The EURO-ART study: an analysis of the initial European experience with the AngioJet rapid thrombectomy catheter. J Am Coll Cardiol 1997;29:186A.

Hosokawa H, Yamaguchi T, Kobayashi T, *et al*. for the REDUCE investigators. Acute results of the Restenosis Reduction by Cutting Balloon Evaluation study. J Am Coll Cardiol 1998;31:315A.

Ischinger TA. A novel device for removal of thrombus from coronary arteries: The X-SIZER Multicenter Trial. J Am Coll Cardiol 2000;35:41A.

Ischinger TA, Reifart N, Mathey D, *et al*. The X-SIZER catheter system: initial multicenter clinical experience of a novel device for removal of occlusive tissue material from coronary arteries. Eur Heart J 1999;20 (Suppl): I-269.

Kern M. Current status of translesional coronary physiology: decisions regarding coronary interventions in the catheterization laboratory. In:

Beyar R, Keren G, Leon MB, Serruys PW. Frontiers in interventional cardiology. London: Martin Dunitz; 1997:307-16.

Kern MJ, Flynn MS. Clinical applications of intracoronary coronary doppler flow velocity in interventional cardiology. In: White CJ, Ramee SR, eds. Interventional cardiology. New York: Marcel Dekker; 1995:39-78.

Kim RH, Fischmann DL, Dempsey CM, Savage MP. Rheolytic thrombectomy of a chronic coronary occlusion. Cathet Cardiovasc Diagn 1998;43:483-9.

King SB III, Williams DO, Chougule P, *et al*. Endovascular beta-radiation to reduce restenosis after coronary balloon angioplasty. Results of the Beta Energy Restenosis Trial (BERT). Circulation 1998;97:2025-30.

Levendag PC, ed. Vascular brachytherapy: new perspectives. London: Remedica Publishing; 1999.

Nakagawa Y, Matsuo S, Yokoi H, *et al*. Stenting after thrombectomy with the AngioJet® catheter for acute myocardial infarction. Cathet Cardiovasc Diagn 1998;43:327-30.

Pimentel CX, Schreiter SW and Gurbel PA. The use of the Tracker® catheter as a guidewire support device in angioplasty of angulated and tortuous circumflex coronary arteries. J Invas Cardiol 1995;7:66-71.

Prpic R, Kwok OH, Goldar-Najafi and Popma JJ. Angiographic outcomes after intracoronary X-Sizer® helical atherectomy: first use in humans. Circulation 1999;100 (Suppl I)I-305.

Ramee SR, Baim DS, Popma JJ, *et al*. A randomized, prospective multi-center study comparing intracoronary urokinase to rheolytic thrombectomy with the Possis AngioJet catheter for intracoronary thrombus: final results of the VEGAS II trial. Circulation 1998;98(Suppl I):I-86.

Serruys PW, di Mario C, Piek J, *et al*. Prognostic value of intracoronary flow velocity and diameter stenosis in assessing the short- and long-term outcomes of coronary balloon angioplasty. The DEBATE study (Doppler Endpoints Balloon Angioplasty Trial Europe). Circulation 1997;96:3369-77.

Waksman R, Serruys PW, eds. Handbook of vascular brachytherapy. London: Martin Dunitz; 1998.

Waksman R. Radiation therapy for restenosis from preclinical studies to human trials. Stent 1997;1:9-13.

White CJ, Jain SP. Intravascular ultrasound. In: Grech ED, Ramsdale DR, eds. Practical interventional cardiology. London: Martin Dunitz; 1997:279-91.

15

Complications after coronary intervention

There is a wide range of complications that can occur after coronary intervention, although these are generally infrequent in experienced hands. Coronary artery dissection, thrombosis and occlusion are perhaps the most serious. Coronary artery perforation is rare but may be seen after laser, directional or Rotablator® atherectomy and occasionally after PTCA itself. Coronary artery spasm is not uncommon after Rotablator® atherectomy, but it is usually reversible with intracoronary nitrates. Specific complications are associated with coronary artery stent implantation and include stent loss, strut damage, stent jail and intra-stent restenosis.

Although coronary stents have reduced the need for emergency CABG surgery in the event of acute closure caused by dissection or thrombosis after PTCA, surgical back-up is still important if extensive myocardial infarction and death are to be avoided when a complication such as perforation or mechanical device failure cannot be solved by transcatheter therapeutics.

A plan of management should always be anticipated, depending on the anatomical problem, the amount of myocardium at risk, the importance of the vessel being addressed and the clinical status of the patient. An understanding with the cardiac surgeons should always be obtained. Although it is not feasible and indeed it is unnecessary to have a cardiac theatre standing empty in today's very demanding environment, a 'next available theatre' strategy is required and, if necessary, emergency CABG surgery in the catheter laboratory should be possible in the event of haemodynamic collapse after a major complication and cardiac arrest.

Complications after PTCA
Coronary artery dissection

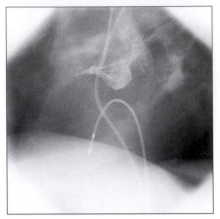

a

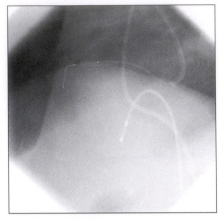

b

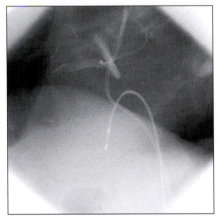

c

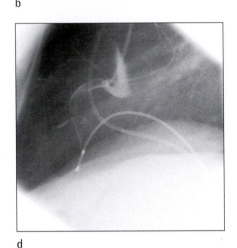

d

Figure 15.1

(a) A proximal RCA occlusion (1988). A guidewire crossed the occlusion but was not advanced into the distal vessel.
(b) The balloon catheter was inflated in occlusion but the guiding catheter was unstable and disengaged.
(c, d) Local dissection, which extended backwards into the aortic root, resulted from the balloon dilatation. This is an unusual occurrence.

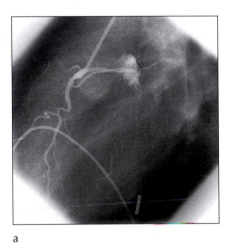

a

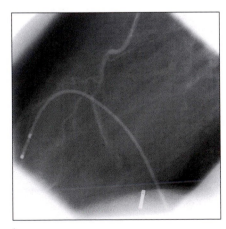

b

Figure 15.2

(a) A proximal RCA occlusion. Absence of a tapered tip and a side branch at the point of occlusion are unfavourable features for successful recanalization.
(b) Attempts to cross the lesion with a 0.014-inch Intermediate® guidewire caused dissection and a parallel false lumen.

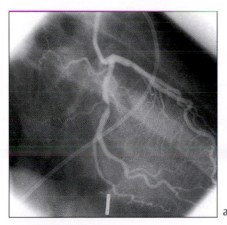
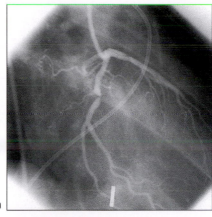

Figure 15.3
(a) This LCx stenosis could not be crossed with one of the early generation balloons (1983).
(b) Forceful guide catheter back-up caused dissection of the left main coronary artery.

This required emergency CABG surgery.

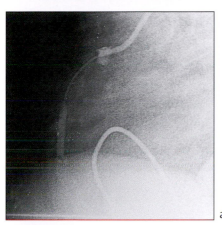
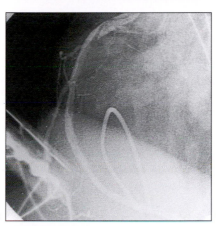

Figure 15.4
(a) Guiding catheter tip trauma can cause dissection.
(b) Dissection extended down the RCA in a spiral fashion in this case.

Modern guiding catheters have soft tips to reduce the likelihood of dissection of the coronary ostium or proximal coronary artery during deep engagement.

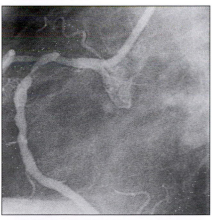
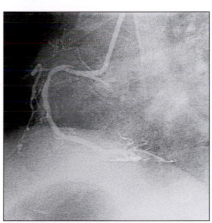

Figure 15.5
(a) A severe stenosis in proximal RCA in a 52-year-old woman with uncontrolled angina required guiding catheter support to enable crossing.
(b) Trauma from the guiding catheter tip caused dissection of the ostium of the RCA.

After reopening the RCA with a 2.0mm, 40mm long Rally™ (Scimed), prolonged balloon inflation at the site of dissection using a 2.5mm RX® Perfusion balloon (c) resulted in sealing of the tear and an acceptable angiographic improvement (d).

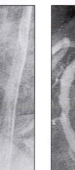
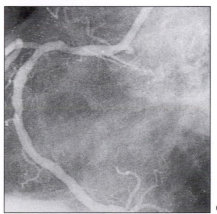

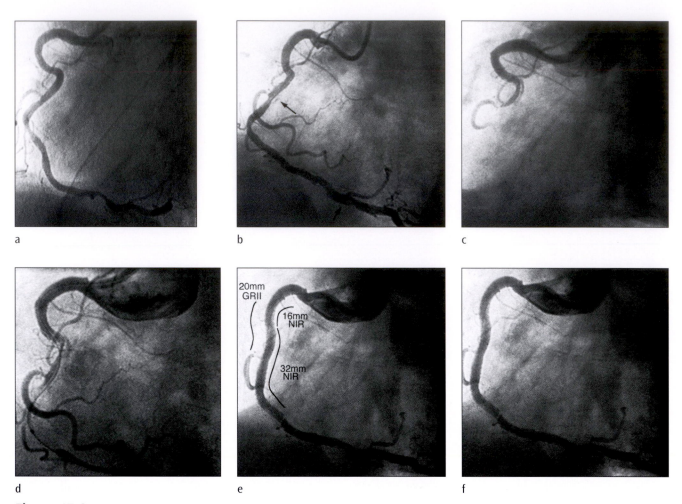

a   b   c

d   e   f

Figure 15.6

Tortuous 'shepherd's crook' RCAs remain a challenge to the coronary interventionist. Excellent guide catheter support is essential for successful delivery of guidewires, balloon catheters and stents, but such support carries the risk of guide catheter-induced dissection and acute closure, as demonstrated here. Once this complication occurs, it can be extremely difficult or impossible to re-establish guidewire position in the true lumen in order to salvage the situation.

(a) A 50% stenosis in the middle third of the RCA and a 75% eccentric stenosis just proximal to the PDA in a 64-year-old man.

A 6F Amplatz Left I guide catheter was chosen to give extra support and facilitate deep engagement if necessary. A 0.014-inch Floppy® guidewire was passed with some difficulty into the distal RCA and a 3.0mm Europass™ balloon catheter was used to dilate both lesions.

(b) Linear dissections were visible (arrow) at the proximal and distal lesion sites and persisted after further dilatation.

A 3.0mm, 15mm long Multilink™ stent could not be advanced beyond the proximal bend and the post-PTCA result was accepted.

Two hours later, the patient developed severe chest pain and inferior ST-segment elevation, owing to (c) occlusion of the proximal RCA and extensive spiral dissection down the vessel.

This was thought to be due to deep guide catheter engagement during attempted stent delivery. An 8F Amplatz Left I guide catheter was chosen for added support. A 3.0mm Olympix II™ balloon catheter was used to facilitate guidewire exchanges, alternating between a 0.014-inch high torque Floppy™ wire and a Choice PT™ wire (Scimed) until the the distal vessel was reached through the true lumen (d).

A 3.5mm, 40mm long Viva™ balloon was then used to perform sequential dilatations from the crux backwards to the proximal RCA. A 32mm NIR™ stent was then mounted on to the long Viva™ balloon and advanced down the RCA. Because of the tortuosity of the vessel, the stent could not be advanced across the distal lesion and so it was deployed proximal to it at a pressure of 14 atmospheres. A 16mm NIR™ stent could not be advanced through the first stent and had to be deployed proximally too.

A further attempt to reach the distal lesion with a 4.0mm, 20mm long Gianturco-Roubin II™ stent failed, again because of the tortuosity of the vessel and 'stent-stent interaction'.

(e) Therefore, this stent was deployed between the first two stents.

The distal lesion was therefore redilated with a 3.5mm balloon and the final angiographic result was satisfactory, with TIMI III flow (f).

The creatine phosphokinase level rose to 770 U per litre, but the patient was discharged 48 hours later on aspirin and ticlopidine.

Stent delivery in such cases may be aided by exchanging the guidewire for an extra-support guidewire and by the use of multiple short, flexible stents deployed in turn from the distal extent of the dissection backwards to its origin. High-pressure dilatation of the stented segment to increase lumen size and improve strut apposition may also help with the passage of a stent through a stent, as may the use of a second (or 'buddy') guidewire.

Courtesy of Drs I Penn and J Rankin, Vancouver General Hospital and Health Sciences Centre, Vancouver, British Columbia, Canada.

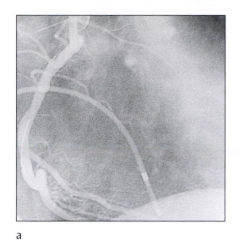

a

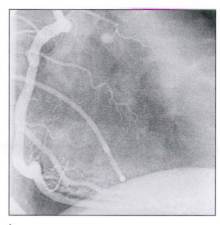

b

Figure 15.7
A proximal RCA dissection after a PTCA
(a) can be successfully treated by stent
implantation – as was done in this case
with a 3.5mm Microstent II™ (b).

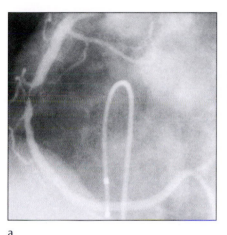

a

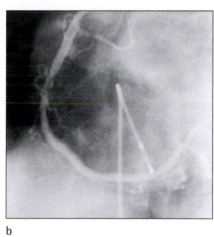

b

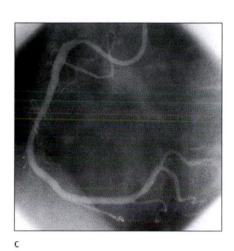

c

Figure 15.8
This RCA stenosis (a) was dilated in 1985, resulting in a non-occlusive local dissection, which was treated conservatively (b).
(c) A restudy at 6 months showed a normal angiographic appearance.
Courtesy of Dr DH Bennett, Wythenshawe Hospital, Manchester, UK.

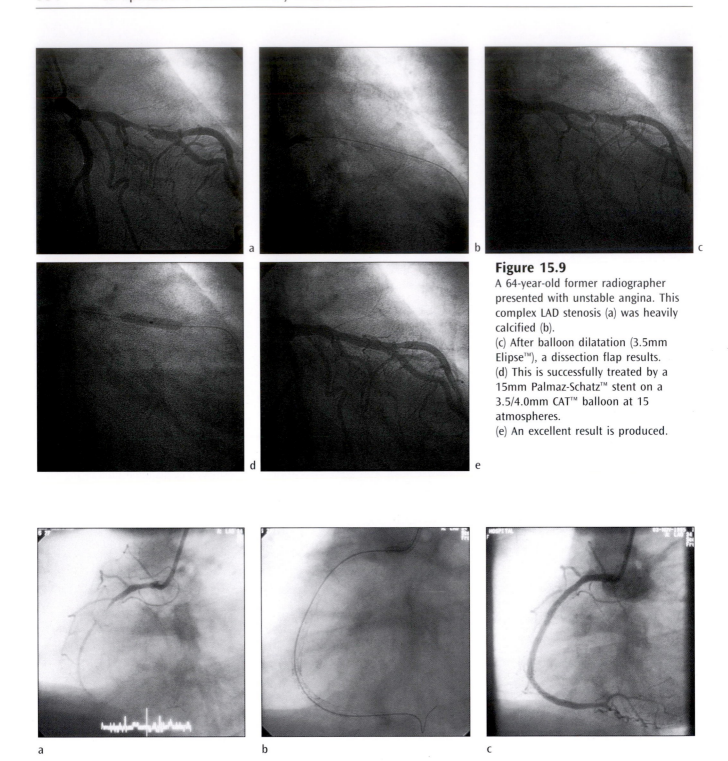

Figure 15.9
A 64-year-old former radiographer presented with unstable angina. This complex LAD stenosis (a) was heavily calcified (b).
(c) After balloon dilatation (3.5mm Elipse™), a dissection flap results.
(d) This is successfully treated by a 15mm Palmaz-Schatz™ stent on a 3.5/4.0mm CAT™ balloon at 15 atmospheres.
(e) An excellent result is produced.

Figure 15.10
A 55-year-old man with stable angina had a significant stenosis in the proximal third of the RCA. (a) PTCA produced an occlusive dissection.

After deployment of a 3.0mm, 15mm long Palmaz-Schatz™ stent, the vessel occluded completely, which necessitated deployment of a series of more distal stents in order to rescue the situation.

(b) Four 3.0mm coronary stents (one 16mm long Wiktor®, one 18mm long Microstent II™ and two 18mm long GFX™ stents) were deployed between the crux and the most proximal stent.

(c) Final result.

Such multi-stent deployment, including stent-through-stent passage, can be very difficult and is expensive. This procedure was performed before long stents were available.

Courtesy of Dr A Gershlick, Glenfield Hospital, Leicester, UK.

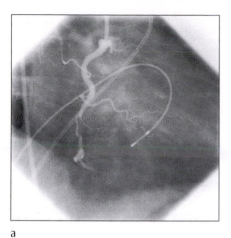 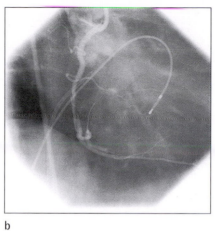 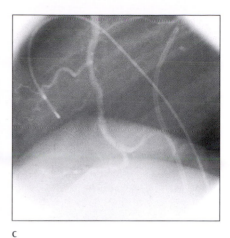

a   b   c

Figure 15.11
(a) This severely diseased RCA is occluded distally.
(b) The vessel was opened by PTCA, but local dissection is visible.
(c) Final result after perfusion balloon treatment (pre-stent era).

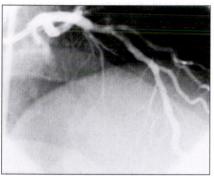 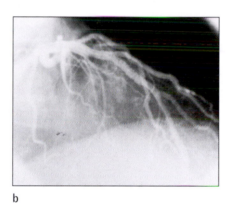

a   b

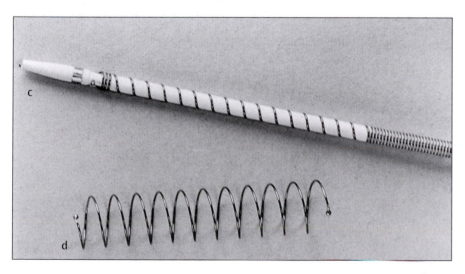

c

d

Figure 15.12
(a) PTCA produced dissection in this mid-LAD just beyond a DG branch.
(b) The radio-opaque, self-expanding, nitinol Cardiocoil™ stent (Medtronic) is positioned across the ostium of the diagonal branch, producing an excellent angiographic result.

The DG was dilated through the side wall of the stent.

The Cardiocoil stent can be seen (c) on and (d) off its delivery catheter. It is no longer available.
Courtesy of Dr R Beyar, Rambam Medical Center, Haifa, Israel.

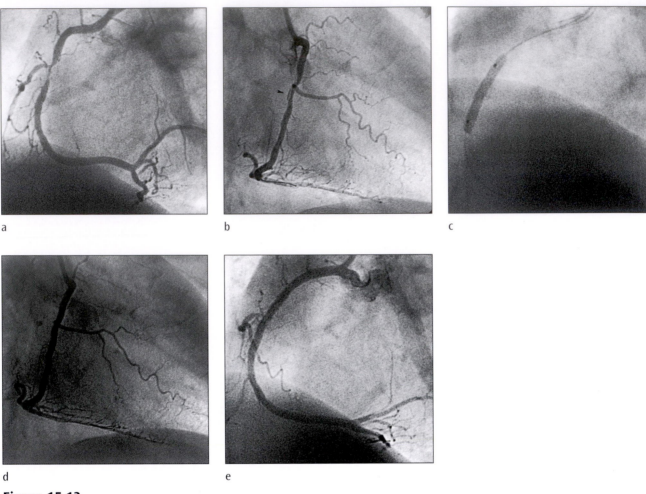

a   b   c

d   e

Figure 15.13
(a) Stenosis in the RCA.
(b) The stenosis was dilated with a 3.0mm Rocket™ balloon, which produced a local dissection (arrowhead).
(c) A 3.0mm, 18mm long GFX™ stent was deployed.
(d, e) This gave a good final result, and there were no further complications.

Coronary artery spasm

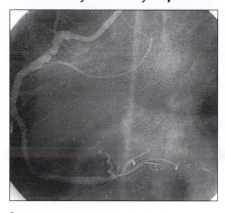

a

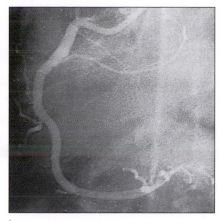

b

Figure 15.14
(a) A distal stenosis in this RCA had undergone successful PTCA, but spasm was apparent in the proximal third immediately after dilatation.
(b) This spasm settled rapidly after intracoronary glyceryl trinitrate.

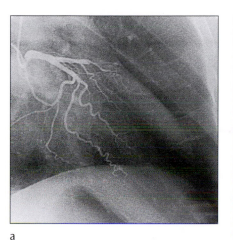

a

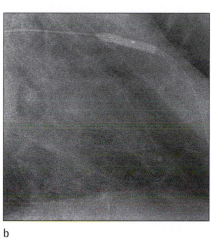

b

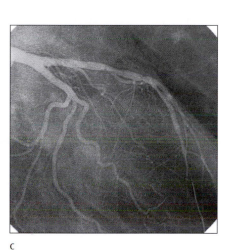

c

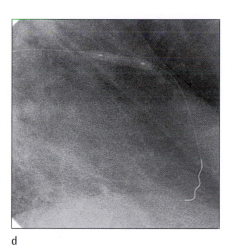

d

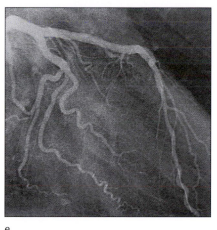

e

Figure 15.15
(a) The proximal LAD remains occluded in a 62-year-old man with anterior myocardial infarction despite treatment with rtPA and subsequently intracoronary streptokinase.
(b) The LAD was recanalized by PTCA with a 3.0mm Cheetah™ balloon over a 0.014-inch Floppy® guidewire.
(c) This revealed a significant underlying stenosis. Note the presence of spasm in the distal vessel immediately after reperfusion. This soon disappeared with improved flow and intracoronary glyceryl trinitrate.
(d) A 3.5mm, 15mm long Multilink™ stent was implanted at the site of residual stenosis.
(e) This produced an excellent result.

Spasm in gastroepiploic arterial grafts

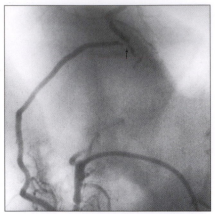

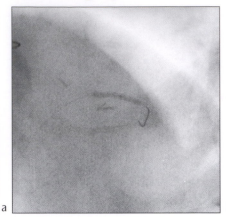

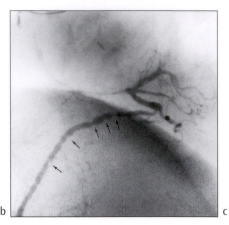

a

b

c

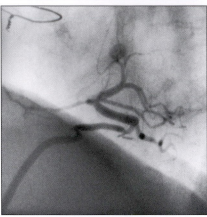

Figure 15.16

A 53-year-old man developed (a) an asymptomatic severe stenosis at the distal insertion of the gastroepiploic artery into the posterior descending branch of the RCA (arrow).

(b) A 2.5mm fixed-wire Orion™ balloon catheter (Cordis) was used via a 7F El Gamal guide catheter.

(c) Although the lesion site was satisfactorily dilated, diffuse segmental spasms with a 'string-of-beads' appearance occurred along the graft (arrows).

The spasm was relieved by 2mg of isosorbide dinitrate, which was given down the graft. In order to prevent such spasm, adequate amounts of calcium channel blockers or nitrates, or both, should be administered intravenously or directly into the graft before, during and after PTCA. Balloon-oversizing should be avoided.

(d) Result at 6 months.

d   **Courtesy of Dr N Komiyama, Department of Cardiovascular Medicine, Toranomon Hospital, Tokyo, Japan.**

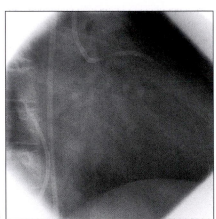

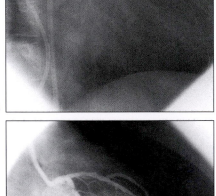

Acute coronary artery occlusion

a

b

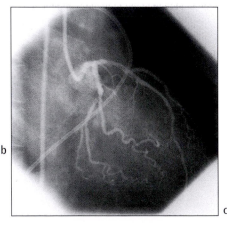

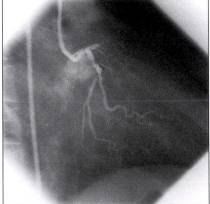

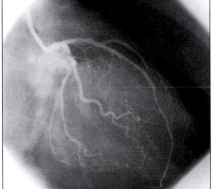

c

Figure 15.17

(a) Severe proximal LAD stenosis in a 47-year-old woman who presented with acute anterior myocardial infarction and was treated with intravenous streptokinase.

(b) PTCA produced a good result (c).

(d) However, 14 hours later an acute occlusion of the LAD occured.

d   e   (e) This was successfully redilated by PTCA.

Recurrent occlusion

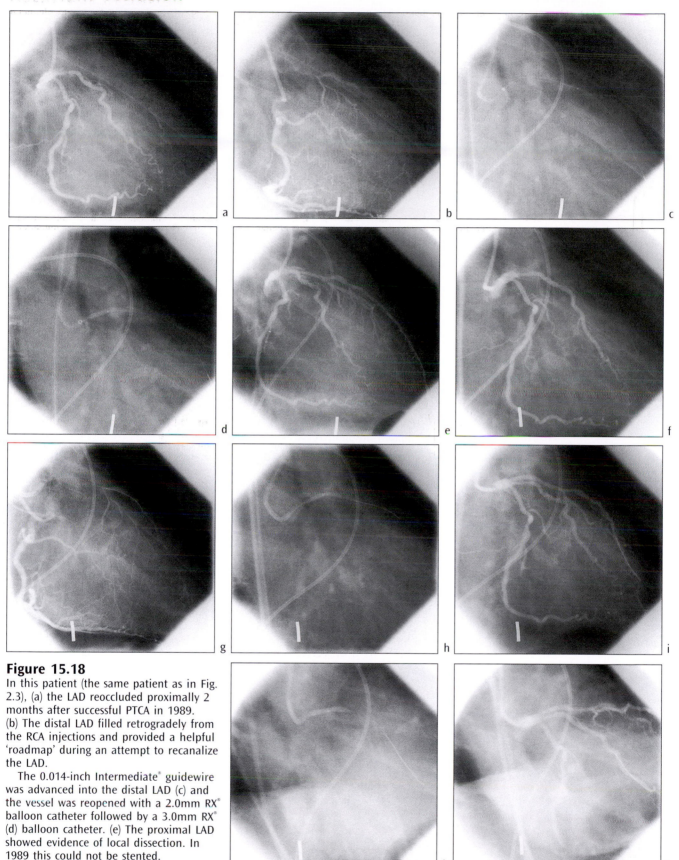

Figure 15.18

In this patient (the same patient as in Fig. 2.3), (a) the LAD reoccluded proximally 2 months after successful PTCA in 1989.

(b) The distal LAD filled retrogradely from the RCA injections and provided a helpful 'roadmap' during an attempt to recanalize the LAD.

The 0.014-inch Intermediate® guidewire was advanced into the distal LAD (c) and the vessel was reopened with a 2.0mm RX® balloon catheter followed by a 3.0mm RX® (d) balloon catheter. (e) The proximal LAD showed evidence of local dissection. In 1989 this could not be stented.

(f) Two months later, the proximal LAD reoccluded. (g) Once again, the distal LAD is visualized from the RCA. Once a 0.014-inch Intermediate® guidewire was advanced through the occlusion, a 2.5 RX® balloon followed by a 3.0RX® balloon (h) was used to reopen the LAD. A good angiographic result was achieved (i) and the stenosed intermediate artery was dilated with the 3.0mm RX® balloon (j) with an excellent final result (k).

Coronary artery thromboembolism

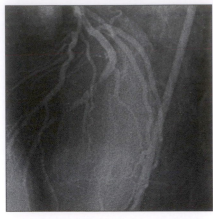

a

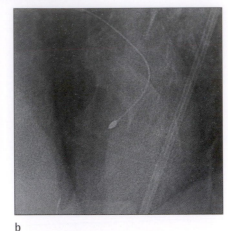

b

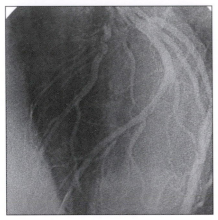

c

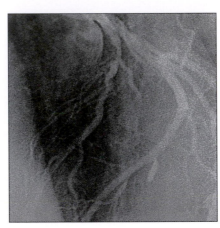

d

Figure 15.19
(a) This distal LCx has a complex, bulky, calcified stenosis.

Rotablator® atherectomy (b) resulted in improvement but with residual plaque/thrombus (c) at a side branch.

(d) Result after PTCA showed that the plaque/thrombus has embolized down and occluded the side branch, which could not be recanalized.

Two further examples of coronary artery thromboembolism after coronary intervention are shown in Fig. 5.6 and Fig. 13.43.

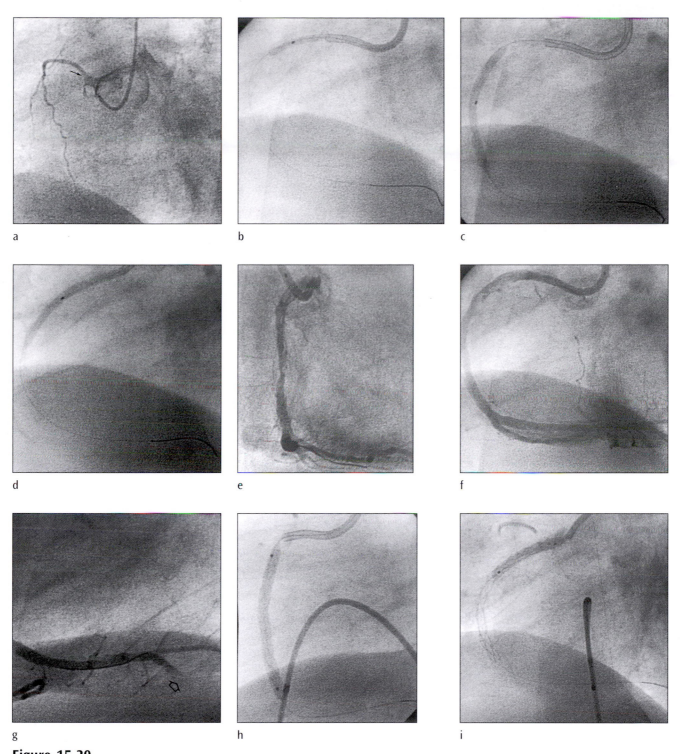

Figure 15.20

A 65-year-old retired teacher presented with a 2-week history of angina and was found to have small Q waves in leads II, III and aVF. (a) Coronary arteriography showed proximal occlusion of a dominant RCA. There was retrograde filling of the distal vessel from the normal left coronary artery.

(b) The lesion was crossed with a 0.014-inch Intermediate® guidewire and the RCA reopened with a 2.5mm Worldpass™ balloon. This revealed much thrombus within the vessel.

(c, d) The clot-filled vessel was dilated with a 3.0mm, 40mm long Elipse™ balloon.

(e, f) This dramatically improved flow; however, there was evidence of thrombus and dissection.

(g) Moreover, thrombus had embolized and occluded the posterior descending branch (open arrow).

The RCA was stented with a 3.5mm, 39mm long Microstent™ in the middle third (h) and with a 3.5mm, 24mm long Microstent™ in the proximal third (i).

continued

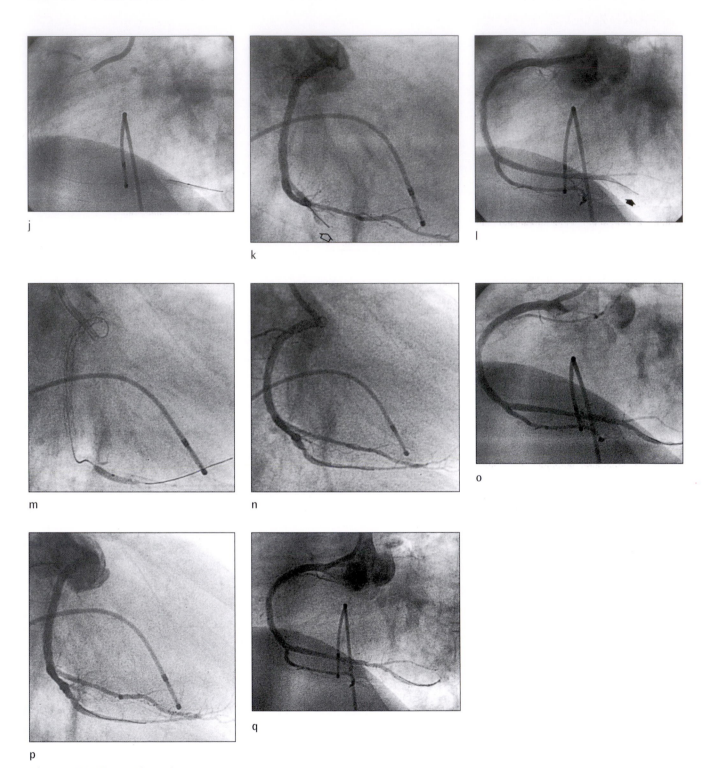

Figure 15.20 *continued*

Boluses of 5mg of rtPA were injected down the RCA at 10 minute intervals (total infusion – 25mg).

(j–m) The thrombus in the posterior descending branch was mechanically disrupted by PTCA with a 2.0mm Elipse™ balloon (arrow).

The final angiographic appearance was satisfactory and no thrombus was visible – (n, p) RAO projection; (o, q) LLAT projection. No rise in cardiac enzymes occurred.

Coronary artery perforation

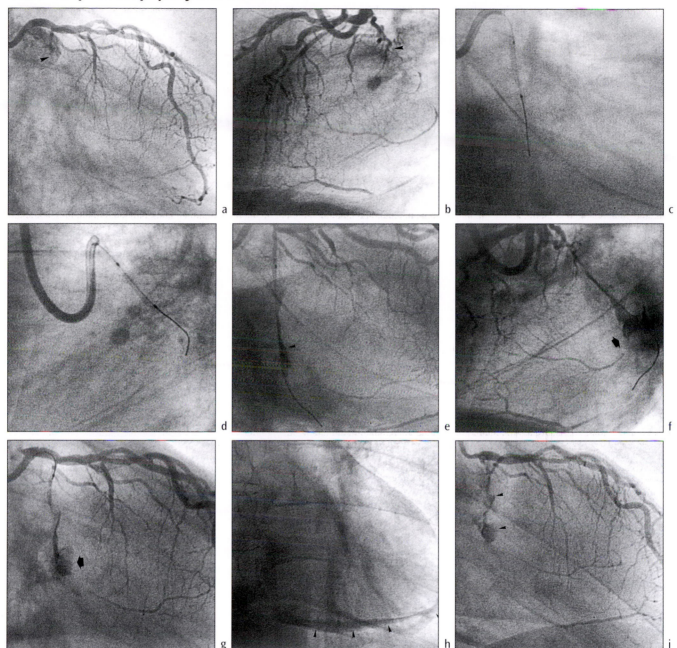

Figure 15.21

(a, b) A 56-year-old man with angina and significant three-vessel coronary artery disease had a proximal occlusion of the LCx (arrowhead), which was thought to be of more than 8 years' duration.

Some distal retrograde filling of two marginal branches was apparent, but the occlusion was estimated to be more than 7cm long. The strategy was to proceed to PTCA of the RCA and LAD at another session if the LCx procedure was successful.

The occlusion could not be crossed with a 0.014-inch Intermediate® guidewire, even with balloon support.

(c, d) A 0.014-inch Standard™ guidewire could be advanced distally fairly easily with balloon support, although the guidewire did not appear to be aligned exactly with the distal marginal as seen on the road map.

(e, f) After balloon dilatation in the proximal vessel, contrast injection showed more distal dissection and perforation of the coronary artery, (arrow) confirming that the guidewire had entered the pericardial space.

(g) With the guidewire and balloon withdrawn, the perforation was clearly significant (arrow).

At this point, there was little chance of ever entering the true lumen. Echocardiography showed a small amount of pericardial fluid, and (h) fluoroscopy also demonstrated contrast surrounding the heart (arrows).

However, the right atrial pressure remained at 3mmHg.

Heparinization was reversed with protamine sulphate and (i) the LCx reoccluded. Contrast extravasation is visible (arrows).

There were no signs of cardiac tamponade, although the patient complained of intermittent sharp precordial chest pain over the following 2 hours. The patient was referred for elective CABG surgery.

Complications after Rotablator® atherectomy
Coronary artery perforation

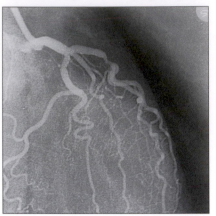

a

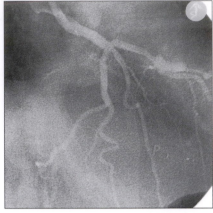

b

Figure 15.22

Significant stenosis between two bends in an LAD of a 63-year-old retired female teacher (a) was treated with a single 2.25mm Rotablator® burr. The procedure was associated with significant slowing of the burr, subsequent coronary artery spasm and progressive 'dilatation' of the lesion site (b). This LAD perforation was not associated with any haemodynamic instability or pain. The patient was sent for emergency CABG surgery when the roof of the LAD appeared to be absent under bruised epicardial fat. This is a rare occurrence after Rotablator® atherectomy and was almost certainly caused by oversizing the burr, not using a 'step-up' burr technique and allowing the rotational speed to slow.

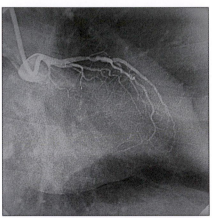

a

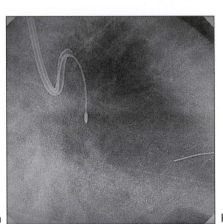

b

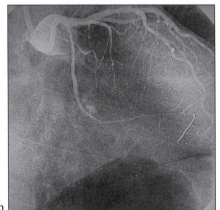

c

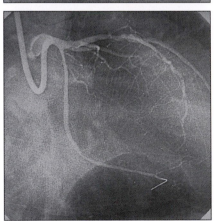

d

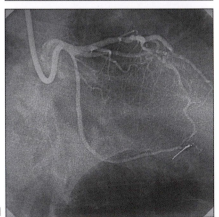

e

Figure 15.23

A 60-year-old insurance agent with angina had (a) a severe eccentric RCA stenosis and an occluded LCx.

The RCA stenosis was pre-dilated with a 3.0mm Express™ balloon and a 3.5mm, 25mm long Multilink™ was implanted with a good result.

An Amplatz guiding catheter was inserted into the LCx and a 0.014-inch Intermediate® guidewire was used to enter the distal LCx. However it proved impossible to cross the LCx with a 2.0mm Samba™ balloon.

(b) The guidewire was exchanged for a 0.009-inch Rotawire® and a 1.25mm Rotablator® burr used to create a channel along the occluded vessel.

A 1.75mm burr would not advance into the distal third of the vessel and caused sharp chest pain.

(c) Angiography showed a pin-point perforation.

(d) This perforation was sealed with a 2.5mm, 40mm long Elipse™ balloon along the length of the vessel.

(e) Final result.

Guidewire fracture

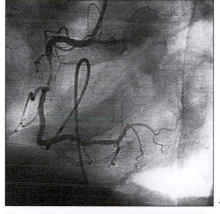

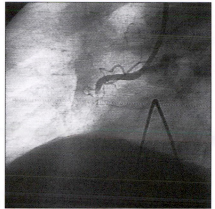

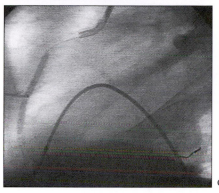

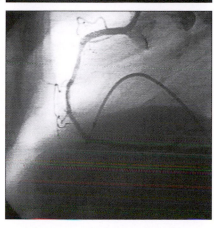

Figure 15.24

(a) Guidewire fracture, which is a rare complication of Rotablator® atherectomy, occurred during an attempt to ablate the long severe stenosis in an angulated RCA in a 72-year-old man with severe angina and obstructive airways disease. (b) The 1.5mm burr crossed the lesion but caused acute occlusion.

During an attempt to reopen the RCA by PTCA along the C-wire™, the balloon appeared to travel down a side branch and not down the main RCA. As the balloon catheter was withdrawn, it was not on the guidewire, which confirmed the diagnosis of guidewire fracture.

The situation was retrieved by crossing the occluded RCA with a 0.014-inch high-torque Floppy® guidewire and PTCA was performed using a 3.5mm, 30mm long Express™ balloon (c). The opaque distal segment of the fractured C-wire™ can be seen as well as the floppy guidewire.

(d) The final result was acceptable. The patient was treated with warfarin for 3 months and there were no sequelae.

Side branch occlusion

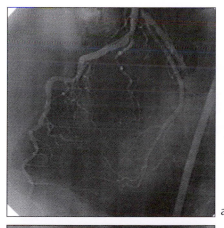

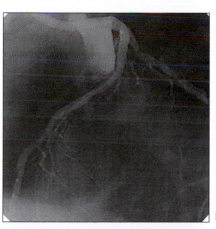

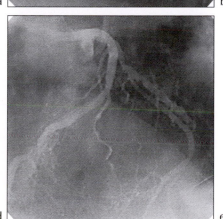

Figure 15.25

(a) This severe calcific stenosis in the mid-LAD at its bifurcation with the DG involved the ostium of the branch. (b) The DG occluded after Rotablator® atherectomy of the LAD stenosis with a 1.5mm burr and a 2.0mm burr followed by PTCA. (c, d) The DG was easily entered with a guidewire and, after PTCA had been performed to the LAD with a 3.0mm balloon, simultaneous inflations were performed with a 2.5mm balloon catheter (in the DG) and a 3.0mm (in the LAD) balloon catheter ('kissing-balloon' technique). (e) Result after PTCA.

Complications after DCA

Occlusive dissection

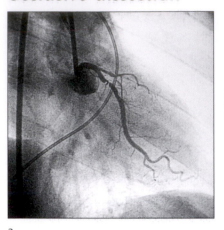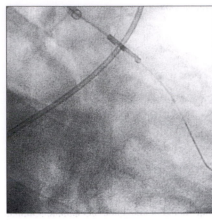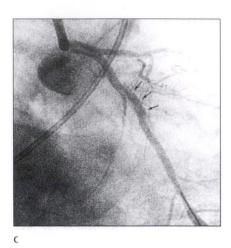

a   b   c

Figure 15.26
This DCA procedure was performed in 1991 with a SCA-1® device in a 63-year-old man with moderate angina. The LCx had a severe eccentric stenosis (a), which was not pre-dilated before crossing with the device (b).
(c) This caused a traumatic dissection. The patient underwent successful urgent CABG surgery in this pre-stent period.

Guiding catheter dissection

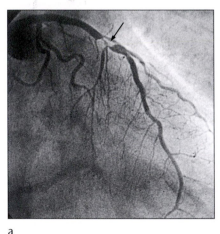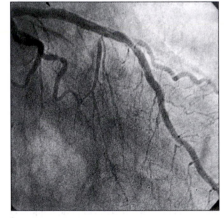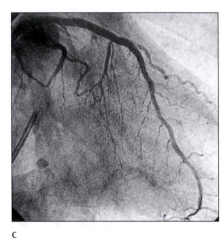

a   b   c

Figure 15.27
DCA demands the use of large guide catheters. Until recently, only the stiff DVI® guide catheters were able to offer sufficient support to deliver the Atherocath® into the coronary artery.

A 69-year-old retired telephone engineer with moderate angina, hypertension and hypercholesterolemia had (a) a severe bulky stenosis in the middle third of the LAD and a less severe stenosis just beyond this.

The lesion was crossed with a 0.014-inch Floppy® guidewire via a 10F FL5 Medtronic guide catheter. A 7F Bantam Atherocath™ was used to remove nine pieces of atheromatous tissue from the proximal lesion, and both lesions were adjunctively dilated with a 3.0mm, 30mm long Elipse™ balloon. The lesions were stented with a 3.0mm, 25mm Multilink™ stent.

(b) There appeared to be a small dissection proximally (arrowhead) as a result of deep engagement of the guide catheter tip in order to deliver the Atherocath® from this dilated and unfolded ascending aorta.

A 3.5mm, 25mm long Multilink™ stent was therefore placed in the proximal LAD to overlap the first stent and then the junction was post-dilated with the 3.5mm, 30mm balloon.

(c) This gave an excellent final result.

Complications after coronary stenting
Acute occlusion

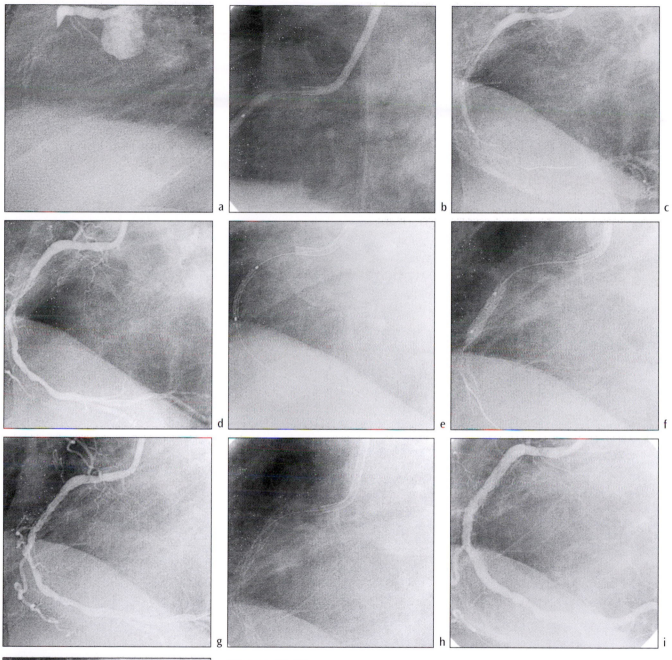

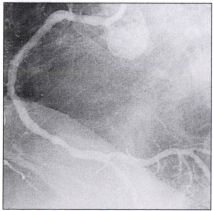

Figure 15.28

This RCA received a 3.5mm Microstent II™ to its middle third following dissection after PTCA. Thirty-six hours later, severe chest pain in the patient was associated with inferior ST-segment elevation on the ECG. (a) Repeat angiography showed acute thrombotic occlusion of the stent.

(b–d) Flow was re-established by PTCA and intracoronary rtPA but with a suboptimal result.

A further 3.0mm Microstent II™ was implanted over an apparent dissection (e, f) and a 3.5mm Microstent II™ was placed more distally over a further dissected segment (g, h).

(i, j) The final result was reasonably satisfactory.

It is important to ensure that the separate stents overlap and that no 'gaps' are left unstented in such difficult situations. Long stents should be preferred whenever possible.

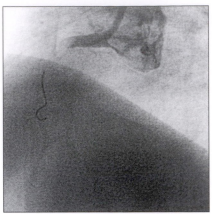

a

Figure 15.29

A 60-year-old man with unstable angina and an occluded LAD had a severe RCA stenosis dilated by PTCA. A dissection was treated successfully by a 32mm long NIR™ stent on a 3.5mm balloon. Two weeks later he developed severe chest pain caused by stent thrombosis (a), which was associated with extensive inferolateral ST-segment elevation and hypotension.

It proved impossible to reach the distal RCA through the central lumen of the stent and cardiac arrest occurred in the catheter laboratory. Full cardiopulmonary resuscitation was required until the patient was placed on bypass and underwent emergency CABG surgery. The patient survived without complication. Such a case should probably be regarded as a contraindication to PTCA even in this era of stents.

Courtesy of Dr J Morris, Cardiothoracic Centre, Liverpool, UK.

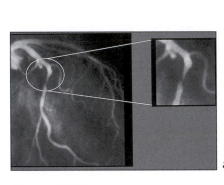

a

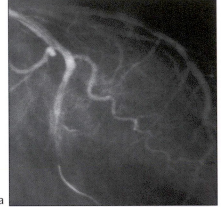

b

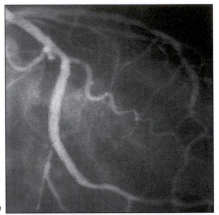

c

Figure 15.30

A 55-year-old woman who had severe unstable angina underwent coronary arteriography via the left brachial approach and was found to have (a) a severe stenosis in the mid-LCx.

PTCA was performed with a 3.0mm, 30mm long Bandit™ balloon up to 12 atmospheres.

(b) This caused severe dissection of the LCx.

(c) A 3.0mm, 39mm long Microstent™ was deployed with an excellent angiographic result. The patient received aspirin, ticlopidine and heparin.

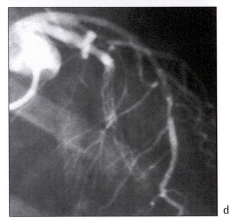

d

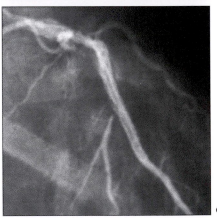

e

Four hours later, the patient's left arm was noted to be cold, cyanotic and pulseless and emergency embolectomy was organized. On the way to the operating room, the patient developed severe chest pain, with ST-segment elevation in leads V1-V4 that was consistent with anterior myocardial infarction. The patient was returned to the catheter laboratory.

(d) Angiography revealed total occlusion of the recently stented LCx artery.

Intravenous abciximab was administered according to standard protocols.

(e) The occlusion was crossed with a guidewire and flow adequately restored after PTCA with the 3.0mm balloon up to 18 atmospheres.

During the procedure, the patient's left arm reperfused spontaneously, with resolution of the cyanosis and return of pulses. The patient received a 12-hour infusion of abciximab and her recovery was uneventful. Creatine phosphokinase values were not elevated. Lysis and potential disaggregation of arterial thrombi after intracoronary abciximab have been described previously.

Courtesy of Drs NAF Chronos, ME Leimbach, SB King III and DC Morris, Andreas Gruentzig Cardiovascular Center, Emory University Hospital, Atlanta, Georgia, USA.

Coronary artery dissection
PTCA through the side wall of a stent for stent jail

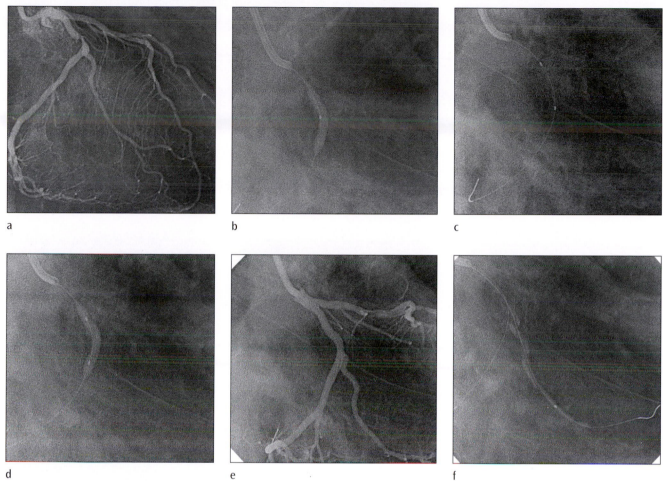

a b c

d e f

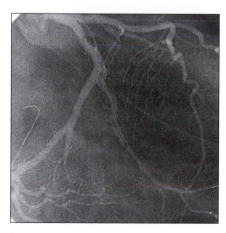

g

Figure 15.31

A 69-year-old insulin-dependent diabetic woman had (a) a second restenosis in this LCx, just above the origin of the first OMCx (RAO projection). The two previous procedures included PTCA and Rotablator® atherectomy.

After pre-dilatation with a 3.5mm Elipse™ balloon (b), elective coronary stent implantation using a 3.5mm, 18mm long Multilink™ stent produced a perfect angiographic result (c–e) (LAO projections).

Four hours later, however, acute chest pain was associated with inferolateral ST-segment elevation and subtotal occlusion of the obtuse marginal by a local dissection.

(f) The vessel was reopened by PTCA through the stent struts.

(g) The spiral dissection that was produced did not impair antegrade flow (RAO projection).

Stents advanced through a stent

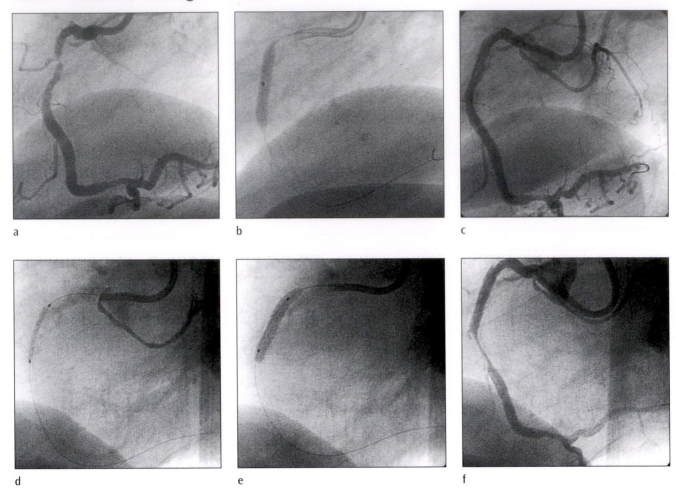

Figure 15.32

A 63-year-old lady had (a) a severe stenosis in the proximal third of a large, dominant and tortuous RCA. There was a less severe stenosis at the crux.

(b) PTCA was performed with a 3.5mm Passage™ balloon.

(c) This produced lesion rupture at 7.5 atmospheres and an improved result with local dissection.

However deployment of a 3.5mm, 18mm long GFX™ stent at 10 atmospheres (d, e) produced extensive dissection towards the crux of the RCA (f, g).

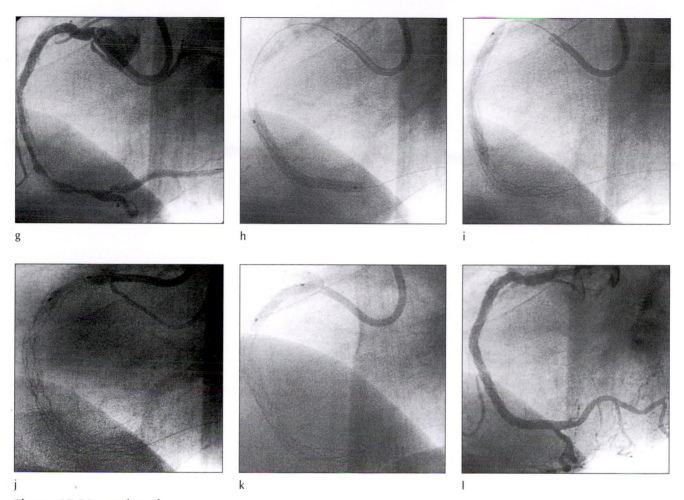

g

h

i

j

k

l

Figure 15.32 *continued*

(h) The situation was rescued by passing a 3.5mm, 39mm long Microstent™ through the first stent and deploying it distally at the crux (h).

The balloon was used to dilate the two stents and the RCA between them (i) before a third Microstent™ (3.5mm, 18mm long) was placed between the first two stents. A 3.5mm, 12mm long Microstent™ was then placed proximal to the first stent (j, k).

(l) This produced a satisfactory final result.

Altogether, 87mm of stent was deployed in this rescue procedure but emergency CABG surgery was avoided.

Multiple short stents deployed in series

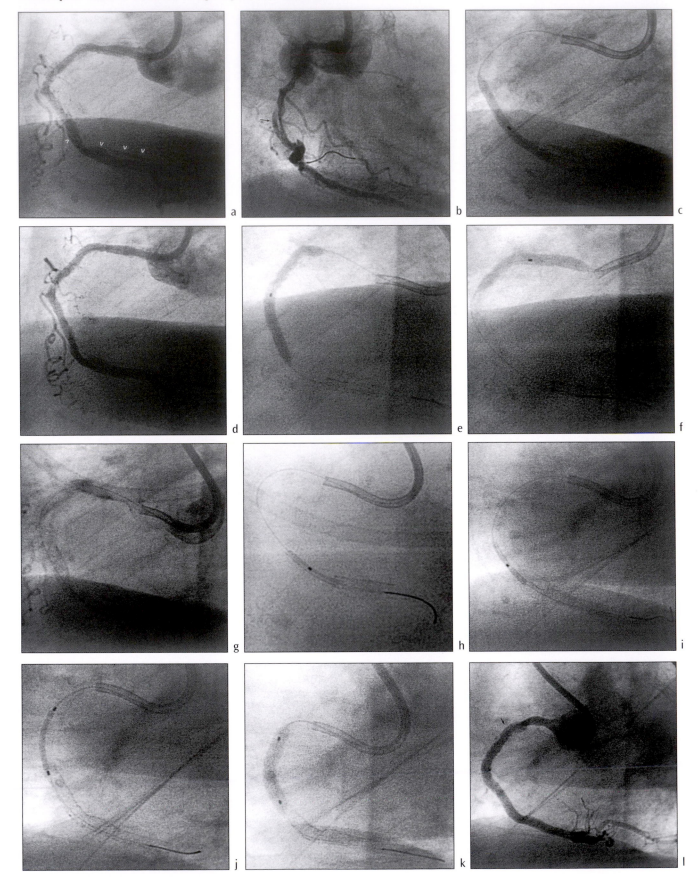

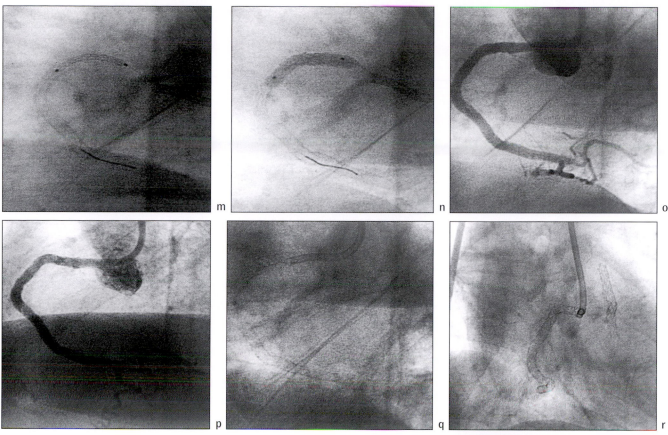

Figure 15.33

When extensive coronary artery dissection in a severely diseased or tortuous vessel prevents delivery of a long stent, the problem can be overcome by delivery of multiple short and flexible stents, as in this case, but the cost of the procedure is significantly increased.

This female patient had previously undergone PTCA to the LCx, which had necessitated stenting because of dissection.

(a, b) PTCA and implantation of a 3.0mm, 15mm long Paragon™ stent to a severe lesion above the crux of the RCA caused extensive retrograde dissection and much contrast extravasation (arrows and arrowheads).

(c) A 32mm long NIR™ stent would not advance beyond the proximal bend in the RCA even after pre-dilatation with a 3.5mm, 30mm long balloon.

(d) The appearance was still unsatisfactory.

After further dilatations along its length with the long balloon (e, f), local dissection resulted in dye extravasation (g).

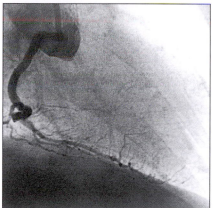

(h, i) Two 3.0mm, 16mm long Crossflex™ stents were easily delivered in turn (in series and overlapping), with the first Crossflex stent overlapping the distal Paragon stent.

(j, k) A second 3.0mm, 16mm long Paragon™ stent was then implanted more proximally.

(l) However, there was residual dissection proximally (arrow).

(m, n) Therefore, a 3.0mm, 24mm long GFX™ stent was implanted most proximally.

(o, p) The final result was satisfactory. There were no further complications.

(q, r) The five stents placed in the vessel can be clearly seen on fluoroscopy as giving the typical 'metal artery' appearance.

(s) The RAO view shows that the dissection has been adequately sealed.

Courtesy of Dr JL Morris, Cardiothoracic Centre, Liverpool, UK.

Temporary occlusion of a side branch after stenting

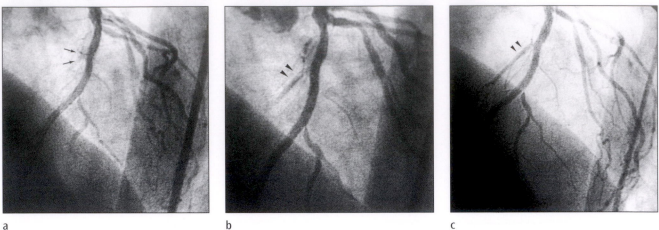

a   b   c

Figure 15.34

A 46-year-old banker (the same patient as in Fig. 10.51) who had extensive LAD disease had multiple stents placed along its length. (a) One of the stents covered and temporarily occluded a septal branch (arrows), which itself had an ostial stenosis. (b, c) Ten minutes after intracoronary glyceryl trinitrate, the septal branch slowly reappeared.

It proved impossible to enter this septal branch (before or after stent deployment) because of a 'Z' bend tortuosity beginning at its origin.

Stent jail of side-branch ostial lesion: escape using Rotablator®-assisted PTCA

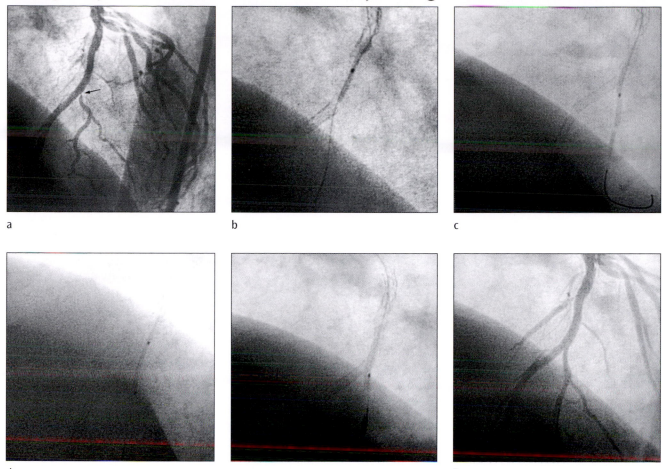

a   b   c

d   e   f

Figure 15.35

The 46-year-old man discussed in Fig. 15.34 had persisting angina 2 weeks after multiple stents were implanted in series in the LAD. The distal Paragon™ stent covered the diagonal branch, which had a severe ostial stenosis. It was felt that the branch was not large enough to give rise to troublesome angina.

(a) At repeat angiography, the stents appeared satisfactory but the ostial diagonal lesion remained severe.

(b) A 1.5mm Worldpass™ and 1.5mm Rocket™ balloon would not pass and clearly inflated above the lesion.

The 0.014-inch Floppy® guidewire was exchanged for a 0.009-inch Rotawire™ using a Transit™ catheter (Cordis) placed up to the ostium. A 1.25mm Rotablator® would not pass the obstructed ostium either.

(c) However, after six failed passes, the 1.5mm Worldpass™ balloon crossed the lesion.

(d) The balloon ruptured at 3 atmospheres, as did the double-marker Rocket™ balloon. It appeared that the balloon had been cut in half by a sharpened strut.

(e) A 2.5mm Cruiser® II balloon was inflated to 6 atmospheres without rupture.

(f) This gave a good result. This procedure was successful in relieving the patient's angina.

Occlusion of a side branch after stenting

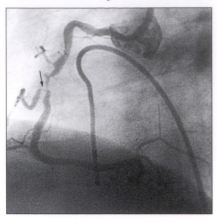

a

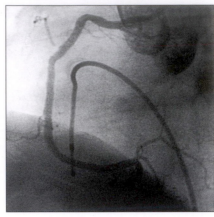

b

Figure 15.36
(a) This dominant RCA has a severe, complex lesion in its proximal third, from which exits a right ventricular branch with ostial disease (arrow).
(b) After PTCA with a 3.0mm balloon, the flow in the side-branch became impaired and the vessel became occluded immediately after stenting with a 3.5mm, 15mm long Multilink™ stent.

No attempt was made to recanalize this side-branch and there were no clinical sequelae and no rise in cardiac enzymes.

Side-branch 'jailing' after stenting seems to be more common with tubular stents than with coil stents. Periprocedural complications are uncommon if jailed side branches are left untreated when the flow appears to be unobstructed.

Coronary artery perforation

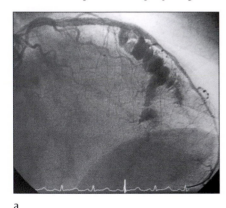

a

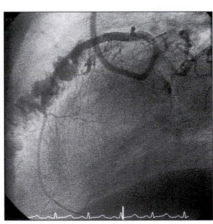

b

Figure 15.37
A 60-year-old woman underwent PTCA to a long segment of diffuse disease in the proximal LAD with a 3.0mm Adante™ balloon. The lesion was then stented with a 3.0mm, 23mm long Multilink Duet™ stent and a 3.0mm, 32mm long NIRoyal™ stent in series. After post-dilatation with a 3.5mm, 12mm long Seajet® balloon, the patient experienced sudden chest pain as a result of rupture of the coronary artery.
(a, b) Much contrast extravasation occurred into the pericardium.

This resulted in cardiac tamponade and hypotension. Despite the insertion of a pericardial drain, the patient required emergency CABG surgery, which had a successful outcome. Rupture of the LAD in this case was almost certainly due to oversizing of the stent by too large a balloon at too high a pressure.
Courtesy of an anonymous colleague!

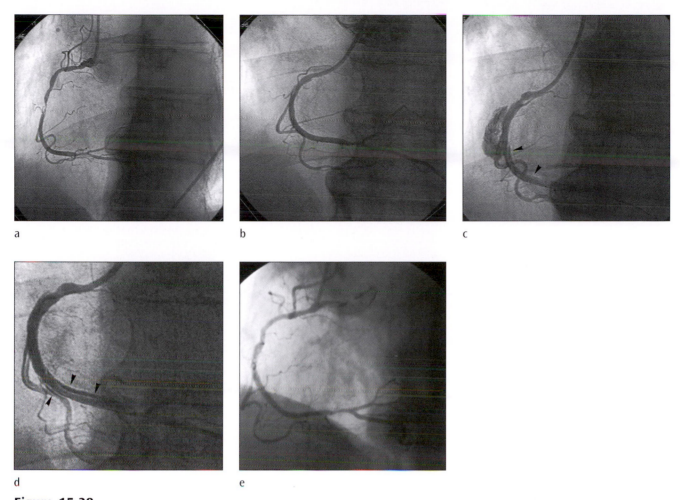

a   b   c

d   e

Figure 15.38

A 78-year-old man with angina had (a) a significant stenosis in the middle third of the RCA.

A 6F guiding catheter was used and a 0.014-inch Floppy ExtraSupport™ guidewire crossed the stenosis.

A 3.0mm Bonnie™ balloon (Schneider) was used to dilate the lesion at 8 atmospheres.

(b) This produced a local dissection. Prolonged inflations were made but the dissection persisted.

A 3.5mm, 12mm long Microstent™ was therefore implanted.

(c) After stent deployment, a type III coronary rupture occurred with extravasation of contrast into the pericardium. The patient complained of chest pain and ST-segment elevation appeared. The systolic blood pressure fell to 60mm Hg. A prolonged balloon inflation for 5 minutes sealed the perforation, but a long dissection extended (arrowheads) down the entire length of the RCA.

However, the patient's blood pressure and chest pain improved.

A second NIR™ stent (3.5mm, 16mm long) was inserted distal to the first stent. (d) After multiple inflations proximal and distal to the two stents, the appearance of the perforation was improved, but the posterior right ventricular branch was occluded at the end of the procedure and a long dissection persisted (arrowheads).

Abciximab was administered in an attempt to aid recanalization of the posterior right ventricular branch. The outcome was uneventful and the patient was discharged 2 days later.

(e) At 1 year, the appearance of the RCA was satisfactory.

This case illustrates the way in which long dissections can heal adequately with conservative treatment as long as the dissection is not flow-limiting. A covered stent may be useful for treating coronary artery perforation.

Courtesy of Drs JJ Goy, P Urban and E Eeckhout, University Hospital, Lausanne, Switzerland. Published in Stent 1998;4:141-2.

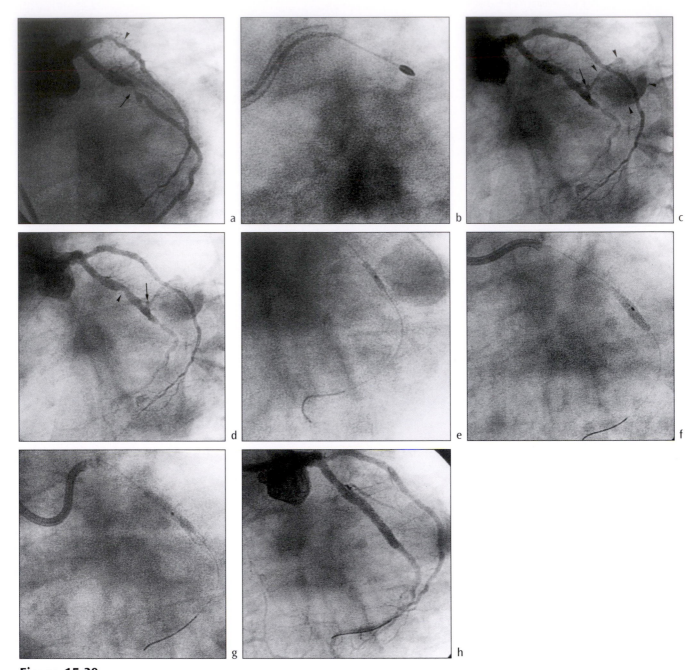

Figure 15.39
The patient in this case had uncontrolled angina 8 years after CABG surgery.
   (a) The LCx (arrow) and the intermediate (arrowhead) artery had undilatable, calcified stenoses.
   The intermediate artery was successfully treated by Rotablator® atherectomy and stent implantation (see c).
   However, after Rotablator® atherectomy to the LCx lesion (b), a 3.5mm, 15mm long Multilink™ stent was implanted.
   On stent deployment, the vessel perforated at the distal end of the stent on a bend point in the artery.
   (c) A false aneurysm is outlined by contrast (arrowheads) and the perforation point is easily visible (arrow).
   (d) After high-pressure dilatation of the lesion within the stent (arrowhead) was carried out, a 12mm JoStent® PTFE-Covered Stent Graft was deployed initially at the perforation point (e, f). However, since the flow into the false aneurysm persisted, a further 9mm JoStent® PTFE-Covered Stent Graft was then placed between the two stents (g).
   (h) This obliterated flow into the false aneurysm.
   Angiography at 6 weeks showed that the aneurysm was closed.

In-stent restenosis

In-stent restenosis occurs in at least 15% of patients and, depending on lesion and patient factors, this figure may be much higher. If it occurs in its diffuse form, the use of balloon redilatation may result in 're-restenosis' rates of 80%.

Treatment by PTCA

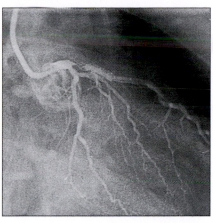
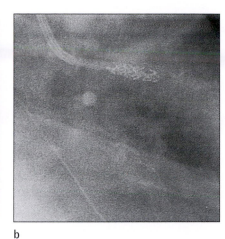
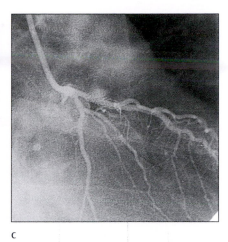

a   b   c

Figure 15.40
A 44-year-old patient developed severe angina and (a) restenosis proximal to and within a 3.5mm Wiktor® stent placed in the proximal LAD 4 months after it had been implanted.
(b) The lesion was redilated by a 3.0mm Samba™ balloon.
(c) A satisfactory result was obtained.

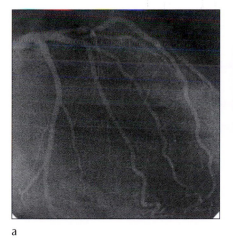
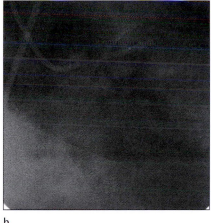
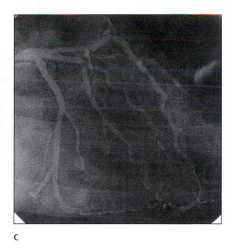

a   b   c

Figure 15.41
A 57-year-old man presented with severe unstable angina 3 months after DCA and Palmaz-Schatz™ stent implantation to the proximal LAD. (a) Angiography showed a stenosis of more than 50% within the stent and a tight concentric stenosis beyond the stent at the origin of the septal perforating artery.
(b) PTCA was performed with a 3.0mm Passage® balloon at 9 atmospheres.
(c) This gave a good angiographic result.

   The assessment of restenosis is easier in the non-radio-opaque Palmaz-Schatz™ stent than in a densely radio-opaque stent such as the Wiktor® stent. However, the latter is more flexible and, being radio-opaque, it is easier to position during deployment.

Treatment by rotational atherectomy

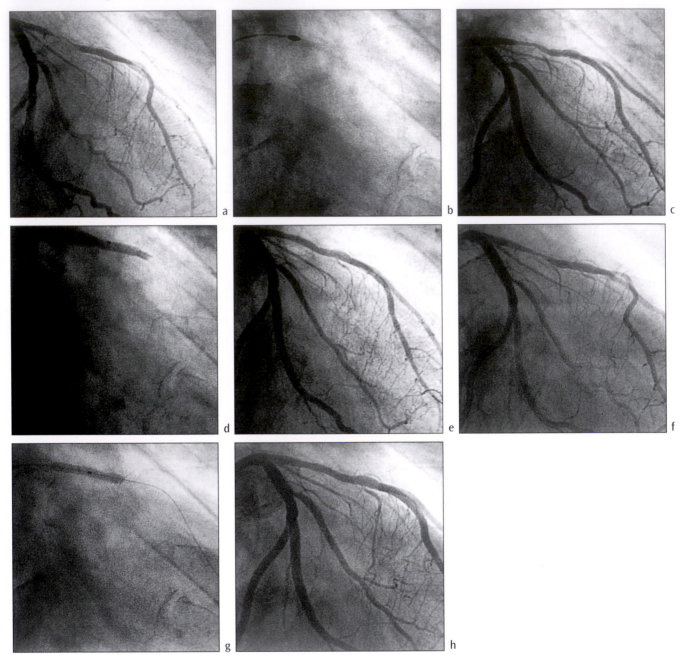

Figure 15.42

A 73-year-old man developed recurrent angina 5 months after Rotablator® atherectomy had been performed for restenosis inside a Multilink™ stent in the proximal LAD. (a) A second restenosis was found at angiography.

(b) The lesion was treated again with a 1.75mm followed by a 2.25mm burr.

(c) This produced some improvement.

(d) Adjunctive PTCA with a 3.0mm Bonnie™ balloon was performed.

(e) A satisfactory angiographic and clinical result was obtained.

  Five months later, the patient's exercise stress test showed ST-segment depression of 2.0mm in lead V6 after 7 minutes of the Bruce protocol, with mild angina.

(f) Repeat angiography showed a third intrastent restenosis, although this was not as severe as previously.

(g) It was treated successfully by PTCA with a 3.5mm LOGO™ balloon (JoMed).

(h) This gave an excellent final result without further restenosis.

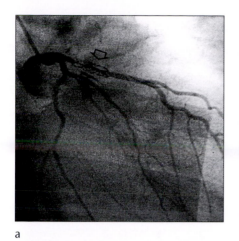

a

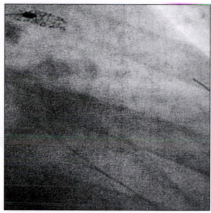

b

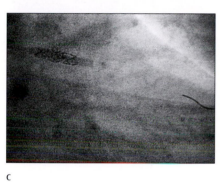

c

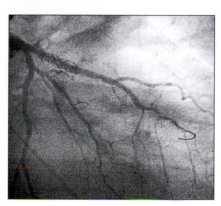

d

Figure 15.43
A 45-year-old man (the same patient as in Figs 7.23 and 15.48) developed (a) a third restenosis inside a 3.5mm Wiktor® stent in the LAD.
(b) The lesion was ablated with a 1.75mm and a 2.25mm Rotablator® burr.
(c) It was then dilated with a 3.5mm Elipse™ balloon.
(d) Final result.

The ARTIST randomized trial (in Europe) and the ROSTER randomized trial (in the USA) examined whether Rotablator® atherectomy was better than PTCA for treating in-stent restenosis. In the ROSTER trial, rotational atherectomy resulted in a lower incidence of stent use and lower clinical restenosis compared to PTCA. Results from the ARTIST trial were less encouraging.

Treatment by PTCA and stenting

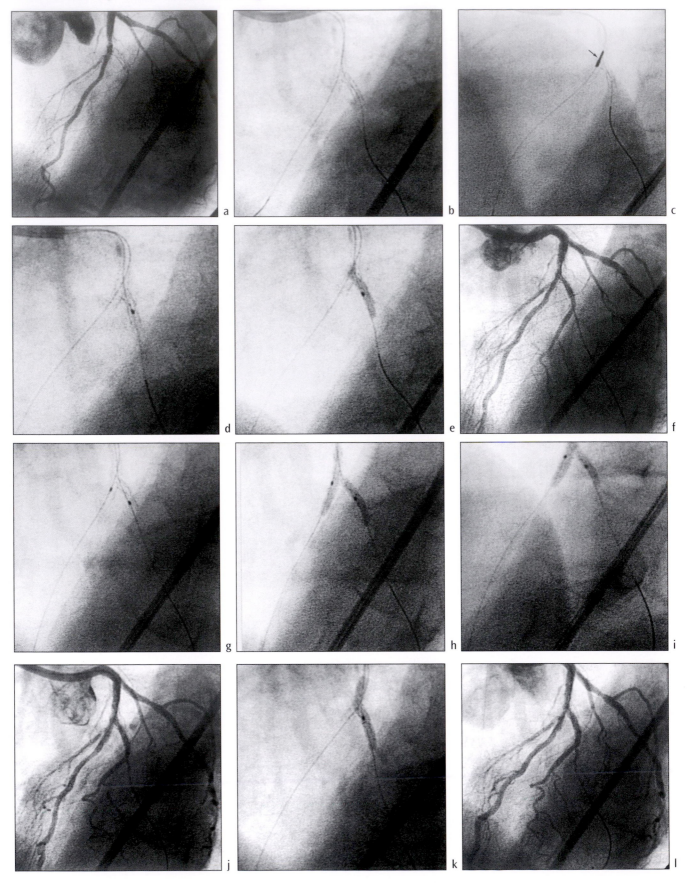

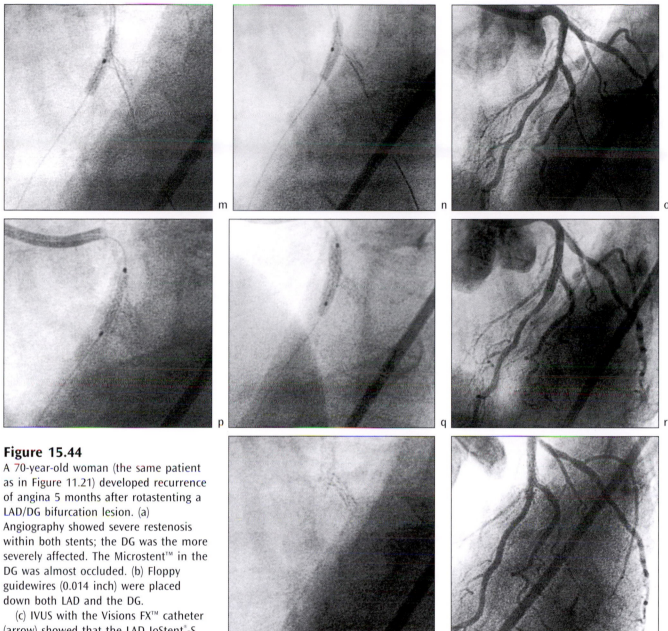

Figure 15.44
A 70-year-old woman (the same patient as in Figure 11.21) developed recurrence of angina 5 months after rotastenting a LAD/DG bifurcation lesion. (a) Angiography showed severe restenosis within both stents; the DG was the more severely affected. The Microstent™ in the DG was almost occluded. (b) Floppy guidewires (0.014 inch) were placed down both LAD and the DG.

(c) IVUS with the Visions FX™ catheter (arrow) showed that the LAD JoStent®-S side-branch stent also had dense in-stent restenosis.

(d, e) The stent in the DG was first dilated with a 2.0mm Worldpass balloon and then a 2.5mm Cruiser II balloon.

(f) Result.

(g–i) The LAD was dilated with a 3.0mm balloon and the 'kissing balloon' technique was applied to the bifurcation (a 3.0mm balloon in the LAD at 9 atmospheres and a 2.0mm balloon in the DG at 11 atmospheres).

(j) Result.

(k) A 3.0mm balloon is then placed through the side wall of the LAD stent and dilated across the ostium of the DG.

(l) Result.

(m, n) The LAD was then further dilated.

(o) The result was inadequate.

(p, q) The LAD was therefore stented with a 3.0mm, 18mm long Microstent™ placed inside the JoMed stent.

(r) This gave a good final angiographic result.

(s) The bifurcation stents are moderately radio-opaque.

(t) The angiographic result 6 months later, when the patient was asymptomatic.

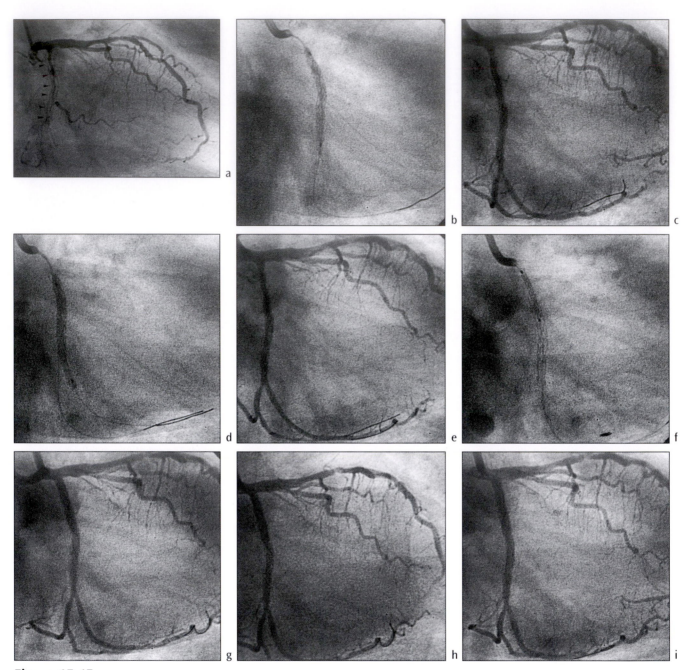

Figure 15.45

A 56-year-old female general practitioner (the same patient as in Fig. 11.5) developed (a) severe restenosis (arrows) within a 3.0mm, 39mm long Microstent™ that had been implanted 4 months earlier into the LCx. The vessel was virtually occluded.
(b) The long lesion was dilated with a 3.0mm, 36mm long Viva Primo™ balloon.
(c) This gave a good result.
(d) The severe stenoses at the distal bifurcation point were dilated with the distal end of the balloon after repositioning the guidewire tip.
(e) This gave significant improvement.
(f) A 3.0mm, 18mm long Microstent™ was implanted at the proximal end of the stent.
(g) This produced an excellent result.
(h, i) A 3.0mm Passage® balloon was finally used to dilate both the ostia of the PLCx and OMCx branches in turn.
  The LAD and the RCA appeared unchanged.

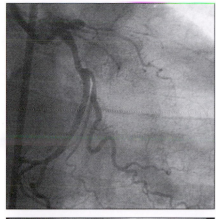

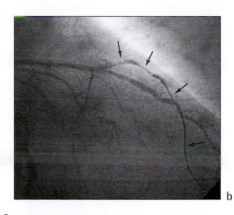

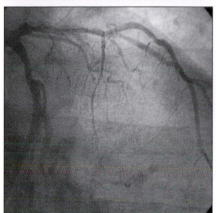

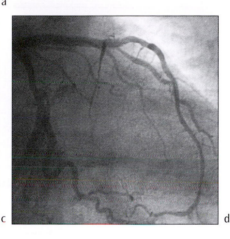

a

b

c

d

Figure 15.46
A 48-year-old airline technician presented with recurrent angina 6 months after a 3.0mm, 18mm long GFX™ stent had been placed in the proximal LAD. (a) Angiography showed that the LAD was totally occluded just proximal to the stent as a result of dense restenotic tissue within the stent. (b) It was possible to cross the occlusion with a 0.014-inch Intermediate® guidewire and reopen the vessel with a 2.0mm Adante™ and then a 3.0mm Freeway™ balloon. The distal LAD initially appeared thin, owing to spasm along the length of the vessel (arrows), which is not infrequent in this situation.

After intracoronary glyceryl trinitrate, the mid- and distal LAD opened satisfactorily (c).

A 3.5mm, 28mm long Multilink Duet™ stent was then deployed along the long segment of disease, both within and beyond the implanted stent, and a 3.5mm, 13mm long Multilink Duet™ stent was deployed more proximally, almost extending back to the ostium.

(d) The result was excellent.

Treatment by cutting balloon

Figure 15.47
A 52-year-old journalist developed recurrence of angina as a result of recurrent in-stent restenosis. The LAD had been stented with a 3.0mm, 30mm long AVE GFX stent 13 months earlier. In-stent restenosis had occurred at 3 months, and this had been treated successfully by rotational atherectomy as

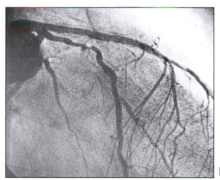

a

b

part of the ARTIST trial. Four months later, a recurrence of angina was caused by virtual occlusion of the stent from further in-stent restenosis. This was treated by PTCA using a 3.25mm, 10mm long Cutting Balloon™.

However, 6 months later angina recurred. (a) The angiogram showed mild diffuse in-stent restenosis with a more focal severe stenosis as shown (arrow).

The lesion was crossed with a 0.014-inch Floppy® guidewire and dilated with a 3.25mm Barath™ Cutting Balloon™. The rest of the stented segment was similarly dilated with the same balloon.

(b) The final result was excellent.

Although these techniques may well reduce the rate of 're-restenosis' inside the stent (to 30-40%), the recurrence rate is still high and has significant cost implications. Attention has therefore turned to preventing in-stent restenosis by:
* *radiation delivered either endovascularly or on the stent itself;*
* *the incorporation of drugs on to the stent itself which will inhibit the biological reaction of the smooth muscle cells to PTCA and stenting; or*
* *the development of an inert or non-reactive stent.*

Plaque prolapse through stent struts of a coil stent

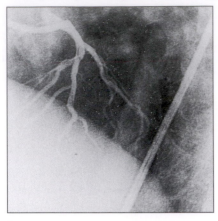

a

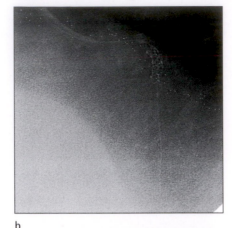

b

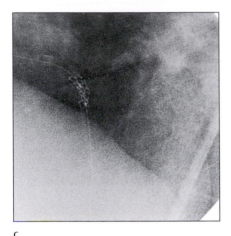

c

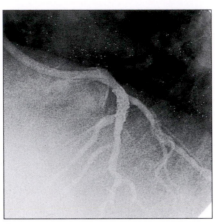

d

Figure 15.48
After DCA and adjunctive PTCA to a proximal LAD lesion (a) in this patient (the same patient as in Figs 7.23 and 15.43), a loose flap dissection was evident.
(b) A Wiktor® stent was implanted but the flap appeared to prolapse through the splayed coils of the stent.
(c) A Microstent II™ was placed inside the Wiktor® stent with a satisfactory result (d).

Coil stent disruption

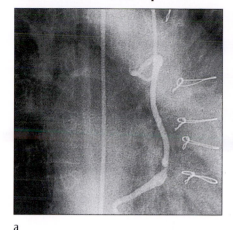

a

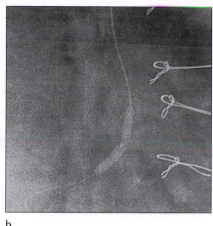

b

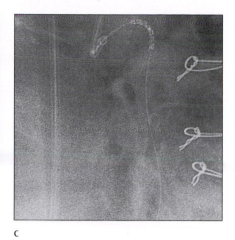

c

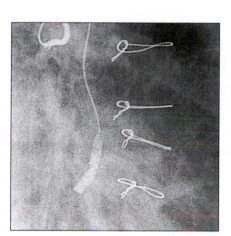

d

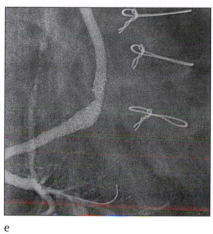

e

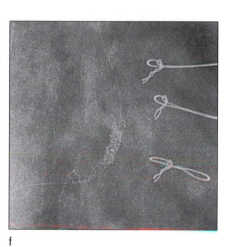

f

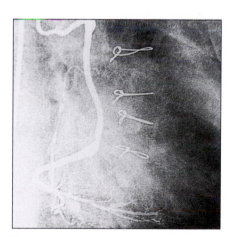

g

Figure 15.49

(a) A severe, eccentric stenosis in the distal body of a 10-year-old RCA SVG in a 72-year-old man with severe angina.

(b) PTCA with a 3.5mm Gold Ex™ balloon showed a hard stenosis that indented the balloon at 12 atmospheres.

(c) A 4.0mm Wiktor® stent was chosen because of its flexibility around sharp bends.

(d) This stent was deployed at the lesion site.

(e) However, a persistent eccentric defect was still visible despite a high inflation pressure.

(f) A 10mm long Finale™ balloon was inflated at 20 atmospheres to the 'defect'; this produced disruption or unravelling of the distal stent.

(g) Final result with residual eccentric stenosis.

This patient also had an LCx SVG stented at the same procedure with a 3.5mm Wiktor® stent and he was rendered asymptomatic.

PTCA through side wall of stent for side-branch ostial restenosis

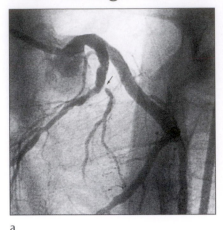 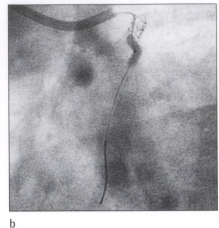 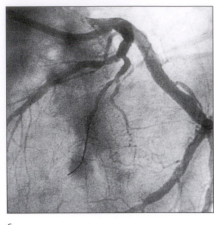

a   b   c

Figure 15.50

A 57-year-old man had undergone multivessel PTCA and stenting 5 months earlier. The proximally occluded LAD had been reopened by PTCA and stented with a 3.5mm, 18mm long Microstent™ proximally overlapping a 3.0mm, 25mm long Multilink™ stent that was placed over and beyond a DG. The DG had had a stenosis in its middle third, which had been dilated and stented with a 2.5mm, 9mm long NIR™ stent before LAD stent deployment.

Angina recurred 5 months after the initial procedure. (a) Although there was some in-stent restenosis in the Multilink™ stent, a severe stenosis was evident at the ostium of the DG (arrow).

(b) This was crossed with a 0.014-inch Floppy® guidewire and dilated with a 2.0mm and then a 2.5mm Worldpass balloon.

The final result (c) resulted in the abolition of symptoms.

Failure to deliver a stent

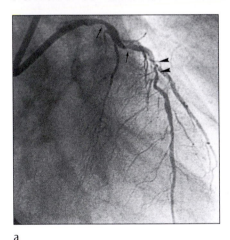 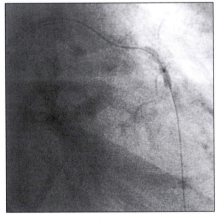 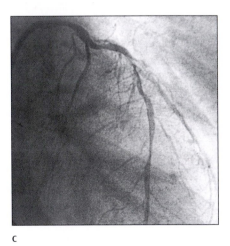

a   b   c

Figure 15.51

(a) This tortuous calcified LAD had two stenoses (small arrows) before a sharp bend and a severe, long lesion beyond the bend (arrowheads).

The LAD could only be accessed with a left Amplatz guide catheter and a 7F size was necessary because of occlusion of the left main stem with an 8F guide catheter.

(b) The distal lesion was dilated first with a 3.0mm balloon.

(c) This produced a poor angiographic result and dissection.

continued

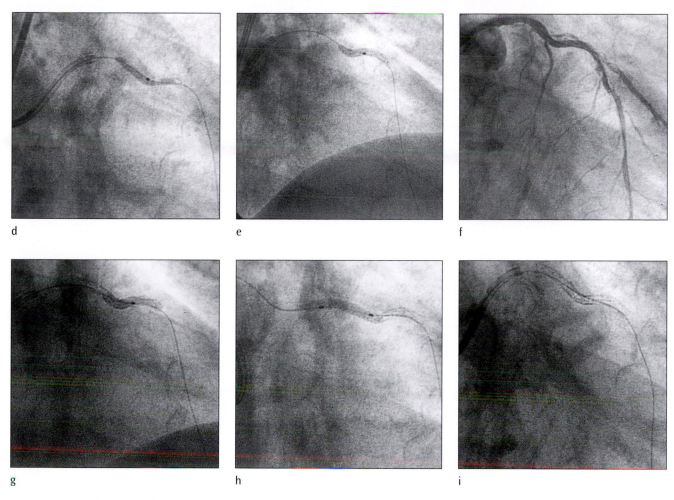

d   e   f

g   h   i

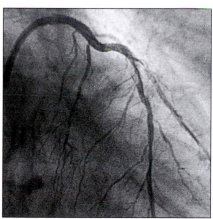

j

Figure 15.51 *continued*

Despite pre-dilatation of the proximal vessel with a 3.0mm balloon (d), a 2.5mm Microstent™ could not be delivered beyond the sharp bend in LAD and was therefore deployed proximal to the most severe lesion (e, f).

A second 2.5mm Microstent™ could not be advanced through the first stent and an attempt to bring back the stent into the guide catheter dislodged it from the balloon.

(g) The stent was engaged back on to the balloon by simply advancing the balloon into the LAD and the stent was then deployed as close to the sharp bend as possible.

Further attempts to advance stents through the first also failed (h), which had to be deployed proximally (i).

(j) The proximal vessel looked good angiographically but the vessel remained unsatisfactory beyond the bend.

The strategy of multivessel PTCA and stenting was abandoned and although the patient was stable he underwent multivessel CABG surgery. There were no further sequelae.

Stent loss from balloon and stent retrieval

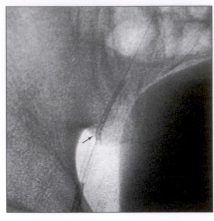 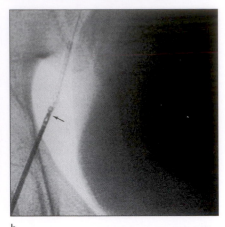

a   b

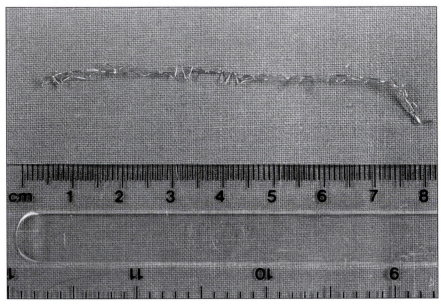

c

Figure 15.52

A 32-year-old man underwent successful PTCA to the RCA but 9 days later the vessel occluded. It was successfully reopened by PTCA and stented with a 3.0mm, 39mm long Microstent™. However, 7 days later the RCA reoccluded at the proximal end of the stent. Although it was possible to reopen the RCA with a 2.5mm balloon, a 3.0mm, 30mm long Microstent™ would not advance beyond the previous stent and was displaced from the balloon by the tip of the guiding catheter on attempted withdrawal. (a) The guide catheter, guidewire and stent (arrow) were withdrawn into the right external iliac artery.

A 5.4F (1.8mm) endomyocardial biopsy forceps catheter was used to capture the stent (b) and to withdraw it into the femoral artery sheath for removal.

(c) The stent completely unravelled during removal.

Courtesy of Dr L Morrison, Cardiothoracic Centre, Liverpool, UK.

The RCA was successfully stented with a 3.0mm, 16mm long NIR™ with a good angiographic result.

Other techniques that use guidewires, snares and grasping forceps can be used for stent retrieval, but this is only possible with high-quality fluoroscopy and a radio-opaque stent.

Because stent embolization outside the coronary artery circulation has a good prognosis and that inside it is poor, every effort should be made to deploy the stent properly or to retrieve it at least into the aortic root.

Stent displacement and distortion after recrossing stent with a guidewire and balloon

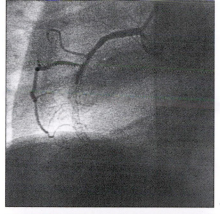

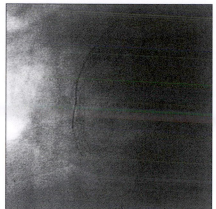

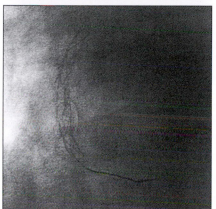

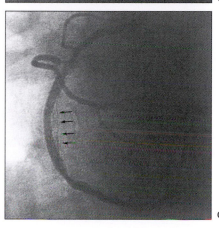

a   b   c   d

Figure 15.53

The same patient as in Fig. 15.52. (a) This RCA reoccluded.

Although the occlusion was crossed with an Intermediate® guidewire (b, c) and the vessel was reopened with PTCA, it is clearly apparent that (d) the guidewire had travelled from a without-within-without-within stent track, thereby causing displacement and distortion of the Microstent™ (arrows).

This problem is difficult to avoid during the first 2-3 months after stent implantation. It can be suspected by a 'gritty' feel – a feeling of slight resistance during the passage of the guidewire, a lack of torquability of the guidewire or a tendency for the guidewire to 'hug' the lateral wall of the coronary artery. It may possibly be avoided by attempting to cross the occlusion with a preshaped 'J' on the guidewire. Once the balloon catheter is advanced along such a misplaced guidewire, stent distortion is almost inevitable and subsequent traverse of the true lumen is virtually impossible.

Courtesy of Dr L Morrison, Cardiothoracic Centre, Liverpool, UK.

Late coronary aneurysm formation

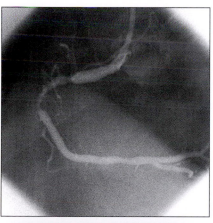

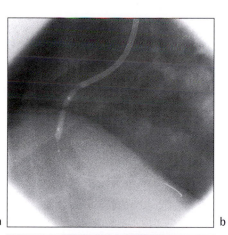

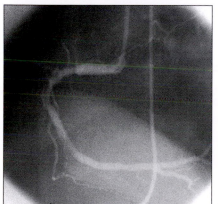

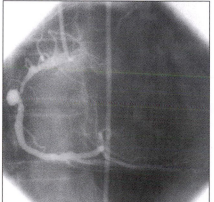

a   b   c   d

Figure 15.54

(a) This balloon-resistant stenosis in the RCA was treated with (b) PTCA up to 15 atmospheres.

However, at this pressure the balloon ruptured.

(c) As this occurred in the pre-stent era, this angiographic result was accepted.

(d) When the angiogram was repeated 10 months later, a large aneurysm was demonstrated at the site of severe restenosis.

The patient was referred for CABG surgery.

Courtesy of Dr DH Bennett, Regional Cardiac Unit, Wythenshawe Hospital, Manchester, UK.

Restenosis

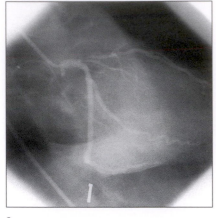

a

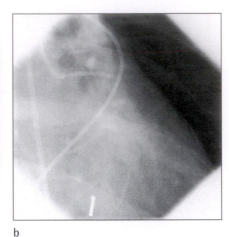

b

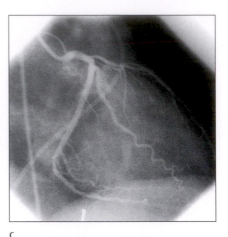

c

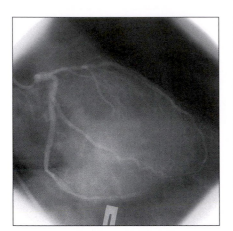

d

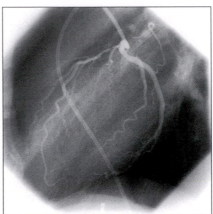

e

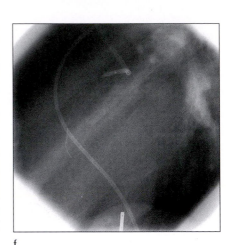

f

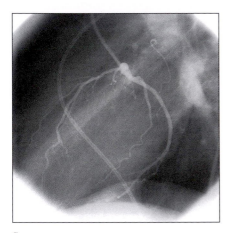

g

Figure 15.55

(a) A second restenosis in an ostial LAD lesion of a 46-year-old man.

(b) PTCA was performed with a 2.5mm balloon.

(c, d) A good angiographic result was obtained.

(e) A further restenosis had produced recurrence of angina within 5 months (LLAT projection).

(f) PTCA with a 2.5mm balloon was performed.

(g) A good result was obtained. The patient remains asymptomatic 8 years on.

The REST trial (of stent versus PTCA for restenosis) showed a significant reduction in the need for target-vessel revascularization (10% in stented patients versus 27% in PTCA patients) and angiographic restenosis (18% in stented patients versus 32% in PTCA patients) in favour of stenting.

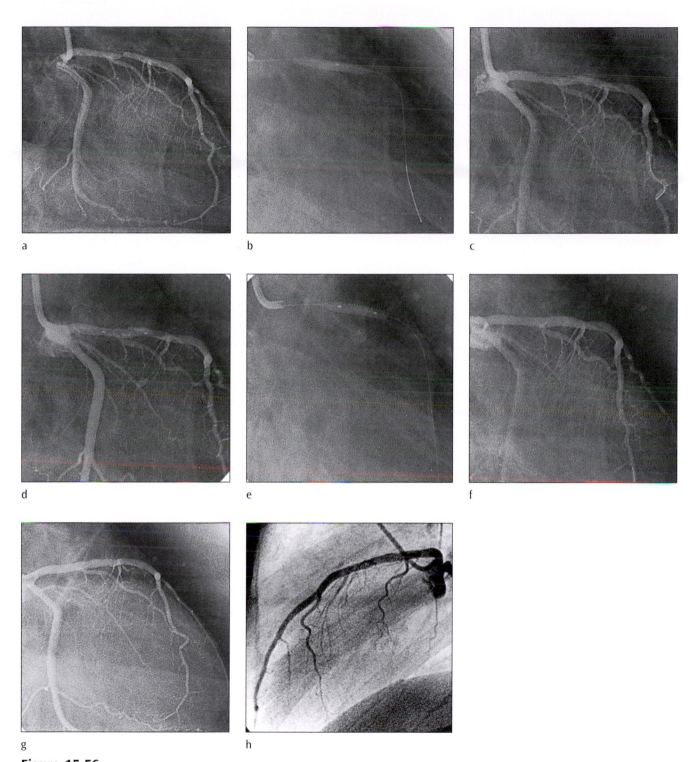

a

b

c

d

e

f

g

h

Figure 15.56
Restenosis occurred 4 months after DCA in this 46-year-old woman, causing frequent angina. (a) Angiography showed a severe, discrete lesion in the proximal LAD.
(b, c) A 3.5mm Cheetah™ balloon caused significant intimal disruption.
(d, e) This required implantation of a 3.5mm, 15mm long Multilink™ stent.
(f) This gave a good final result.
   Result at 6 months – (g) RAO projection; (h) LLAT projection.

Recurrent restenosis or reocclusion

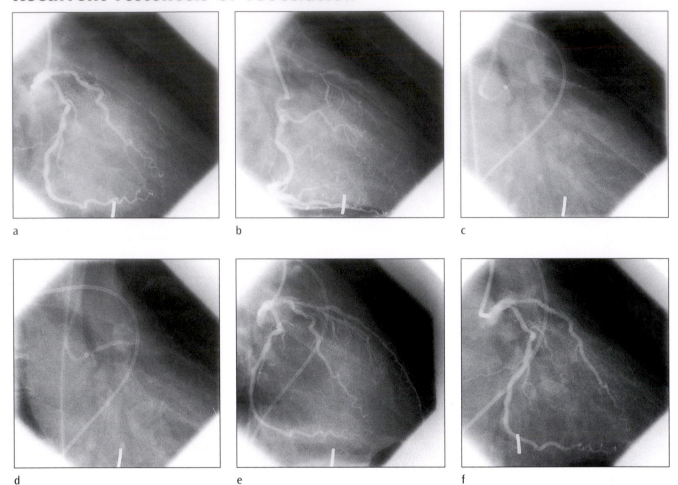

a   b   c

d   e   f

Figure 15.57

A 63-year-old man (the same patient as in Fig. 2.3 and 15.18) presented with chest pain 2 months after successful PTCA to an occluded LAD (see Fig. 2.3). (a) The LAD was reoccluded proximally.

(b) The LAD filled retrogradely from the RCA.

(c) The guidewire crossed the occlusion into the distal vessel.

(d) A 3.0mm balloon was used to reopen the LAD.

(e) Local dissection was left alone – this was in 1987.

(f) Two months later the patient presented again with acute chest pain caused by LAD occlusion.

(g) Similarly, the LAD filled retrogradely from the RCA and allowed confirmation that the guidewire was in the LAD.

(h, i) The LAD was reopened by PTCA.

(j, k) The intermediate artery stenosis was also dilated.

Three months later, the patient presented again with angina.

(l) Restudy showed a significant restenosis at the distal end of the previous occlusion point.

(m, n) PTCA was again performed with a good final result.

(o) Routine angiography at 6 months showed no restenosis. The patient remained asymptomatic 10 years later.

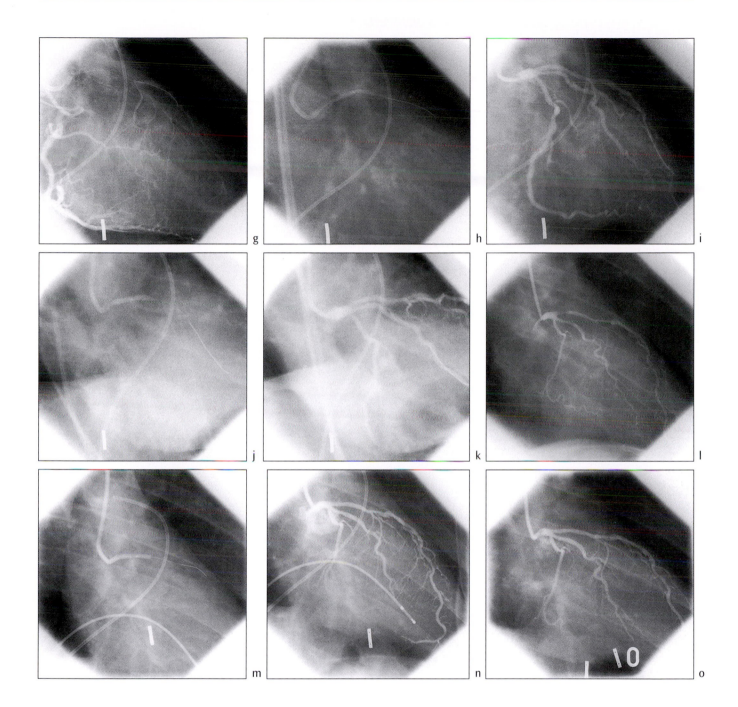

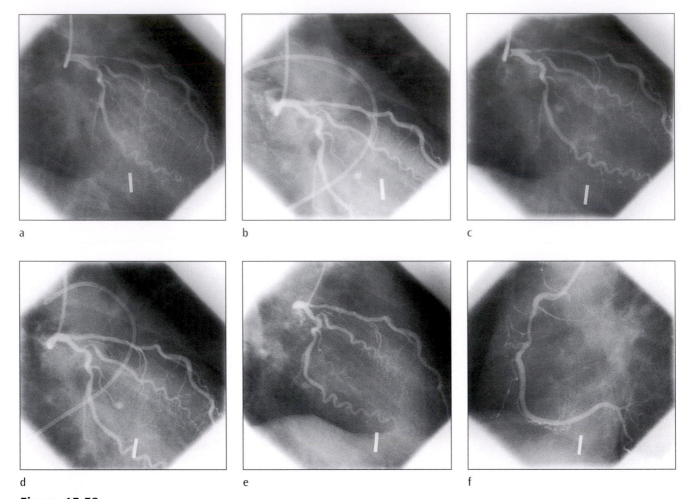

a   b   c

d   e   f

Figure 15.58
A 46-year-old man developed (a) restenosis in the proximal LAD 5 months after three-vessel PTCA, which included reopening of an occluded LAD (see Figure 2.2).
(b) PTCA produced a satisfactory result.
(c) However, the vessel restenosed again 4 months later.
(d) PTCA again produced an excellent angiographic result.
(e) This result persisted at 6 months.
(f) The RCA remained satisfactory 15 months after initial PTCA.

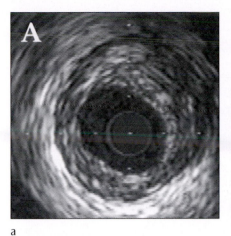

a

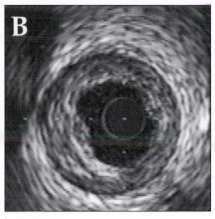

b

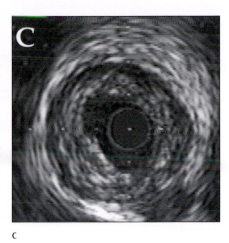

c

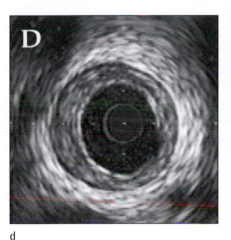

d

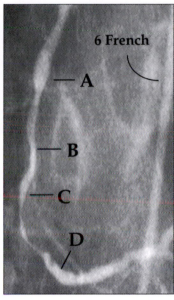

e

Figure 15.59

Over an 18 month period, a 62-year-old man had undergone three repeat PTCA procedures to this RCA because of recurrent restenosis. The vessel was thought to be only 2.0mm in diameter by angiography. However, progressively larger balloons were used in the repeat procedures, although the largest was only 3.0mm diameter.

(a–e) When the patient presented with restenosis for the fourth time, IVUS demonstrated a significantly larger vessel than had been observed from the angiogram. Plaque was distributed in both a concentric and an eccentric manner along its length.

Aggressive PTCA with a 4.0mm balloon was followed by deployment of a 4.0mm stent with both a good angiographic and IVUS result (not shown).

Courtesy of Dr P Fitzgerald, Stanford University School of Medicine, Stanford, California, USA.

Although other devices, including stents, are now available to help to reduce the frequency of recurrent restenosis and occlusion, interventional cardiologists (and their patients) are at present often rewarded only by sheer persistence. This situation will remain until a practical solution is found to the restenosis phenomenon.

Reading

Abbo KM, Dooris M, Glazier S, et al. Features and outcome of no-reflow after percutaneous coronary intervention. Am J Cardiol 1995;75:778-82.

Arora R, Raymond R, Dimas A, et al. Side-branch occlusion during coronary angioplasty: incidence, angiographic characteristics and outcome. Cathet Cardiovasc Diagn 1989;18:210-12.

Baim DS, Carrozza JP Jr. Understanding the 'no-reflow' problem. Cathet Cardiovasc Diagn 1996;39:7-8.

Bal ET, Plokker HWT, van den Berg EMJ, et al. Predictability and prognosis of PTCA-induced coronary artery aneurysms. Cathet Cardiovasc Diagn 1991;22:85-8.

Bauters C, Hubert E, Prat A, et al. Predictors of restenosis after coronary stent implantation. J Am Coll Cardiol 1996;31:1291-8.

Black AJR, Anderson HV, Ellis SG, eds. Complications of Coronary Angioplasty. New York: Marcel Dekker; 1991.

Califf R, Fortin D, Frid D, et al. Restenosis after coronary angioplasty: an overview. J Am Coll Cardiol 1991;17:2B-13B.

Carozza JP, Baim DS, Safian RD. Risks and complications of coronary atherectomy. In: Holmes DR, Garratt KN, eds. Atherectomy. Boston: Blackwell Scientific; 1992:132-48.

Collins TJ. Adjunctive thrombolysis in angioplasty. In: White CJ, Ramee SR, eds. Interventional Cardiology. New York: Marcel Dekker; 1995:227-41.

de Belder A, Thomas MR. The pathophysiology and treatment of in-stent restenosis. Stent 1998;1:74-82.

de Feyter PJ, Ruygrok PN. Coronary intervention: risk stratification and management of abrupt coronary occlusion. Eur Heart J 1995;16:97-103.

Ellis SG, Tamai H, Nobuyoshi M, et al. Contemporary percutaneous treatment of unprotected left main coronary stenoses. Initial results from a multicenter registry analysis 1994-1996. Circulation 1997;96:3867-72.

Fischman DL, Savage MP, Leon MB, et al. Fate of lesion-related side branches after coronary artery stenting. J Am Coll Cardiol 1993;22:1641-6.

Gershlick AH, Baron J. Dealing with in-stent restenosis. Heart 1998;79:319-23.

Hays J, Stein B, Raizner A. The crumpled coronary: an enigma of arteriographic pseudopathology and its potential for misinterpretation. Cathet Cardiovasc Diagn 1994;31:293-300.

Holmes DR Jr, Garratt KN, Popma J. Stent complications. J Invas Cardiol 1998;10:385-95.

Hong MK, Popma JJ, Baim DS, et al. Frequency and predictors of major in-hospital ischemic complications after planned and unplanned new-device angioplasty from the New Approaches to Coronary Intervention (NACI) Registry. Am J Cardiol 1997;80:40K-49K.

Iniguez A, Macaya C, Alfonso F, et al. Early angiographic changes of side branches arising from a Palmaz-Schatz™ stented coronary segment. J Am Coll Cardiol 1994;23:911-15.

Kent KM. Restenosis after percutaneous transluminal coronary angioplasty. Am J Cardiol 1988;67G-70G.

Kher N, Ling FS. Successful unplanned Palmaz-Schatz™ stenting of a compromised side branch through a previously deployed Palmaz-Schatz™ stent. J Invas Cardiol 1997;9:192-6.

Kuntz R, Baim D. Defining coronary restenosis: newer clinical and angiographic paradigms. Circulation 1993;88:1310-23.

Laird JR, Wortham DC. Salvaging failed coronary angioplasty. In: White CJ, Ramee SR, eds. Interventional Cardiology. New York: Marcel Dekker; 1995:317-42.

Lansky AJ, Popma JJ, Mintz GS, et al. Frequency and prognostic importance of creatine phosphokinase myocardial isoforms after successful balloon and new device coronary angioplasty. J Invas Cardiol 1996;8 (Suppl C):3C-9C.

Leroy O, Martin E, Prat A, et al. Fatal infection of coronary stent implantation. Cathet Cardiovasc Diagn 1996;39:168-70.

Mak KH, Belli G, Ellis SG, et al. Subacute stent thrombosis: evolving issues and current concepts. J Am Coll Cardiol 1996;27:494-503.

Moussa I, Di Mario C, Reimers B, et al. Subacute stent thrombosis in the era of intravascular ultrasound-guided coronary stenting without anticoagulation: frequency, predictors and clinical outcome. J Am Coll Cardiol 1997;29:6-12.

Muhlestein JB, Karagounis LA, Treehan S, et al. 'Rescue' utilization of abciximab for the dissolution of coronary thrombus as a complication of coronary angioplasty. J Am Coll Cardiol 1997;30:1729-34.

O'Murchu B, Myler RK. Percutaneous transluminal coronary angioplasty: history, techniques, indications and complications. Unstable angina: pathophysiology and treatment with angioplasty. In: Grech ED, Ramsdale DR, eds. Practical Interventional Cardiology. London: Martin Dunitz; 1997:31-48.

Pan M, Medina A, Suarez-de-Lezo J, et al. Follow-up patency of side branches covered by intracoronary Palmaz-Schatz™ stent. Am Heart J 1995;129:436-40.

Rath PC, Tripathy MP. Management of coronary artery dissection and perforation following coronary angioplasty by intra coronary stent. J Invas Cardiol 1997;9:197-9.

Riessen R, Karsch KR. Cellular biology of restenosis. Int Cardiol Monitor 1995;2:29-35.

Satler L, Leon M, Kent K, Pichard A. Strategies for acute occlusion after coronary angioplasty. J Am Coll Cardiol 1992;19:936-8.

Seckler JI, Butte A, Harrell L, et al. Acute occlusion during coronary interventions: the changing pattern in the era of stents. J Invas Cardiol 1998;10:208-12.

Singh B, Kaul U, Thatai D. Crimped stent-induced pin hole rupture of balloon resulting in extensive coronary dissection. J Invas Cardiol 1997;9:432-4.

Topaz O, Cowley M, Vetrovec G. Coronary perforation during angioplasty: angiographic detection and demonstration of complete healing. Cathet Cardiovasc Diagn 1992;27:284-8.

Waller B, Orr C, Pinkerton C, et al. Coronary balloon angioplasty dissections: the good, the bad and the ugly. J Am Coll Cardiol 1992;20:701-6.

Yip ASB, Chow WH. Spontaneous resolution of pseudo-narrowing after coronary artery stenting. J Invas Cardiol 1996;8:263-5.

Appendix

Trials in coronary intervention

ABACAS
Adjunctive Balloon Angioplasty Coronary Atherectomy Study.
J Am Coll Cardiol 1997;29:281A.
J Am Coll Cardiol 1999;34:1028–35.

ACCESS
A randomized comparison of transradial, brachial and femoral coronary angioplasty with 6F guiding catheters.
J Am Coll Cardiol 1997;29:1269–75.

ACME
Angioplasty Compared to MEdicine study.
N Engl J Med 1992;326:10–16.

ACUTE
Analysis of Coronary Ultrasound Thrombolysis Endpoints in acute myocardial infarction (ACUTE) trial. Results of the feasibility phase.
Circulation 1997;95:1411–16.

ADMIRAL
Abciximab before direct angioplasty and stenting in myocardial infarction.
Circulation 1999;100(Suppl I):I–86, 87.
Eur Heart J 1999;20 (Suppl):170.

AIR PAMI
Randomized trial of thrombolysis vs transfer for primary PTCA in high risk AMI patients.
J Am Coll Cardiol 2000;35:376A.

ALKK
Primary angioplasty versus thrombolysis in the treatment of acute myocardial infarction (Angioplasty vs Lysis study of Kardiologie Klinikum).
Am J Cardiol 1997;79:264–69.

AMIGO
Atherectomy before Multilink Improves lumen Gain Outcome.
Principal investigator: A Colombo, Centro Cuore Columbus, Milan, Italy.

AMRO
AMsterdam ROtterdam trial (ELCA vs PTCA).
Lancet 1996;347:79–84.

APLAUSE
Anti-PLatelet treatment After intravascular Ultrasound guided optimal Stent Expansion.
Circulation 1995;92(Suppl I):I–795.
Circulation 1996;94(Suppl I):I–686.

ARREST
Angiorad Radiation for RESTenosis in un-stented native vessel.
Principal investigator: R Waksman, Washington Hospital Center, Washington, DC, USA.
J Am Coll Cardiol 1999;33:56A.

ARTIST
Angioplasty versus Rotablation for Treatment of Intra-STent stenosis/occlusion.
Principal Investigators: HG Klues and J vom Dahl, Universitaetsklinikum der RWTH Aachen, Aachen, Germany.
J Am Coll Cardiol 2000;35:7A–8A.
J Am Coll Cardiol 2000;35:83A.

ARTISTIC	Angiorad Radiation Therapy for In-STent restenosis Intra-Coronary. Principal investigator: R Waksman, Washington Hospital Center, Washington, DC, USA. Circulation 1998;98(Suppl I):I-442. J Am Coll Cardiol 1999;33:56A.
ARTS	Artery Revascularization Therapy Study. Principal investigator: P Serruys, Thoraxcenter, Rotterdam, The Netherlands. Circulation 1998;98(Suppl I):I-498. Eur Heart J 1998;19(Suppl):137. Int J Cardiovasc Interventions 1999;2:41–50.
ASCENT	ACS Multilink stent trial. Principal investigator: DS Baim, Beth Israel-Deaconess Medical Center, Boston, Massachusetts, USA. J Am Coll Cardiol 1998;31:139A.
ATLAS	Acolysis During Treatment of Lesions Affecting SVGs. Principal investigator: MB Leon, Washington Hospital Center, Washington, DC, USA.
AVERT	Atorvastatin VErsus Revascularization Treatments. Principal investigator: DM Black, University of Michigan Medical Center, Ann Arbor, Michigan, USA. J Am Coll Cardiol 1999;33:341A. N Engl J Med 1999;341:70–6.
AVID	Angiography Vs Intravascular ultrasound Directed coronary stent placement. Principal investigator: R Russo, Scripps Clinic Research Foundation, La Jolla, California, USA. Circulation 1999;100(Suppl I):I-234. J Am Coll Cardiol 2000;35:45A.
BARASTER registry	Balloon Angiopasty and Rotational Atherectomy for in-STEnt Restenosis. Principal investigator: SL Goldberg, UCLA Medical Center, Los Angeles, California, USA. Circulation 1997;96(Suppl I):I-80. Circulation 1998;98(Suppl I):I-363.
BARI	Bypass Angioplasty Revascularization Investigation. N Engl J Med 1996;335:217–24.
BAROCCO	Balloon Angioplasty versus ROtational angioplasty in Chronic Coronary Occlusions. Am J Cardiol 1995;75:330–4.
BENESTENT I	BElgium-NEtherland STENT I. N Engl J Med 1994;331:489–95. Eur Heart J 1999;20(Suppl):136. Circulation 1999;100(Suppl I):I-233.
BENESTENT II pilot study	BElgium-NEtherland STENT II: heparin coated Palmaz-Schatz™ stents in human coronary arteries. Circulation 1996;93:412–22.
BENESTENT II	BElgium-NEtherland STENT II: heparin coated Palmaz-Schatz™ stents in human coronary arteries. Principal investigator: P Serruys, Thoraxcenter, Rotterdam, The Netherlands. Circulation 1995;92(Suppl I):I-279,542. Lancet 1998;352:673–81.
BERT	Beta Energy Restenosis Trial. Circulation 1998;97:2025–30.

BESMART	BEstent in SMall ARTeries study. J Am Coll Cardiol 1999;33:95A. Eur Heart J 1999;20(Suppl):383. Circulation 1999;100(Suppl I):I-503.
BESSAMI	BErlin Stent Study in Acute Myocardial Infarction trial. Eur Heart J 1999;20(Suppl):170.
BEST	BE STent trial. Principal investigator: J Brinker, Johns Hopkins University, Baltimore, Maryland, USA.
BETA WRIST	BETA-Washington Radiation for In-Stent restenosis Trial. Principal investigator: R Waksman, Washington Hospital Center, Washington, DC, USA. J Am Coll Cardiol 1999;33:19A. Circulation 1999;100(Suppl I):I-75. J Am Coll Cardiol 2000;35:21A.
BETA CATH	BETA CATH Trial. Principal investigator: R Kuntz, Beth Israel-Deaconess Medical Center, Boston, Massachusetts, USA.
BOAT	Balloon versus Optimal Atherectomy Trial. Circulation 1998;97:322–31. Circulation 1999;100(Suppl I):I-779.
BOSS	Balloon Optimization vs Stent Study. Circulation 1997;96(Suppl I):I-592.
BRIE	Beta Radiation In Europe. Principle Investigator: P Serruys. Circulation 1997;96(Suppl I):I-592.
CABRI	Coronary Angioplasty vs Bypass Revascularization Investigation. Lancet 1995;346:1179–84.
CADILLAC	Controlled Abciximab and Device Investigation to Lower Late Angioplasty Complications. Principal investigator: GW Stone, Washington Hospital Center, Washington, DC, USA.
CAPARES	Coronary AngioPlasty Amlodipine REStenosis Study. Eur Heart J 1999;20(Suppl):285. J Am Coll Cardiol 2000;35:592–9.
CAPAS	Cutting balloon Angioplasty vs Plain old balloon Angioplasty randomized Study in type B/C lesions. J Am Coll Cardiol 1997;28:458A. J Am Coll Cardiol 1998;31:315A. J Am Coll Cardiol 1999;33:47A.
CAPTURE	Chimeric c7E3 AntiPlatelet Therapy in Unstable REfractory angina. Lancet 1997;349:1429–35.
CARAT I and II	Coronary Angioplasty and Rotational Atherectomy Trial I and II. J Am Coll Cardiol 1998;31:378A.
CARPORT	Coronary Artery Restenosis Prevention On Repeated Thromboxane antagonism study. Circulation 1991;84:1568–80. Circulation 1993;88:975–85.
CART	Coronary Angioplasty Restenosis Trial. J Am Coll Cardiol 1991;33:1619–26.

CAVEAT I	A Comparison of directional Atherectomy VErsus coronary Angioplasty Trial in patients with coronary artery disease. N Engl J Med 1993;329:221–7. Circulation 1995;91:2158–66.
CAVEAT II	A multicenter randomized trial of Coronary Angioplasty VErsus directional ATherectomy for patients with saphenous bypass vein graft lesions. Circulation 1995;91:1966–74.
CBBEST	Cutting Balloon BEfore STent in native coronary arteries. Principal investigator: MB Leon, Washington Hospital Center, Washington, DC, USA.
CCAT	Canadian Coronary Atherectomy Trial. N Engl J Med 1993;329:228–33.
CLAPT	Cholesterol Lowering Atherosclerosis PTCA Trial. Principal investigator: A Kleeman, University of Munster, Germany.
CLASSICS	CLopidogrel ASpirin Stent International Co-operative Study. Circulation 1999;100(Suppl I):I-379. Circulation 2000; 102: 624–9.
CLOUT	CLinical Outcomes with Ultrasound Trial. Circulation 1997;95:2044–52. J Am Coll Cardiol 1999;33:81A.
COBRA	COmparison of Balloon vs Rotational Angioplasty. Principal investigator: U Dietz, University Hospital, Mainz, Germany. Circulation 1997;96(Suppl I):I-80,324.
CORAMI II	Cohort Of Rescue Angioplasty in Myocardial Infarction. Circulation 1997;96(Suppl I):I-532.
CORSICA	Chronic Occlusion Revascularization with Stent Implantation versus Coronary Angioplasty trial. Eur Heart J 1997;18(Suppl):382. Eur Heart J 1998;19(Suppl):471.
COURT	A randomized trial of COntrast media Utilization in high Risk PTCA. J Am Coll Cardiol 1999;33:11A.
CROSSFLEX	CROSSFLEX stent for the treatment of native coronary disease. Principal investigator: JE Sousa, São Paolo, Brazil.
CROWN	Palmaz-Schatz™ CROWN balloon expandable stent with PowerGrip™ over the wire delivery system. Principal investigator: DO Williams, Rhode Island Hospital, Providence, Rhode Island, USA.
CRUISE	Can Routine Ultrasound Influence Stent Expansion. Circulation 1996;95(Suppl I):I-422. Circulation 1997;96(Suppl I):I-222. J Am Coll Cardiol 1998;31:396A.
CRUSADE	Coronary Reserve Utilization for Stent and Angiography: the Doppler Endpoint study. Principal investigator: JD Joyce, Allegheny Hospital, Pittsburgh, Pennsylvania, USA.
CUBA	CUtting balloon versus conventional Balloon Angioplasty. Circulation 1997;96:223A. Eur Heart J 1998;19(Suppl):48. J Am Coll Cardiol 1999;33:48A.
CURE	Columbia University Restenosis Elimination safety trial. J Am Coll Cardiol 1999;33:94A. Circulation 1999;100(Suppl I):I-75.

CUTTING BALLOON RCT	The international **CUTTING BALLOON** Randomized Clinical Trial. Principal investigator: R Bonan, The Montreal Heart Institute, Montreal, Canada. Circulation 1997;96(Suppl I):I-324.
DANAMI	**DAN**ish trial in **A**cute **M**yocardial **I**nfarction. Circulation 1997;96(Suppl I):I-596. Circulation 1997;96:748–55.
DART	**D**ilation vs **A**blation **R**evascularization **T**rial. Principal investigator: M Reisman, Swedish Medical Center, Seattle, Washington, USA. Circulation 1997;96(Suppl I):I-467.
DEBATE I	**D**oppler **E**ndpoint **B**alloon **A**ngioplasty **T**rial **E**urope. Circulation 1997;96:3369–77.
DEBATE II	**D**oppler **E**ndpoint **B**alloon **A**ngioplasty **T**rial **E**urope II. Principal investigator: PW Serruys, Thoraxcenter, Rotterdam, The Netherlands. Circulation 1998;98(Suppl I):I-499. Eur Heart J 1999;20(Suppl):371,372.
DEFER	**DEFER**ral versus performance of PTCA based on coronary pressure derived fractional flow reserve. J Am Coll Cardiol 1999;33:89A. Eur Heart J 1999;20(Suppl):371.
DESIRE	**DE**bulking and **S**tenting **I**n **R**estenosis **E**limination (DCA + stent vs stent) J Am Coll Cardiol 2000;35:94A.
DESTINI	**D**oppler **E**ndpoint **ST**enting **IN**ternational **I**nvestigation of coronary flow reserve. Principal investigator: A Colombo, Centro Cuore, Columbus, Milan, Italy. Circulation 1998;98(Suppl I):I-499. J Am Coll Cardiol 1999;33:47A.
DIRECT	**DIRECT** stenting vs stenting with pre-dilation in selected coronary lesions. J Am Coll Cardiol 2000;35:35A.
DOUBTLESS	**DO**ppler and **U**ltrasound guided **B**alloon **T**herapeutics for coronary **LES**ion**S**. Principal investigator: A Pichard, Washington Hospital Center, Washington, DC, USA.
EASI	The **E**uropean **A**ntiplatelet **S**tent **I**nvestigation. Principal investigator: M Rothman, Cardialysis, Rotterdam, The Netherlands.
EAST	**E**mory **A**ngioplasty versus **S**urgery **T**rial. N Engl J Med 1994;331:1044–50. Circulation 1995;92:2831–40.
EDRES	The **E**ffects of **D**ebulking on **RES**tenosis. Principal investigator: B Dunn, King Faisal Hospital, Riyadh, Saudi Arabia. Circulation 1997;96(Suppl I):I-709.
EPIC	**E**valuation of 7E3 for the **P**revention of **I**schemic **C**omplications. N Engl J Med 1994;330:956–61. Lancet 1994;343:881–6. J Am Coll Cardiol 1997;30:149–56.
EPILOG	**E**valuation in **P**TCA to **I**mprove **L**ong term **O**utcome with Abciximab **G**PIIb/IIIa blockade. Circulation 1997;96(Suppl I):I-162. N Engl J Med 1997;336:1689–96. Circulation 1999;99:1951–8.

EPISTENT	Evaluation of Platelet IIb/IIIa Inhibitor for STENTing trial Lancet 1998;352:87–92. J Am Coll Cardiol 1999;33:32A. Lancet 1999;354:2019–24.
ERACI	Argentine randomized trial of coronary angioplasty vs bypass surgery in multivessel disease. J Am Coll Cardiol 1993;22:1060–7.
ERACI II	Argentine randomized study optimal balloon angioplasty and stenting vs coronary bypass surgery in multiple vessel disease (ERACI II). J Am Coll Cardiol 1999;33:33A. Eur Heart J 1999;20(Suppl):137. Circulation 1999;100(Suppl I):I-234. J Am Coll Cardiol 2000;35:3A,8A,9A.
ERASER	Evaluation of Reopro And Stenting to Eliminate Restenosis. Principal investigator: S Ellis, Cleveland Clinic Foundation, Cleveland, Ohio, USA. Circulation 1997;96(Suppl I):I-87. Circulation 1999;100:799–806.
ERBAC	Excimer laser, Rotational atherectomy and Balloon Angioplasty Comparison study. Circulation 1997;96:91–8.
ESCOBAR	Emergency Stenting compared to COnventional Balloon Angioplasty Randomized trial. Principal investigator: H Suryapranata, Hospital de Weezenlanden, Zwolle, The Netherlands.
ESPRIT	Elimination of restenosis by Stenting after Plaque Reduction with platelet Inhibitor Trial. J Am Coll Cardiol 2000;35:8A.
ESSEX	European Scimed Stent EXperience. Principal investigator: PW Serruys, Thoraxcenter, Rotterdam, The Netherlands.
EURO-ART	EUROpean experience with the Angiojet Rapid Thrombectomy catheter. J Am Coll Cardiol 1997;29:186A.
EUROCARE	A European multicentre randomised double-blind placebo controlled trial to evaluate the efficacy of carvedilol after successful directional coronary atherectomy in the prevention of late restenosis. Circulation 1998;98(Suppl I):I-513. Circulation 2000;101:1512–18.
EXACTO	EXcimer laser Angioplasty in Coronary Total Occlusion. Principal investigator: R Simon, Klinik Fur Kardiologie, Kiel, The Netherlands. Eur Heart J 1999;20(Suppl):270.
EXCITE	Evaluation of oral Xemilofiban in ControllIng Thrombotic Events. Principal investigator: WW O'Neill, William Beaumont Hospital, Royal Oak, Michigan, USA.
EXTRA	Evaluation of the XT stent for Restenosis in native Arteries. Principal investigator: J Carrozza, Beth Israel Deaconess Hospital, Boston, Massachusetts, USA.
FANTASTIC	Full ANticoagulation versus Ticlopidine plus Aspirin after STent Implantation in Coronary arteries. Principal investigator: M Bertrand, Université de Lille, France. Circulation 1998;98:1597–603.
FAST	Fujigaoka Antiplatelet Stent Trial in acute myocardial infarction. Eur Heart J 1999;20(Suppl):285.

FINESS I	The NIR Stent European Registry: First INternational Endovascular Stent Study. Eur Heart J 1997;18:156. J Am Coll Cardiol 1997;30:847–54.
FINESS II	The NIR Stent European Registry: the Second INternational Endovascular Stent Study. Principal investigator: PW Serruys, Thoraxcenter, Rotterdam, The Netherlands.
FLARE	FLuvastatin Angioplasty REstenosis. Principal investigator: PW Serruys, Thoraxcenter, Rotterdam, The Netherlands. Eur Heart J 1999;20:58–69.
FLEXOR	Focused Lesion EXpansion Optimizes Results. Principal investigator: L Cannon, Thomas Jefferson University, Philadelphia, Pennsylvania, USA.
FREEDOM	European FREEDOM Stent Registry. Principal investigator: I de Scheerder, University Hospital Leuven, Belgium.
FRESCO	Florence Randomized Elective Stenting in acute Coronary Occlusions. Circulation 1997;96(Suppl I):I-327. J Am Coll Cardiol 1998;31:1234–9. Circulation 1999;100(Suppl I):I-855.
FRISC II	FRagmin and fast revascularisation during InStability in Coronary artery disease. Lancet 1999;354:701–7;708–15. Circulation 1999;100:(Suppl I):I-497–8.
FROST	French Randomized Optimal Stenting Trial. Principal investigator: PG Steg, Hospital Bichat, Paris, France. J Am Coll Cardiol 1998;31:317A. J Am Coll Cardiol 1999;33:89A.
GABI	German Angioplasty Bypass surgery Investigation. N Engl J Med 1994;331:1037–43.
GABI-II	German, prospective, multicenter study for the treatment of patients with symptomatic multivessel disease. Circulation 1998;98(Suppl I):I-498. Eur Heart J 1998;19(Suppl):136. Eur Heart J 1999;20(Suppl):137.
GAMMA I	A multicenter randomized trial of localized radiation therapy to inhibit restenosis after stenting. Principal investigator: MB Leon, Washington Hospital Center, Washington, DC, USA. J Am Coll Cardiol 1999;33:19A. Circulation 1999;100(Suppl I):I-75.
GAMMA II	A multicenter randomized trial of localized radiation therapy to inhibit restenosis after stenting. Principal investigator: MB Leon, Washington Hospital Center, Washington, DC, USA. J Am Coll Cardiol 2000;35:50A.
GAMMA WIRE	Effect of iridium[192] administered by a wire in coronary restenosis after PTCA. Circulation 1997;96:727–32.
GENEVA	Intracoronary beta-irradiation to reduce restenosis after balloon angioplasty. Circulation 1997;95:1138–44.
GISSOC	Gruppo Italiano di Studio Sullo Stent Nelle Occlusion Coronariche. J Am Coll Cardiol 1998;32:90–6.

GRII	Gianturco-Roubin II stent. Principal investigator: MB Leon, Washington Hospital Center, Washington, DC, USA. Eur Heart J 1998;19(Suppl):47. J Am Coll Cardiol 1999;33:61A.
GRACE	Gianturco-Roubin stent Acute Closure Evaluation. J Interven Cardiol 1994;7:333–9.
GRAMI	GRII stent in Acute Myocardial Infarction. J Am Coll Cardiol 1998;30:64A. Am J Cardiol 1998;81:1286–91.
GRAPE	Glycoprotein Receptor Antagonist Patency Evaluation pilot study. Circulation 1997;96(Suppl I):I-474. J Am Coll Cardiol 1999;33:1528–32.
GUIDE II	Guidance by Ultrasound Imaging for Decision Endpoints. Principal Investigators: P Fitzgerald and P Yock, Stanford University, Palo Alto, California, USA.
GUSTO I angiographic substudy	Global Utilization of Streptokinase and Tissue plasminogen activator for Occluded coronary arteries trial. Circulation 1998;97:1549–56.
GUSTO IIb Primary Angioplasty Substudy	Global Use of Strategies To Open occluded coronary arteries in acute coronary syndromes. N Engl J Med 1997;336:1621–8.
GUSTO III substudy	Global Use of Strategies To Open occluded coronary arteries in acute coronary syndromes III. J Am Coll Cardiol 1998;842A.
HAPI	Heparin After Percutaneous Intervention. J Am Coll Cardiol 1999;34:461–7.
HEAP	High dose heparin as pretreatment for primary angioplasty in acute myocardial infarction: the Heparin in EArly Patency randomized trial. J Am Coll Cardiol 1998;31:289–93. J Am Coll Cardiol 2000;35:600–4.
HELVETICA	Hirudin in a European triaL Versus HEparin in The prevention of RestenosIs after PTCA trial. Principal investigator: P Serruys, Thoraxcenter, Rotterdam, The Netherlands.
HEROICS	How Effective are Revascularization Options In Cardiogenic Shock? Principal investigator: M Walters, Hull Royal Infirmary, UK. Circulation 1997;96(Suppl I):I-31.
HIPS	Heparin Infusion Prior to Stenting. Circulation 1997;96(Suppl I):I-710. J Am Coll Cardiol 1998;31:457A. Eur Heart J 1998;19(Suppl):49.
IMPACT I	Integrilin to Minimize Platelet Aggregation and prevent Coronary Thrombosis. Circulation 1995;91:2151–7.
IMPACT II	Integrilin to Minimize Platelet Aggregation and prevent Coronary Thrombosis. Lancet 1997;349:1422–8.
IMPACT AMI	CombIned accelerated tissue plasMinogen activator and PlAtelet glycoprotein IIb/IIIa integrin reCeptor blockade with InTegrilin in Acute Myocardial Infarction. Circulation 1997;95:846–54.

IMPRESS	Prevention of neo-intimal proliferation after stent implantation by local delivery of low-molecular-weight heparin randomized trial. Eur Heart J 1998;19(Suppl):50.
INHIBIT	**INHIBIT** restenosis with beta radiation. Principal investigator: R Waksman, Washington Hospital Center, Washington, DC, USA.
IRIS	Isostent for Restenosis Intervention Study. Eur Heart J 1998;19(Suppl):457. J Am Coll Cardiol 1998;31:350A. J Am Coll Cardiol 1999;33:21A.
ISAR	Intracoronary Stenting and Antithrombotic Regimen trial. Circulation 1997;95:2015–21. Circulation 1997;96:462–7.
ITALICS	Investigation by the Thoraxcenter on Antisense DNA given by Local delivery and assessed by Intravascular ultrasound after Coronary Stenting. Principal investigator: P Serruys, Thoraxcenter, Rotterdam, The Netherlands. Eur Heart J 1998;19(Suppl):569. Circulation 1998;98(Suppl I):I-363.
JIMI	Japanese Intervention trial in Myocardial Infarction. Circulation 1997;96(Suppl);I-536.
LARS (European surveillance study)	Laser Angioplasty for Restenosed Stents. J Am Coll Cardiol 1998;31:143A.
LARS (randomized, multicenter)	Laser Angioplasty for Restenosed Stents. Principal Investigators: MB Leon, Washington Hospital Center, Washington, DC, USA and P Serruys, Thoraxcenter, Rotterdam, The Netherlands.
LARS (retrospective USA registry)	Laser Angioplasty for Restenosed Stents. J Am Coll Cardiol 1998;31:142A.
LAVA trial	Laser facilitated balloon Angioplasty Versus Angioplasty. J Am Coll Cardiol 1997;30:1714–20.
LOCAL PAMI	**LOCAL** heparin delivery after Primary PTCA in Acute Myocardial Infarction. Principal investigator: C Grines, William Beaumont Hospital, Royal Oak, Michigan, USA.
LONG WRIST	**LONG** lesions: Washington Radiation for In-Stent restenosis Trial. Principal investigator: R Waksman, Washington Hospital Center, Washington, DC, USA.
MAJIC	MAyo-Japan Investigation for Chronic total occlusion. Circulation 1998;98(Suppl):I-639.
MARCATOR	Multicenter American Research trial with Cilazapril after Angioplasty to prevent Transluminal coronary Obstruction and Restenosis. J Am Coll Cardiol 1995;2:362–9.
MASS	The Medicine, Angioplasty or Surgery Study. J Am Coll Cardiol 1995;26:1600–5. J Am Coll Cardiol 1999;33:349A.
MATE	Medicine versus Angiography in Thrombolytic Exclusion Trial Circulation 1997;96(Suppl I):I-595–6. J Am Coll Cardiol 1998;32:596–605.
MATTIS	Multicenter Aspirin and Ticlopidine Trial after Intracoronary Stenting. J Am Coll Cardiol 1998;31:397A. Circulation 1998;98:2126–32.
MENTOR	MEdtroNic WikTOR GX/heparinized Stent study in single de novo lesions. Principal investigator: MC Vrolix, Heart Center Limberg, Genk, Belgium.

MERCATOR	Multicenter European Research trial with Cilazapril after Angioplasty to prevent Transluminal coronary Obstruction and Restenosis. Circulation 1992;86:100–10.
MILAN	Intravascular ultrasound (IVUS) analysis of beta-particle emitting radioactive stent implantation in human coronary arteries: preliminary, immediate and intermediate-term results of the MILAN study. Circulation 1998;98(Suppl I):I-780.
MUSCAT	One balloon approach for optimized Palmaz–Schatz™ stent implantation: The MUSCAT trial. Cathet Cardiovasc Diagn 1997;42:130–6.
MUSIC	Multicenter Ultrasound Stenting In Coronary arteries. J Am Coll Cardiol 1996;29:137A. Eur Heart J 1998;19:1214–23.
MUST	The MUlticenter Stent Trial. J Am Coll Cardiol 1997;29:93A. J Invas Cardiol 1998;10:457–63.
NACI: excimer laser	New Approaches to Coronary Interventions: registry of excimer laser coronary angioplasty (ELCA). Am J Cardiol 1997;80:99K–105K.
NACI: Gianturco-Roubin	New Approaches to Coronary Interventions: registry of Gianturco-Roubin stents. Am J Cardiol 1997;80:89K–98K.
NACI: Palmaz-Schatz	New Approaches to Coronary Interventions: registry of Palmaz-Schatz™ stents. Am J Cardiol 1997;80:78K–88K.
NACI: rotational atherectomy	New Approaches to Coronary Interventions: registry of rotational atherectomy. Am J Cardiol 1997;80:60K–67K.
NIRVANA	NIR Vascular Advanced North American trial. Circulation 1997;96(Suppl I):I-594. J Am Coll Cardiol 1998;31:80A.
OARS	Optimal Atherectomy Restenosis Study. Circulation 1998;97:332–9.
OCBAS	Optimal Coronary Balloon Angioplasty versus Stent. J Am Coll Cardiol 1997;29:311A. Circulation 1997;96(Suppl I):I-593. J Am Coll Cardiol 1999;32:1351–7.
OPTICUS	OPTimization with ICUS to reduce stent restenosis. Circulation 1997;96(Suppl I):I-582. J Am Coll Cardiol 1998;31:494A. Circulation 1998;98(Suppl I):I-363. Eur Heart J 1999;20(Suppl):370.
OSTI-I	Optimal STent Implantation trial: I. J Am Coll Cardiol 1997;29:369A.
OSTI-IIA	Optimal STent Implantation trial: IIA. Circulation 1997;96(Suppl I):I-402. J Am Coll Cardiol 1998;31:16A.
OSTI-IIB	Optimal STent Implantation trial: IIB. Principal investigator: GW Stone, El Camino Hospital, Mountain View, California, USA.
PACT	Plasminogen activator Angioplasty Compatibility Trial. J Am Coll Cardiol 1999;34:1954–62.

PAIR	<u>P</u>ullback <u>A</u>therectomy for <u>I</u>n-stent <u>R</u>estenosis trial. Circulation 1999;100(Suppl I):I-307.
PAMI	<u>P</u>rimary <u>A</u>ngioplasty in <u>M</u>yocardial <u>I</u>nfarction. N Engl J Med 1993;328:673–9. J Am Coll Cardiol 1995;25:370–7.
PAMI II	Second <u>P</u>rimary <u>A</u>ngioplasty in <u>M</u>yocardial <u>I</u>nfarction. J Am Coll Cardiol 1997;29:1459–67.
PAMI NO SOS	<u>P</u>rimary <u>A</u>ngioplasty for acute <u>M</u>yocardial <u>I</u>nfarction with <u>NO</u> <u>S</u>urgery <u>O</u>n <u>S</u>ite. Circulation 1998;98(Suppl I):I-306. J Am Coll Cardiol 1999;33:352A.
PAMI stent pilot	<u>P</u>rimary stenting in <u>A</u>cute <u>M</u>yocardial <u>I</u>nfarction. J Am Coll Cardiol 1998;31:23–30. Eur Heart J 1998;19(Suppl):59.
PAMI stent	<u>P</u>rimary stenting in <u>A</u>cute <u>M</u>yocardial <u>I</u>nfarction. J Am Coll Cardiol 1999;33:361A,379A. N Engl J Med 1999;341:1949–56.
PARAGON	<u>P</u>latelet IIb/IIIa <u>A</u>ntagonism for the <u>R</u>eduction of <u>A</u>cute coronary syndrome events in a <u>G</u>lobal <u>O</u>rganization <u>N</u>etwork. Circulation 1997;96(Suppl I):I–474. Circulation 1998;97:2386–95.
PARK	<u>P</u>ost-<u>A</u>ngioplasty <u>R</u>estenosis <u>K</u>etanserin study. Circulation 1993;88:1588–1601.
PAS	<u>P</u>aragon elective or <u>A</u>cute <u>S</u>tent. Principal investigator: D Holmes Jr, The Mayo Clinic, Rochester, Minnesota, USA.
PASTA	<u>P</u>rimary <u>A</u>ngioplasty and <u>ST</u>ent implantation in <u>A</u>cute myocardial infarction. Circulation 1997;96(Suppl I):I-595. Cathet Cardiovasc Intervention 1999;48:262–8.
PELCA	The <u>P</u>ercutaneous <u>E</u>xcimer <u>L</u>aser <u>C</u>oronary <u>A</u>ngioplasty. J Am Coll Cardiol 1995;26:1264–9.
PICTURE	<u>P</u>ost-<u>I</u>ntra<u>C</u>oronary <u>T</u>reatment <u>U</u>ltrasound <u>R</u>esults <u>E</u>valuation. Circulation 1997;95:2254–61.
PILOT	<u>P</u>olish <u>I</u>ntramural <u>L</u>ow molecular weight heparin <u>O</u>utpatient stent <u>T</u>rial. Principal investigator: E Deutsch, Temple University, Philadelphia, Pennsylvania, USA.
POLONIA	Local delivery of enoxaparin to decrease restenosis rate after coronary stenting. J Am Coll Cardiol 2000;35:9A.
POST	<u>P</u>redictors and <u>O</u>utcomes of <u>S</u>ubacute <u>T</u>hrombosis. J Am Coll Cardiol 1997;29:60A.
PRAGUE	Transport for angioplasty vs thrombolysis vs both in acute myocardial infarction in community hospitals in Prague. Eur Heart J 1998;19(Suppl):56.
PREDICT	Prevention of restenosis by pravastatin after PTCA. J Am Coll Cardiol 1997;30:863–9.
PRESTO	<u>P</u>revention of <u>RES</u>tenosis with <u>T</u>ranilast and its <u>O</u>utcomes: a placebo-controlled trial. Multicentre study sponsored by SmithKline Beecham. Chairman of Steering Committee: D Holmes, Mayo Clinic, Rochester, Minnesota, USA.

PREVENT
Proliferation REduction with Vascular ENergy Trial.
Principal investigator: A Raizner, Baylor College of Medicine, Houston, Texas, USA.
Circulation 1999;100(Suppl I): I-75, 517.

PRISAM
PRImary Stenting for Acute Myocardial infarction.
Circulation 1997;96(Suppl I):I-397, 531.
Circulation 1999;100(Suppl I):I-856.

PRISM
Platelet Receptor Inhibition for ischemic Syndrome Management.
N Engl J Med 1998;338:1498–505.

PRISM-PLUS
Platelet Receptor Inhibition for ischemic Syndrome Management in Patients Limited by Unstable Signs and symptoms.
Circulation 1997;96(Suppl I):I-474.
N Engl J Med 1998;338:1488–97.

PRISON
PRImary coronary Stent deployment in Occlusive Native coronary artery disease.
Circulation 1999;100(Suppl I):I-504..

PSAAMI
Primary Stenting vs Angioplasty in Acute Myocardial Infarction.
J Am Coll Cardiol 1999;33:29A.
Circulation 1999;100(Suppl I):I-87.

PURSUIT
Platelet glycoprotein IIb/IIIa in Unstable angina: Receptor Suppression Using Integrilin Therapy trial.
N Engl J Med 1998;339:436–43.
J Am Coll Cardiol 1999;33:72A.

RAPPORT
Reopro for Acute myocardial infarction and Primary PTCA Organization and Randomized Trial.
Circulation 1997;96(Suppl I):I-473.
Circulation 1998;98:734–41.
Circulation 1998;98(Suppl I):I-22.
J Am Coll Cardiol 1998;31:237A.

RAVES
Reduced Anticoagulation VEin graft Study.
Principal Investigator: MB Leon, Washington Hospital Center, Washington, DC, USA.
J Am Coll Cardiol 1999;33:37A.

REDUCE (Germany)
Low molecular weight heparin, reviparin, in the prevention of restenosis after PTCA.
J Am Coll Cardiol 1996;27:113A.
J Am Coll Cardiol 1996;28:1437–43.

REDUCE (Japan)
Restenosis reduction by cutting balloon evaluation.
J Am Coll Cardiol 1998;31;315A.
J Am Coll Cardiol 1999;33:101A.

REFLEX
REstenosis Rates with FLEXible GFX Stents.
Principal Investigators: N Reifart and C Vallbracht, Verum Mirai, Amsterdam, The Netherlands.

REGRESS
REgression GRowth Evaluation Statin Study.
Eur Heart J 1998;19(Suppl):569.
J Am Coll Cardiol 1999;33:79A.

RENEWAL
A randomised trial of endoluminal reconstruction using the NIR stent or Wallstent in angioplasty of long segment native coronary disease.
Circulation 1998;98(Suppl I):I-662.
Eur Heart J 1998;19(Suppl):48.

RESIST	REStenosis after Intravascular ultrasound STenting. J Am Coll Cardiol 1998;32:320–8. Eur Heart J 1999;20(Suppl):371. Circulation 1999;100(Suppl I):I-467. J Am Coll Cardiol 2000;35:3A.
REST	REstenosis STent study. J Am Coll Cardiol 1996;28:139A.
RESTORE	Randomized Efficacy Study of Tirofiban for Outcomes and REstenosis. Circulation 1997;96(Suppl I):I-648. Circulation 1997;96:1445–1453. J Am Coll Cardiol 1999;34:1061–6.
RITA	Randomized Intervention Treatment of Angina trial. Lancet 1993;341:573–80. Lancet 1994;344:927–30. Circulation 1996;94:135–42. Eur Heart J 1998;19(Suppl):473. Lancet 1998;352:1419–25.
RITA-2	The second Randomized Intervention Treatment of Angina trial. Lancet 1997;350:461–8. Eur Heart J 1998;19(Suppl):473.
RITA-3	The third Randomized Intervention Treatment of Angina trial. Principal investigator: K Fox.
ROSE	Registry for Optimal beStent Evaluation. Principal investigator: PW Serruys, Thoraxcenter, Rotterdam, The Netherlands.
ROSTER	ROtablator® vs Balloon for STEnt Restenosis. J Am Coll Cardiol 1998;40:142A. Circulation 1998;98(Suppl I):I-511. Eur Heart J 1998;19(Suppl):115. J Am Coll Cardiol 1999;33:49A. Eur Heart J 1999;20(Suppl):24.
R and R	Restenosis following minimally traumatic Rotational atherectomy. Principal investigator: G Braden, Bowman Gray School of Medicine, Winston-Salem, North Carolina, USA. J Am Coll Cardiol 1998;31:378A. J Am Coll Cardiol 2000;35:94A.
r-UK	Initial recanalization of occluded vein bypass grafts with intracoronary infusion of Recombinant UroKinase. Principal investigator: P Teirstein, Scripps Clinic, La Jolla, California, USA.
SAFE	The SAFE Study. Multicenter evaluation of a protection catheter system for distal embolization in coronary venous bypass grafts (SVGs). J Am Coll Cardiol 1999;33:37A. J Am Coll Cardiol 2000;35:41A.
SALTS	Strategic ALternatives with Ticlopidine in Stenting study. J Am Coll Cardiol 1998;40:352A.
SARECCO	Stent implantation after successful balloon angioplasty of a chronic coronary occlusion. Eur Heart J 1999;20(Suppl):137.
SAVED	SAphenous VEin De novo trial. J Am Coll Cardiol 1997;29:17A. N Engl J Med 1997;337:740–7.

SCORES	Scimed stent COmparative REStenosis trial. Circulation 1997;96(Suppl I):I-584,654. J Am Coll Cardiol 1998;31:314A.
SCRIPPS	Scripps Coronary Radiation to Inhibit Proliferation Post Stenting. N Engl J Med 1997;336:1697–703. Circulation 1999;99:243–7.
SCRIPPS II	Gamma radiotherapy for diffuse coronary restenosis. J Am Coll Cardiol 1998;31:238A.
SCRIPPS III	Gamma radiotherapy for diffuse coronary restenosis. Status: triple-centre, single-arm study; enrolling.
SHARP	The Subcutaneous Heparin and Angioplasty Restenosis Prevention trial. J Am Coll Cardiol 1995;26:947–54.
SHOCK	Should we emergently revascularize occluded coronaries for cardiogenic shock? Circulation 1999;100(Suppl I):I-87. Am Heart J 1999;137:313–21. N Engl J Med 1999;341:625–34.
SICCO	Stenting In Chronic Coronary Occlusion. J Am Coll Cardiol 1996;28:1444–51. Eur Heart J 1998;19(Suppl):472.
SIMA	Stent vs LIMA for proximal LAD stenosis. Principal investigator: U Kaufmann, Division of Cardiology, Berne, Switzerland. Circulation 1998;98(Suppl I):I-349.
SIPS	Strategy of ICUS guided PTCA and Stenting trial. Circulation 1997;96(Suppl I):I-222,582. J Am Coll Cardiol 1997;29:96A. Eur Heart J 1998;19(Suppl):136.
SISA	Stenting In Small Arteries study. J Am Coll Cardiol 1999;33:28A. Eur Heart J 1999;20(Suppl):386. J Am Coll Cardiol 2000;35:8A.
SLIDE	Selected Lesion Indication for Direct stEnting. Principal investigator: Dr B Chevalier, Centre Cardiologique du Nord, Paris, France.
SMART	Study of AVE-Microstent Ability to limit Restenosis Trial. J Am Coll Cardiol 1998;31:65A. J Am Coll Cardiol 1998;31:80A.
SMASH	The Swiss eMergency revascularization for Acute myocardial infarction with SHock. Principal investigator: JC Stauffer, University Hospital, Lausanne, Switzerland. Eur Heart J 1999;20:1030–8.
SOLD	Stenting after Optimal Lesion Debulking. Circulation 1997;96(Suppl I):I-81. Circulation 1998;98:1604–9.
SOPHOS	Study Of PHosphorylcholine coating On Stents. Eur Heart J 1999;20(Suppl):272,273.
SOS Europe	Stent Or Surgery trial Europe for multivessel disease. Principal investigator: U Sigwart, Royal Brompton Hospital, London, UK.

SPACTO

Stent vs PTCA After Chronic Total Occlusion.
Circulation 1997;I-268.
Eur Heart J 1998;19(Suppl):47.
J Am Coll Cardiol 1999;34:722–9.

SPORT

Stenting POst Rotational atherectomy Trial.
Principal Investigators: MB Leon, Washington Hospital Center, Washington, DC, USA
and M Buchbinder, Sharp Memorial Hospital, San Diego, California, USA.
J Am Coll Cardiol 2000;35:8A.

STARC

Studio Trapidil versus Aspirin nella Restenosi Coronarica.
Circulation 1994;90:2710–15.

STARS

STent Anti-thrombotic Regimen Study.
Principal investigator: MB Leon, Washington Hospital Center, Washington, DC, USA.
Circulation 1997;96(Suppl I):I-594.
N Engl J Med 1999;339:1665–71.

START

STent versus directional coronary Atherectomy Randomized Trial.
Circulation 1997;96(Suppl I):I-81.
J Am Coll Cardiol 1998;31:315A,379A.
Eur Heart J 1998;19(Suppl):47.
J Am Coll Cardiol 1999;33:15A.
J Am Coll Cardiol 1999;34:1050–7.
J Am Coll Cardiol 1999;34:1498–506.
Circulation 1999;100(Suppl I):I-727.

STAT

Stents versus Thrombolytics in Acute myocardial infarction Trial.
Circulation 1999;100(Suppl I):I-86.

STELLA

Stenting of long coronary lesions. A prospective 6-month quantitative angiographic study.
J Am Coll Cardiol 2000;35:62A.

STENT-BY

Comparison of acute and long-term safety and efficacy of bailout STENTing vs PTCA and
urgent CABG for patients with acute closure.
Principal investigator: R Erbel, University Hospital, Essen, Germany.

STENTIM I

The French Registry of STENTing In acute Myocardial infarction.
J Am Coll Cardiol 1996;27:68A.
Cathet Cardiovasc Diagn 1997;42:243–8.

STENTIM-2

Elective Wiktor STENT In acute Myocardial infarction.
Principal investigator: L Maillard, CHU, Tours, France.
Circulation 1998;98(Suppl I):I-21.
Eur Heart J 1998;19(Suppl):59.

STENT PAMI

Randomized trial of Primary PTCA versus heparin coated STENT Implantation during
Acute Myocardial Infarction.
Principal investigator: C Grines, William Beaumont Hospital, Royal Oak, Michigan, USA.
Circulation 1998;98(Suppl I):I-22.
Eur Heart J 1999;20(Suppl):31.
Circulation 1999;100(Suppl I):I-87.
J Am Coll Cardiol 2000;35:402A.

STOP

A randomized multicenter Israeli study for Stents in Total Occlusion and restenosis
Prevention.
Eur Heart J 1998;19(Suppl):471.
J Am Coll Cardiol 1999;33:28A.
Eur Heart J 1999;20(Suppl):156.

STRATAS	Study To determine Rotablator® And Transluminal Angioplasty Strategy. J Am Coll Cardiol 1998;98:378A. J Am Coll Cardiol 1998;31:455A.
STRESS	The STent REStenosis Study. N Engl J Med 1994;331:496–501.
STRESS I and II (Small Vessel Substudy)	The STent REStenosis Study group. J Am Coll Cardiol 1998;31:307–311.
STRESS III	STent REStenosis Study III. Principal investigator: D Fischman, Thomas Jefferson Medical College, Philadelphia, Pennsylvania, USA.
STRUT	Stent Treatment Region assessed by Ultrasound Tomography. Principal Investigators: P Fitzgerald and P Yock, Stanford University, Palo Alto, California, USA. Circulation 1995;92(Suppl I):I-546.
SURE	Serial Ultrasound REstenosis trial. Circulation 1997;96:475–83.
SVG WRIST	Saphenous Vein Graft: Washington Radiation for In-Stent restenosis Trial. Principal investigator: R Waksman, Washington Hospital Center, Washington, DC, USA.
SWAP	Stenting Without Angioplasty Pre-dilatation. Eur Heart J 1999;20:504.
SWISSI I	SWiss Interventional Study on Silent Ischemia. J Am Coll Cardiol 1999;33:341A.
SWISSI II	SWiss Interventional Study on Silent Ischemia. J Am Coll Cardiol 1999;33:38A.
TACTICS-TIMI18	The treat angina with aggrastat and determine cost of therapy with an invasive or conservative strategy trial. Am J Cardiol 1998;82:731–6.
TASC I	Trial of Angioplasty and Stents in Canada. Circulation 1995;92(Suppl I):I-279, 475. J Am Coll Cardiol 1995;25:156A. J Am Coll Cardiol 1997;29:17A.
TASC II	Trial of Angioplasty and Stents in Canada. Principal investigator: I Penn, Vancouver Hospital, Canada. Circulation 1995;92(Suppl I):I-475.
TASTE	Ticlopidine Aspirin STent Evaluation study. Circulation 1995;92(Suppl I):I-476. J Am Coll Cardiol 1996;27:139A. Eur Heart J 1996;17:1373–80.
TAUSA	Thrombolysis and Angioplasty in UnStable Angina. Circulation 1994;90:69–77.
TECBEST I and II	Transluminal Extraction Catheter BEfore STenting I and II. Principal investigator: JM Parks, University of Alabama, Birmingham, Alabama, USA.
TIMI IIIB	Thrombolysis In Myocardial Ischemia trial. Circulation 1994;89:1545–56.
TIMI-4 substudy	Thrombolysis In Myocardial Infarction: 4 substudy. Am J Cardiol 1997;80:21–26.

TIMI-10B substudy	Thrombolysis In Myocardial Infarction: 10B substudy. J Am Coll Cardiol 1998;31:231A.
TOPIT	Transluminal extraction atherectomy Or PTCA In Thrombus-containing lesions. Principal investigator: B Kaplan, William Beaumont Hospital, Royal Oak, Michigan, USA. Circulation 1996;94(Suppl I):I-317. J Am Coll Cardiol 2000;35:29.
TOSCA	Total Occlusion Study of CAnada. Principal investigator: CE Buller, Epicore Center, Edmonton, Canada. Circulation 1998;98(Suppl I):I-640. Circulation 1999;100:236–42.
TOTAL surveillance study (Europe)	Total Occlusion Trial with Angioplasty by using Laser guidewire. Am J Cardiol 1997;80:1419–23.
TOTAL	Total Occlusion Trial with Angioplasty by using Laser guidewire. Eur Heart J 1998;19(Suppl):471. J Am Coll Cardiol 1998;30:81A.
TOTAL (registry, USA)	Total Occlusion Trial with Angioplasty by using Laser guidewire. Principal investigator: SN Oesterle, Stanford University Medical Center, Stanford, California, USA.
TRAPIST	TRAPIdil on restenosis after STenting. Principal investigator: PW Serruys, Thoraxcenter, Rotterdam, The Netherlands. Eur Heart J 1998;19(Suppl):568. Circulation 1998;98(Suppl I):I-362.
TREAT	Tranilast REstenosis following Angioplasty Trial. Am Heart J 1999;138:968–75.
ULTIMA GROUP experience	Unprotected Left Main Study Group. Principal investigator: H Tamai, Shiga Medical Center, Moriyama, Japan. J Am Coll Cardiol 1998;31:101A. Eur Heart J 1998;19(Suppl):365.
VANQWISH	Veterans Affairs Non-Q-Wave Infarction Strategies in-Hospital. Circulation 1997;96(Suppl I):I-207. N Engl J Med 1998;338:1785–92.
VEGAS I	VEin Graft Angiojet Study: phase I. Principal investigator: S Ramee, Ochsner Medical Center, New Orleans, Louisiana, USA. Circulation 1997;96(Suppl I):I-216.
VEGAS II	VEin Graft Angiojet Study: phase II. Principal investigator: S Ramee, Ochsner Medical Center, New Orleans, Louisiana, USA. Circulation 1998;98(Suppl I):I-86. J Am Coll Cardiol 1999;33:47A. Circulation 1999;100(Suppl I):I-435, 810. J Am Coll Cardiol 2000;35:75A.
VENESTENT	Comparative analysis between the Wiktor-i stent and PTCA in saphenous vein grafts. Principal Investigators: JJRM Bonnier and JJ Koolen, Cardialysis, Rotterdam, The Netherlands. J Am Coll Cardiol 2000;35:9A.
WALLSTENT NATIVE	The WALLSTENT in NATIVE coronary arteries. Principal investigator: PW Serruys, Thoraxcenter, Rotterdam, The Netherlands.

WALLSTENT SVG study	The **WALLSTENT** in vein graft study. J Am Coll Cardiol 1998;30:216A.
WEST I	**W**est **E**uropean **S**tent **T**rial. Principal investigator: PW Serruys, Thoraxcenter, Rotterdam, The Netherlands.
WEST II	**W**est **E**uropean **S**tent **T**rial **II**. Principal investigator: PW Serruys, Thoraxcenter, Rotterdam, The Netherlands.
WIDEST	**WI**ktor stent in **DE** novo **ST**enosis: Is 'bail-out' stenting the effective option? Circulation 1999;100(Suppl I):I-790.
WIN	**W**allstent **I**n **N**ative vessels. Principal investigator: L Bilodeau, Montreal Heart Institute, Montreal, Canada. Circulation 1997;96(Suppl I):I-592. Eur Heart J 1998;19(Suppl):48.
WINS	**W**allstent **IN** **S**aphenous vein grafts. Principal investigator: R Safian, William Beaumont Hospital, Royal Oak, Michigan, USA. Circulation 1998;98(Suppl I):I-662. J Am Coll Cardiol 1999;33:37A,51A.
WRIST	**W**ashington **R**adiation for **I**n-**S**tent restenosis **T**rial. Principal investigator: R Waksman, Washington Hospital Center, Washington, DC, USA. J Am Coll Cardiol 1999;33:63A. J Am Coll Cardiol 2000;35:10A,21A.
ZWOLLE	A comparison of immediate coronary angioplasty with intravenous streptokinase in acute myocardial infarction. N Engl J Med 1993;328:680–684. Eur Heart J 1999;20(Suppl):32
ZWOLLE 5	A randomized comparison of coronary stenting with balloon angioplasty in selected patients with acute myocardial infarction. Circulation 1998;97:2502–5.

Index